VITAMINS AND HORMONES

VOLUME 44

VITAMINS AND HORMONES
ADVANCES IN RESEARCH AND APPLICATIONS

Editor-in-Chief

G. D. AURBACH

Metabolic Diseases Branch
National Institute of Arthritis,
Diabetes, and Digestive and Kidney Diseases
National Institutes of Health
Bethesda, Maryland

Editor

DONALD B. MCCORMICK

Department of Biochemistry
Emory University School of Medicine
Atlanta, Georgia

Volume 44

ACADEMIC PRESS, INC. Harcourt Brace Jovanovich, Publishers

San Diego   New York   Berkeley   Boston
London   Sydney   Tokyo   Toronto

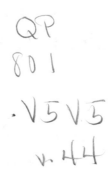

ACADEMIC PRESS, INC.
San Diego, California 92101

United Kingdom Edition published by
ACADEMIC PRESS, INC. (LONDON) LTD.
24-28 Oval Road, London NW1 7DX

LIBRARY OF CONGRESS CATALOG CARD NUMBER: 43-10535

ISBN   0-12-709844-5   (alk. paper)

PRINTED IN THE UNITED STATES OF AMERICA
88 89 90 91   9 8 7 6 5 4 3 2 1

Contents

Inhibins and Activins

NICHOLAS LING, NAOTO UENO, SHAO-YAO YING, FREDERICK ESCH, SHUNICHI SHIMASAKI, MARI HOTTA, PEDRO CUEVAS, AND ROGER GUILLEMIN

Guanine Nucleotide Binding Proteins and Signal Transduction

ALLEN M. SPIEGEL

Insulin-Sensitive Glucose Transport

TETSURO KONO

Calcium Channels

HARTMUT GLOSSMANN AND JÖRG STRIESSNIG

Preface

The revolution that modern protein chemistry and molecular biology have brought to the biological sciences is manifestly evident in the reviews presented in Volume 44 of *Vitamins and Hormones*. In each of the chapters application of these techniques has produced detailed knowledge about the protein structures involved, information that would have been difficult if not impossible to obtain before this revolution came about.

One protein that had eluded endocrinologists for decades is inhibin, initially postulated to be the testicular substance inhibiting FSH secretion in males. Thanks to the technology noted above, the mystery of inhibin has been clarified. N. Ling and associates describe how the protein was isolated, cDNA probes developed, and sequence determined. Inhibin proved to be a dimeric structure (alpha and beta chains), but provided still more surprises. The beta chains show homology to transforming growth factor beta, and dimers of the beta subunit show FSH-releasing activity, an action antagonistic to inhibin itself.

A. M. Spiegel discusses guanine nucleotide regulatory proteins (G-proteins), the membrane-bound proteins that couple signals detected at the cell surface to intracellular effector systems. These proteins are heterotrimers that interact with systems as diverse as the cyclic GMP phosphodiesterase necessary for vision, the adenylate cyclase system, the phospholipase-mediated pathways, and ion channels. One facet of a G-protein interacts with receptors on the cell surface, another with the effector system, and still others represent the sites of binding of guanine nucleotides and the substrate site for the action of certain toxins.

One of the principal functions of insulin is the regulation of glucose transport. T. Kono presents a detailed analysis of the biology and kinetics of the insulin-sensitive glucose transporter whose structure has now been deduced. It proved to be a protein containing 12 membrane-spanning regions.

Another group of proteins, ubiquitously important in the central nervous system, skeletal and smooth muscle function, and secretory processes, is the calcium channel proteins. H. Glossmann and J. Striessnig review the physiology and chemistry of these channel proteins, describe their differential properties, and outline the several classes of ligands that allow dissection of particular calcium channel types.

We thank the staff of Academic Press for expert help in putting together this volume.

G. D. Aurbach
Donald B. McCormick

Inhibins and Activins

NICHOLAS LING, NAOTO UENO, SHAO-YAO YING,
FREDERICK ESCH, SHUNICHI SHIMASAKI, MARI
HOTTA, PEDRO CUEVAS, AND ROGER GUILLEMIN

Laboratories for Neuroendocrinology
The Salk Institute
La Jolla, California 92037

I. Introduction

The concept of gonadal control of pituitary function developed more than 60 years ago with the discovery by Mottram and Cramer that destruction of seminiferous tubules in rats by X-irradiation of the testes caused hypertrophy of the anterior pituitary gland (Mottram and Cramer, 1923). A decade later McCullagh carried this concept further by demonstrating that a water-soluble extract from the testes could prevent hypertrophy of the pituitary in rats after castration, and he named the active principle "inhibin" (McCullagh, 1932). Meanwhile, the two pituitary gonadotropins, luteinizing hormone (LH) and follicle-stimulating hormone (FSH), which regulate the development and maturation of the gonad, were identified by Fevold and co-workers (Fevold *et al.*, 1931). This discovery subsequently led Klinefelter and

1

colleagues to postulate that a testicular factor, inhibin, was responsible for the negative feedback inhibition on pituitary FSH secretion, to account for the clinical observation in patients with gynecomastia (Klinefelter et al., 1942). However, the quest for inhibin did not advance further for three decades until pituitary FSH and LH were purified and isolated in the 1960s (Sairam and Papkoff, 1974) and radioimmunoassays were developed to determine the hormones in tissues and bodily fluids (Midgley, 1966, 1967).

The ability to quantitate FSH and LH in serum immediately revived the inhibin concept, which offered an explanation for the differential regulation of FSH and LH release often observed in humans and experimental animals but not accounted for by interaction between gonadal steroids and gonadotropin-releasing hormone at the pituitary or hypothalamic level (reviewed by Franchimont et al., 1975a, 1979b; Setchell et al., 1977; Main et al., 1979). Moreover, proof of the physiological concept of inhibin offered promise for development as a male contraceptive (Franchimont, 1985). Thus prompted, a heated search for inhibin ensued.

Early work on detection and partial purification of inhibin was confined mainly to materials derived from testes. Numerous reports appeared in the literature in the mid to late 1970s claiming purification of inhibins of widely differing molecular sizes from human (Franchimont et al., 1979a) and bovine seminal plasma (Franchimont et al., 1975b; Chari et al., 1978), ram rete testes fluid (Setchell and Jacks, 1974; Baker et al.. 1976; Davies et al., 1978; Cahoreau et al., 1979), and extracts of spermatozoa (Lugaro et al., 1974) or testes (Keogh et al., 1976). Closer examination of these reports, however, showed that none described homogeneous preparations nor represented the high specific activity expected of true inhibin (reviewed by de Jong, 1979; de Jong et al., 1981). Nevertheless, two polypeptides, named α-inhibin and β-inhibin, were isolated from human seminal plasma and characterized (Seidah et al., 1984; Li et al., 1985) together with two breakdown products of α-inhibin (Ramasharma et al., 1984; Li et al., 1985). Later reports, however, showed α-inhibin to be identical to the major degradation product of the gel-forming protein secreted by seminal vesicles (Lilja and Jeppsson, 1985) and β-inhibin identical to a sperm-coating antigen originating from prostate epithelia (Beksac et al., 1984; Johansson et al., 1984; Akiyama et al., 1985). In addition, synthetic fragments containing the putative biologically active core region of either seminal plasma inhibin were not effective in suppressing FSH secretion from primary cultures of rat anterior pituitary cells (Yamashiro et al., 1984; Kohan et al., 1986). These findings thus raised doubts about the significance of human seminal plasma inhibins α and β.

Arguments for the presence of an inhibin-like substance in ovarian follicular fluid were advocated first by Sherman and Korenman to explain the relative increase in serum FSH versus LH in postmenopausal women (Sherman and Korenman, 1975). Subsequently, de Jong and Sharpe as well as Schwartz and Channing demonstrated that serum FSH could be suppressed by steroid-depleted follicular fluid from bovine and porcine ovaries, respectively (de Jong and Sharpe, 1976; Schwartz and Channing, 1977). The discovery of FSH-suppressing activity in ovarian follicular fluid plus its ready availability prompted many research groups to attempt to purify inhibin from bovine (de Jong et al., 1981), ovine (Dobos et al., 1983), porcine (Lorenzen et al., 1978; Williams et al., 1979; Ward, 1981), and human ovarian fluid (Chari et al., 1979). The best purification method was probably the one devised by de Jong and co-workers, who made use of gel matrix affinity chromatography in early purification steps to selectively adsorb and concentrate inhibin from follicular fluid (Jansen et al., 1981).

In those early days of purification, however, none of the research groups was able to purify ovarian inhibin to homogeneity. The difficulties encountered are best explained by the lack of a reliable and efficient bioassay that could specifically measure the substance throughout the various purification steps, by the apparent self-aggregation or attachment of inhibin to large carrier proteins, as well as by the existence of multiple molecular forms of inhibin. The problem of the bioassay has been adequately reviewed by Baker and co-workers (Baker et al., 1981), who were the first to adapt the rat anterior pituitary cell culture system of Vale and colleagues (Vale et al., 1972) to reliably measure inhibin in gonadal tissue. Most laboratories that eventually succeeded in purifying and isolating inhibin from ovarian follicular fluid used basically the same rat anterior pituitary cell culture system as the assay to monitor the purification. The problem of protein aggregation was solved with the use of denaturing solvents in the purification steps.

With the improved methodologies four research groups finally suceeded in purifying and isolating inhibin from ovarian follicular fluid and determined the amino acid sequence at the amino terminus (Ling et al., 1985; Miyamoto et al., 1985; Rivier et al., 1985; Robertson et al., 1985). Published literature through 1984 on the purification of inhibin and its physiology has been thoroughly reviewed by Channing and co-workers (Channing et al., 1985) and de Jong and Robertson (de

Jong and Robertson, 1985). Thus, we do not include any of this material in this article. Instead, we concentrate on the latest work on the isolation and characterization of inhibins and activins as well as on their biological functions. Data obtained in our laboratory are discussed in more detail, and references to the work of others are included whenever appropriate.

II. Isolation of Inhibin

A. Bioassay

Throughout our purification procedure, inhibin activity was monitored by an *in vitro* bioassay using rat anterior pituitary cells in monolayer culture (Ling *et al.*, 1985). Pituitaries of 22-day-old female Sprague–Dawley rats from Holtzman Co. (Madison, WI) were removed aseptically. The anterior lobes were collected, washed once in sterile 25 mM HEPES buffer, pH 7.4, and dispersed at 37°C in 10 mM HEPES buffer containing collagenase (4 mg/ml), Dispase (2 mg/ml), and DNase (20 μg/ml). After periodic gentle trituration with a Pasteur pipet, the dispersed cells were separated by centrifugation and the pellet resuspended and incubated with neuraminidase (8 μg/ml) in HEPES buffer for 10 min. The cells were subsequently washed twice and plated with Dulbecco's modified Eagle's medium (DMEM) supplemented with 10% fetal bovine serum, HEPES (6 g/liter), and gentamycin (50 mg/liter) onto 24-well Linbro culture plates (Flow Laboratories, McLean, VA). On the second day of culture the medium was removed; samples were dissolved in 1 ml of HEPES–DMEM containing 1% fetal bovine serum, individually sterilized by passing through a 0.22-μm filter (Millipore, Bedford, MA), and added to the cells. After a 48-hour incubation, the medium was harvested and LH and FSH determined by radioimmunoassay, using materials provided by the National Hormone and Pituitary Program of the National Institute of Arthritis, Diabetes, and Digestive and Kidney Diseases.

In this bioassay the inhibin substance inhibits release of FSH but not that of LH; basal release is determined with control cells that receive the incubation medium only. A dose–response curve, determined with raw porcine follicular fluid (PFF), on the release of FSH and LH is presented in Fig. 1. The maximal inhibition of FSH secretion is usually obtained at a concentration of 1.25 μl PFF/ml. For the detection of inhibin activity in the column fractions, aliquots ranging from 0.01 and 0.1% by volume were removed, mixed with 100 μg human serum albumin in 100 μl of water, and dried in a Speed-Vac

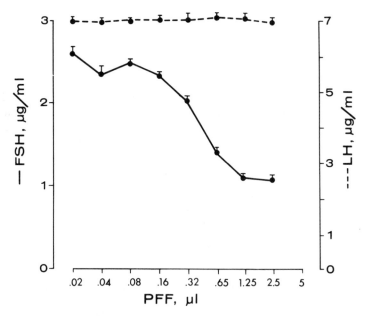

Fig. 1. Dose–response relationship between porcine ovarian follicular fluid (PFF) and the spontaneous release of FSH and LH from rat anterior pituitary monolayer cultures.

concentrator (Savant, Hicksville, NY). The residue was dissolved in 3 ml of 1% fetal bovine serum in HEPES–DMEM, filtered, and assayed in duplicate.

B. Inhibin from Porcine Ovarian Follicular Fluid

In our laboratory we have used a six-step procedure to isolate two inhibins from PFF (Ling *et al.*, 1985). The first is heparin–Sepharose affinity chromatography to concentrate the activity from PFF. Then Sephacryl S-200 gel filtration and four steps of reversed-phase high-performance liquid chromatography (RP-HPLC) are used to yield homogeneous material for chemical characterization.

1. *Heparin–Sepharose Affinity Chromatography*

A bottle containing 500 ml of frozen PFF (collected by J. R. Scientific, Woodland, CA, and generously provided through the Contraceptive Development Branch, Center for Population Research, National Institute of Child Health and Human Development) was defrosted, and the cell debris was sedimented in a Beckman J2-21 centrifuge (Beckman, Palo Alto, CA) in a JA-20 rotor at 10,000 rpm for 30 min.

One-half of the supernatant (250 ml) was diluted to 10 times its volume (2500 ml) with 0.1 M NaCl/10 mM Tris–Cl, pH 7, in a 4-liter Erlenmeyer flask and pumped simultaneously via eight silastic tubings (0.76 mm i.d.) into eight heparin–Sepharose (Pharmacia, Piscataway, NJ) columns (3.5 × 9 cm) by two Rabbit four-channel peristaltic pumps (Rainin Instruments, Emeryville, CA) at 40 ml/hour per column. After all the fluid had been pumped through the heparin–Sepharose matrix, the eight columns were washed simultaneously with 3.5 liters of 0.1 M NaCl/10 mM Tris–Cl, pH 7, in the same manner. The adsorbed proteins were removed by washing the eight columns simultaneously, as above, with 1.3 liters of 1 M NaCl/10 mM Tris–Cl, pH 7. Fractions of 16 ml were collected and monitored by UV absorbance at 280 nm; the inhibin activity was detected by the *in vitro* bioassay. A representative chromatogram of the 1 M NaCl eluate from heparin–Sepharose columns in shown in Fig. 2a. To save time and to simplify the assay, only FSH in the culture medium was measured and plotted in this and subsequent chromatograms. The heparin–Sepharose columns were regenerated by further washing with 1.6 liters of 2 M NaCl/10 mM Tris–Cl, pH 7, and reequilibrated with 3.5 liters of 0.1 M NaCl/10 mM Tris–Cl, pH 7, for purification of the remaining 250 ml of PFF.

2. *Sephacryl S-200 Superfine Gel Filtration*

Fractions containing inhibin activity (denoted by a solid bar in Fig. 2a) eluted from the eight heparin–Sepharose columns were pooled (400 ml) and dialyzed overnight (Spectrapor No. 3 membrane tubing, 28.6 mm cylindrical diameter, molecular weight cutoff 3500; Spectrum Medical Industries, Los Angeles, CA) against 16 liters of 30% (v/v) acetic acid. The retentate was centrifuged (JA-20 rotor, 10,000 rpm, 30 min) to remove a white precipitate, and the supernatant was divided into eight equal portions for application to eight columns (5 × 100 cm) of Sephacryl S-200 Superfine (Pharmacia). Each column was developed with 30% acetic acid at 20 ml/22 min, and fractions were moni-

---

FIG. 2. (a) Heparin–Sepharose affinity chromatography of PFF inhibin proteins, showing the profile of the 1 M NaCl/10 mM Tris–Cl, pH 7, eluate from one of the eight columns. (b) Sephacryl S-200 gel filtration in 30% acetic acid of the inhibin proteins recovered from heparin–Sepharose chomatography (solid bar in a). The profile from one of the eight columns is shown. (c) RP-HPLC purification of the inhibin proteins recovered from gel filtration. The active material (denoted by solid bar in b) was pooled, lyophilized, dissolved in 0.2 N acetic acid, and then applied to a Vydac C$_4$ column and eluted with the indicated gradient of acetonitrile in the Et$_3$NP system. Two zones of inhibin activity (A and B, indicated by solid bars) were recovered.

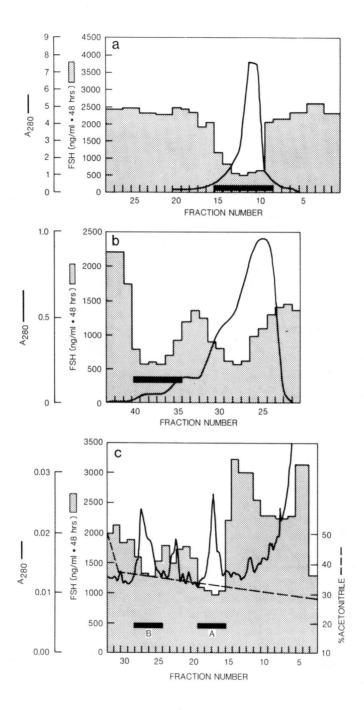

tored by UV absorption at 280 nm and bioassay. A representative
chromatogram from the Sephacryl S-200 gel filtration is shown in Fig.
2b. Two zones of approximately equal activity were detected, one of
apparent molecular weight (M_r) ~30.000 and the other of apparent M_r
~12,000 (see below for further measurement of M_r). However, based
on the protein concentration as determined by UV absorption, the low-
molecular-weight zone contains a much higher specific activity. As a
result, this region (denoted by a solid bar in Fig. 2b) was selected for
further purification.

3. *Reversed-Phase High-Performance Liquid Chromatography*

The RP-HPLC system consisted of a Model 322 gradient liquid chromatography unit (Beckman, Berkeley, CA) equipped with a Spectroflow 757 UV detector (Kratos, Ramsey, NJ), a Soltec 220 recorder
(Soltec, Sun Valley, CA), and a Redirac 2112 fraction collector (LKB,
Gaithersburg, MD). Two RP-HPLC solvent systems were used. In the
ET_3NP system, solvent A consists of 0.25 N phosphoric acid titrated to
pH 3.0 with triethylamine, and solvent B is 80% (v/v) acetonitrile
solvent A. In the TFA solvent system, solvent A contains 1 ml of
trifluoroacetic acid in 999 ml of water, and solvent B is 1 ml of trifluoroacetic acid in 199 ml of water and 800 ml of acetonitrile.

The fractions containing the low-molecular-weight inhibin activity
recovered from the eight Sephacryl S-200 columns were pooled and
lyophilized. The lyophilized material (~40 mg) was dissolved in 40 ml
of 0.2 N acetic acid and filtered through a Millex-HA 0.45-μm filter
(Millipore). The filtrate was applied directly to a Vydac (The Separations Group, Hesperia, CA) 5μ C_4 column (10 × 250 mm) through a
sliding valve (Altex, Berkeley, CA). After all the filtrate had been
loaded, the column was washed with the aqueous solvent A until the
UV absorption reached baseline levels. The inhibin activity was separated by a linear gradient of 28–37% acetonitrile in the Et_3NP system
in 90 min at a flow rate of 3 ml/min. Fractions of 9 ml were collected,
monitored by UV absorption at 280 nm, and bioassayed. As shown in
Fig. 2c, two zones of inhibin were detected, with more activity exhibited by the earlier eluted zone (A) than the later eluted zone (B).

Zones A and B (denoted by the solid bars in Fig. 2c) were separately
pooled and, after being diluted to 2 times their original volume with
0.2 N acetic acid, applied directly onto a Vydac 5μ C_4 column (10 × 250
mm) and eluted with a linear gradient of 29–38% acetonitrile in the
TFA system in 90 min at a flow rate of 3 ml/min. Fractions of 6 ml
were collected, monitored by UV absorption at 210 nm, and bioassayed
as shown in Figs. 3a and 3b, respectively. Active material (denoted by
the solid bars in Figs. 3a and 3b) was pooled, diluted to 2 times its

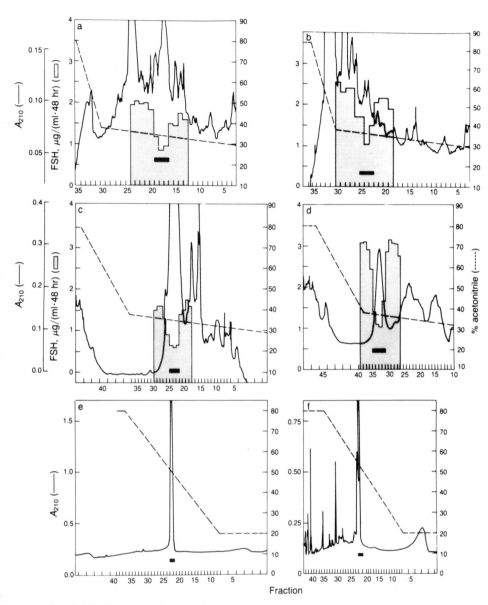

FIG. 3. RP-HPLC purification of inhibin proteins A (left) and B (right). (a, b) Active fractions in zones A and B (solid bars in Fig. 2c), respectively, were pooled and, after being diluted to 2 times their original volume with 0.2 N acetic acid, applied directly onto a Vydac C$_4$ column and eluted with the indicated gradient of acetonitrile in the TFA system. (c, d) The active material (denoted by solid bars in a and b, respectively) was pooled, diluted, and chromatographed on a Vydac phenyl column with the indicated gradient of acetonitrile in the Et$_3$NP system. (e, f) The active material accumulated from 4–10 chromatographic runs identical to those in c and d, respectively, was pooled, diluted, and concentrated by chromatography on an Aquapore RP-300 column, using the indicated gradient of acetonitrile in the TFA system.

original volume and chromatographed as above, using a Vydac 5μ
phenyl column (10 × 250 mm) with a linear gradient of 29–38%
acetonitrile in the Et₃NP system in 90 min at a flow rate of 1 ml/min.
Fractions of 1 ml were collected and monitored similarly. Finally, the
active material accumulated from 4–10 chromatographic runs, identical to those in Figs. 3c and 3d, respectively, was pooled and concentrated by chromatography on an Aquapore (Brownlee, Santa Clara,
CA) 10μ RP-300 column (4.6 × 250 mm), using a linear gradient of 20–
80% acetonitrile in the TFA system in 60 min at a flow rate of 0.5
ml/min. Fractions of 1 ml were collected and monitored by UV absorption only as shown in Figs. 3e and 3f. Altogether, approximately 600
and 60 μg of inhibins A and B, respectively, were purified from 18
liters of PFF.

4. Chemical Characterization of Inhibins A and B

Amino acid analysis (Böhlen and Schroeder, 1982) of inhibin proteins A and B showed that they were closely related but not identical
(Table I). Notable differences were found in the quantities of iso-
leucine, histidine, and lysine. On sodium dodecyl sulfate–polyacrylamide gel electrophoresis (SDS–PAGE) under nonreducing conditions
(Laemmli, 1970), inhibins A and B each showed a single band migrating at M_r 32,000 (Fig. 4a). Under reducing conditions, inhibin A separated into two bands, one migrating at M_r 18,000 and the other at
14,700, while protein B also showed two bands, at M_r 18,000 and
14,000 (Fig. 4b). These data suggest that both inhibins are composed of
two subunits joined together by at least one disulfide bond.

Potency analysis showed that, within experimental error, the two
purified inhibins are about equipotent with half-maximal inhibition of
basal FSH secretion at concentrations of 0.5–1.0 ng/ml (Fig. 5). As
expected, both inhibin proteins inhibit the basal release of FSH but
not that of LH or any other pituitary hormone. Also, reduction of the
proteins to separate the two subunits completely destroys the biological activity.

Microsequence analysis (Esch, 1984) from the amino terminus of
intact inhibin A, using a Model 470A protein sequencer (Applied Bio-
systems, Inc., Foster City, CA), consistently revealed two residues in
approximately equal amounts at each cycle of degradation as shown in
Table II, consistent with the hypothesis that the protein is composed of
two subunits. The same distribution of two residues as in inhitin A
was detected in the Edman degradation when intact inhibin B was
subjected to amino-terminal sequence analysis (Table II). In addition,
the residues identified at the amino termini of intact inhibins A and B

TABLE I
AMINO ACID COMPOSITIONS OF PURIFIED
INHIBIN PROTEINS A AND B FROM PFF[a]

Amino acid	Protein A	Protein B
Asx	18.5 ± 1.6	21.0 ± 1.1
Thr	11.5 ± 0.5	13.5 ± 0.6
Ser	16.3 ± 1.4	18.1 ± 0.7
Glx	21.3 ± 1.4	22.5 ± 0.5
Gly	19.9 ± 1.9	22.4 ± 0.7
Ala	19.7 ± 1.4	22.0 ± 0.6
Val	14.1 ± 1.8	14.4 ± 0.4
Met	6.1 ± 0.4	5.8 ± 0.3
Ile	14.6 ± 1.7	10.3 ± 0.2
Leu	27.3 ± 2.1	27.8 ± 0.8
Tyr	10.7 ± 1.3	11.4 ± 0.4
Phe	11.6 ± 1.4	10.0 ± 0.2
His	14.1 ± 1.2	7.9 ± 0.6
Trp	4.4 ± 0.3	3.9 ± 0.4
Lys	11.9 ± 0.9	5.4 ± 0.2
Arg	13.9 ± 0.6	15.8 ± 0.4
Cys[b]	14.4 ± 0.2	14.2 ± 0.9
Pro	29.2 ± 0.9	29.6 ± 1.1

[a] Values represent means ± SD of four analyses, normalized to a protein of M_r 32,000. Samples were hydrolyzed in 6 N hydrochloric acid plus 5% thioglycolic acid at 110°C for 24 hours.
[b] Determined as cysteic acid after performic acid oxidation.

were almost the same. The only notable differences were in cycles 7, 8, and 10. This suggested that the two inhibins are very closely related in structure.

The two subunits of inhibins A and B were separated by SDS–PAGE under reducing conditions, and the separated subunits were electroblotted onto GF/C paper (Aebersold *et al.*, 1986). After the protein bands were detected with Coomassie blue, they were excised and subjected directly to microsequencing. In addition, the two subunits of inhibin A were also separated by RP-HPLC after reduction and alkylation with iodoacetamide and the separated subunits analyzed by microsequencing. Based on the results from multiple sequence analyses of both intact and reduced inhibin A, the amino-terminal amino acid sequence of the M_r 18,000 α subunit was established as Ser-Thr-Ala-Pro-Leu-Pro-Trp-Pro-Trp-Ser-Pro-Ala-Ala-Leu-Arg-Leu-Leu-Gln-Arg-

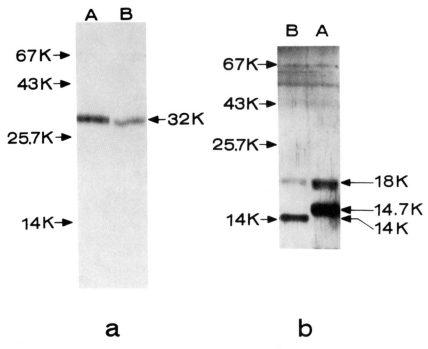

FIG. 4. SDS–PAGE analysis of purified inhibin proteins A and B under nonreducing (a) and reducing conditions (b). Positions of molecular weight standards are indicated at left.

Pro-Pro-Glu-Glu-Pro-Ala-Val and that of the M_r 14,700 β subunit was established as Gly-Leu-Glu-X-Asp-Gly-Lys-Val-Asn-Ile-X-X-Lys-Lys-Gln-Phe-Phe-Val-Ser-Phe-Lys-Asp-Ile-Gly-Trp-Asn-Asp-Trp-Ile-Ile-Ala-Pro. The amino-terminal amino acid sequence of the M_r 18,000 α subunit of inhibin B is identical to that of inhibin A, while the sequence of the M_r 14,000 β subunit was established as Gly-Leu-Glu-X-Asp-Gly-Arg-Thr-Asn-Leu-X-X-Arg-Gln-Gln-Phe-Phe-Ile-Asp-Phe-Arg-Leu-Ile-Gly-Trp. The unidentified residues (X) in the fourth, eleventh, and twelfth positions of the two β subunits are probably cysteines, since at least 14 of these were found by amino acid analyses of the intact molecules (Table I) and no phenylthiohydantoin–amino acid residues could be identified in these cycles. Thus, the tentative structures of the two forms of inhibins (A and B) isolated from PFF are heterodimers of M_r 32,000. Each inhibin is comprised of an identical α subunit of M_r 18,000 and a distinct but related β subunit of M_r 14,000–14,700, linked by interchain disulfide bond(s).

While our work on the isolation of PFF inhibins was in progress,

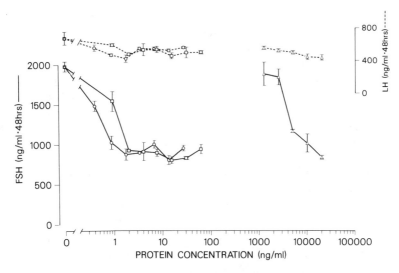

FIG. 5. Dose–response curves for the effect of purified inhibin proteins A (□) and B (○) and the crude PFF standard (△) on basal secretion of FSH and LH from cultured rat anterior pituitary cells. The crude PFF standard was a "charcoal-treated" and 40% saturated ammonium sulfate precipitate of PFF (Schwartz and Channing, 1977).

Miyamoto and co-workers reported the detection of four molecular forms of inhibin in PFF, corresponding to M_r 100,000, 80,000, 55,000, and 32,000 (Miyamoto *et al.*, 1985). The M_r 32,000 form, representing about 70% of the total activity in PFF, was purified to homogeneity, using an assay based on the suppression of spontaneous FSH release from cultured rat anterior pituitary cells. A five-step purification procedure was employed, consisting of Matrex gel Red A (Amicon, Dan-

TABLE II

AMINO-TERMINAL AMINO ACID SEQUENCES OF INHIBINS A AND B
DETERMINED BY MICROSEQUENCING[a]

Inhibin	Cycle									
	1	2	3	4	5	6	7	8	9	10
Inhibin A	S	T	A	P	L	P	W	P	W	S
	G	L	E	X	D	G	K	V	N	I
Inhibin B	S	T	A	P	L	P	W	P	W	S
	G	L	E	X	D	G	R	T	N	L

[a] Amino acids identified are represented by the one-letter abbreviations recommended by IUPAC–IUB. X denotes a residue which was not identified in the analysis.

vers, MA) affinity chromatography, phenyl–Sepharose hydrophobic interaction chromatography, Sephacryl S-200 Superfine gel filtration, DEAE–Sepharose CL6B anion-exchange chromatography, and RP-HPLC. The purified M_r 32,000 inhibin causes half-maximal suppression of FSH release at 0.9 ng/ml, and approximately 1 mg of protein was isolated from 1 liter of PFF. Structural characterization revealed that the isolated inhibin is also comprised of two polypeptide subunits of M_r 20,000 and 13,000, respectively, linked by disulfide bridge(s). Amino-terminal amino acid sequences of the M_r 20,000 and 13,000 subunits were established as Ser-Thr-Ala-Pro and Gly-Leu-Glu-Cys, respectively. These data are in agreement with those of the α and β subunits of porcine inhibin obtained from our laboratory.

Meanwhile, Rivier and colleagues also reported the isolation of a M_r 32,000 inhibin from PFF (Rivier *et al.*, 1985). Their scheme of purification consisted of either 1-propanol or ammonium sulfate precipitation and then preparative gel filtration and RP-HPLC. Inhibin activity was monitored by the suppression of basal FSH release from rat anterior pituitary cell cultures. Final purification was carried out by several steps of RP-HPLC and gel permeation in a FPLC system (Pharmacia). The purified inhibin exhibited half-maximal suppression of FSH release at a concentration of 0.3 ng/ml. Structural characterization revealed that the M_r 32,000 inhibin isolated is also comprised of two subunits of M_r 18,000 and 14,000. The amino-terminal amino acid sequence of the M_r 18,000 subunit was determined as Ser-Thr-Ala-Pro-Leu-Pro, while that of the M_r 14,000 subunit was Gly-Leu-Glu. Again, these results are similar to those obtained by our laboratory. In a more recent paper, the same group (Mayo *et al.*, 1986) published more data on the amino-terminal amino acid sequence of the M_r 14,000 β subunit: Gly-Leu-Glu-Cys-Asp-Gly-Arg-Thr-Asn-Leu-Cys-Cys-Arg-Gln-Gln-Phe-Phe-Ile-Asp-Phe-Arg-Leu-Ile-Gly-Trp. This sequence is identical to that of the M_r 14,000 β subunit from inhibin B determined by us.

C. INHIBIN FROM BOVINE OVARIAN FOLLICULAR FLUID

Robertson and colleagues were the first to report the purification of M_r 56,000 inhibin from bovine follicular fluid (BFF) (Robertson *et al.*, 1985). The purification scheme consisted of successive steps of gel filtration on Sephacryl S-200 Superfine, gel filtration on Sephadex G-100 or G-200, RP-HPLC, and preparative SDS–PAGE. Activity in the column fractions was determined by an *in vitro* bioassay based on the suppression of FSH release from rat anterior pituitary monolayer cultures. The purified inhibin half-maximally suppressed the level of FSH at a concentration of 0.9 ng/ml. The molecule was found to be comprised of two subunits, which dissociated under reducing conditions into an α subunit of M_r 44,000 and a β subunit of 14,000. The amino-terminal amino acid sequence of the α subunit was established as Asn-Ala-Val and that of the β subunit as Tyr-Leu-Glu. Thus, the amino terminus of the bovine M_r 44,000 α subunit is different from that of the porcine M_r 18,000 α subunit, but the second and third residues of the bovine M_r 14,000 β subunit are the same as those of the porcine M_r 14,700 and 14,000 β subunits (see below for further elaboration of the difference between bovine M_r 56,000 and porcine M_r 32,000 inhibins).

Later, a M_r 31,000 inhibin was also isolated from BFF by the same group, using essentially the same purification scheme employed in the isolation of the M_r 56,000 species except that an additional step, i.e., precipitation of the crude inhibin material with 4 M acetic acid at pH 7.5, was added between the Sephacryl S-200 and Sephadex G-100 gel filtration steps (Robertson et al., 1986). The purified material exhibited a half-maximal suppression of FSH levels in the cell culture at a concentration of 1 ng/ml. Interestingly, the M_r 31,000 inhibition was also found to be composed of two subunits of M_r 20,200 and 14,800. These subunit sizes are similar to those of the M_r 32,000 inhibins purified from PFF.

Using the same purification scheme as for the isolation of the M_r 32,000 PFF inhibin, an M_r 32,000 inhibin was also isolated from BFF by Fukuda and co-workers (Fukuda et al., 1986). The purified material could suppress half-maximal FSH release at a concentration of 1.2 ng/ml and was found to be comprised of two polypeptide subunits of M_r 20,000 and 13,000 linked by disulfide bridge(s). The amino-terminal amino acid sequence of the M_r 20,000 subunit was established as Ser-Thr-Pro-Pro, while the M_r 13,000 subunit was Gly-Leu-Glu-Cys. These data, again, are similar to those of the M_r 32,000 inhibins purified from PFF.

III. PRIMARY STRUCTURE OF INHIBIN

A. PORCINE OVARIAN INHIBINS

In collaboration with scientists at Genentech, Inc. (Anthony Mason, Joel Hayflick, Hugh Niall, and Peter Seeburg), we used the information from the amino-terminal amino acid sequences of the α and β subunits of porcine inhibins A and B to identify cloned complementary DNAs, encoding the biosynthetic precursors, from a porcine ovarian cDNA library. From the cDNA sequences, we deduced the corresponding amino acid sequences (Mason *et al.*, 1985).

The precursor of the common α subunit consists of 364 amino acids (M_r ~39,000), of which the carboxyterminal 134 constitutes the α subunit proper (Fig. 6). A pair of arginines preceding these 134 residues is probably the site for proteolytic release of the mature α subunit from its precursor. The proregion of the precursor contains additional arginine pairs at positions 55–56, 59–60, and 68–69, suggesting the possible existence of other bioactive peptides within this precursor. As a matter of fact, cleavage after the arginine pair at positions 59–60 would yield the corresponding porcine M_r 44,000 α subunit of the M_r 56,000 inhibin isolated from BFF (Robertson *et al.*, 1985). The precursor protein sequence also predicts two N-linked glycosylation sites, one within the α subunit proper. Glycosylation would account for the difference in size between that deduced from the amino acid sequence (M_r ~14,500) and the M_r of 18,000 obtained by SDS–PAGE. In addition, the mature α subunit contains seven cysteines. Recently, the complete porcine inhibin α subunit precursor was independently deduced by Mayo and colleagues (Mayo *et al.*, 1986). Their data agree with our findings.

The predicted precursor of the β subunit from inhibin A contains 424 amino acids, of which the carboxy-terminal 116 residues (M_r ~13,400) represents the β subunit proper (Fig. 7). The β_A subunit is preceded by five consecutive arginines, at which it is presumably cleaved proteolytically to generate the mature β subunit. Additional pairs of basic amino acids are found in the proregion of the precursor, suggesting the existence of other peptides derived from the precursor. The deduced amino acid sequence for the mature β subunit of inhibin B is one residue shorter than the β_A subunit and shows 63% similarity with the β_A subunit sequence (Fig. 7). A lesser degree of sequence similarity is also found in the proregion of both precursors. Only one possible N-linked glycosylation site is located in the proregion of both β subunit precursors. Each mature β subunit contains nine cysteine residues at identical positions.

The Northern blot hybridization procedure was used to assess size and relative abundance of mRNAs encoding the peptide subunits of each form of inhibin. The α subunit precursor mRNA was found in at least 10-fold higher abundance than that for the β_A subunit precursor and about 20-fold higher than the β_B precursor mRNA (Mason *et al.*, 1985). In addition, the α precursor mRNA, a single species, was found to be ~1.5 kb long, whereas β_A precursor mRNA sequences were repre-

```
                                                   1                                    10
                                                   met trp pro gln leu leu leu leu leu leu ala pro
  1 TGTGGGGCAGACCCTGACAGAAGGGGCACAGGGCTGGGTGTGGGTTCACCGTTGGCAGGGCCAGGTGAGCT ATG TGG CCT CAG CTG CTC CTC TTG CTG TTG GCC CCA

                        20                                 30                                 40
      arg ser gly his gly cys gln gly pro glu leu asp arg glu leu val leu ala lys val arg ala leu phe leu asp ala leu gly pro
108 CGG AGT GGG CAT GGC TGC CAG GGC CCG GAG CTG GAC CGG GAG CTT GTC CTG GCC AAG GTG AGG GCT CTG TTC CTG GAT GCC TTG GGA CCC

                        50                                 60                                 70
      pro ala val thr gly glu gly gly asp pro gly val arg arg leu pro arg arg his ala val gly gly phe met arg arg gly ser glu
198 CCG GCA GTG ACT GGG GAA GGT GGG GAT CCT GGA GTC AGG CGT CTG CCC CGA AGA CAT GCT GTG GGG GGC TTC ATG CGC AGG GGC TCT GAG

                        80                                 90                                100
      pro glu glu glu asp val ser gln ala ile leu phe pro ala thr gly ala arg cys gly asp glu pro ala ala gly glu leu ala arg
288 CCC GAG GAG GAG GAT GTC TCC CAG GCC ATC CTT TTC CCG GCT ACA GGT GCC CGC TGT GGG GAC GAG CCA GCT GCT GGA GAG CTG GCC CGG

                        110                                120                               130
      glu ala glu glu gly leu thr tyr val phe arg pro ser gln his thr his ser arg gln val thr ser ala gln leu trp phe his
378 GAG GCT GAG GAG GGC CTC TTC ACA TAT GTA TTC CGG CCG TCC CAG CAC ACA CAC AGC CGC CAG GTG ACT TCA GCT CAG CTG TGG TTC CAC

                        140                                150                               160
      thr gly leu asp arg gln gly met ala ala ala asn ser ser gly pro leu leu asp leu leu ala leu ser ser arg gly pro val ala
468 ACG GGA CTG GAC AGA CAG GGG ATG GCA GCC GCC AAT AGC TCT GGG CCC CTG CTG GAC CTG CTG GCA CTA TCA TCC AGG GGT CCT GTG GCT

                        170                                180                               190
      val pro met ser leu gly gln ala pro pro arg trp ala val leu his leu ala ala ser ala leu pro leu leu thr his pro val leu
558 GTG CCC ATG TCA CTG GGC CAG GCG CCC CCT CGC TGG GCT GTG CTG CAC CTG GCC GCC TCT GCC CTC CCT TTG TTG ACC CAC CCA GTC CTG

                        200                                210                               220
      val leu leu leu arg cys pro leu cys ser cys ser ala arg pro glu ala thr pro phe leu val ala his thr arg ala arg pro pro
648 GTG CTG CTG CTG CGC TGT CCT CTC TGT TCC TGC TCA GCC CGG CCC GAG GCC ACC CCC TTC CTG GTG GCC CAC ACT CGG GCC AGG CCA CCC

                        → α subunit               240                               250
      ser gly gly glu arg ala arg arg ser thr ala leu pro pro trp pro trp ser pro ala ala leu arg leu leu gln arg pro pro glu
738 AGC GGA GGG GAG AGG GCC CGA CGC TCC ACC GCC CCT CTG CCC TGG CCT TGG TCC CCC GCC GCG CTG CGC CTG CTG CAG AGG CCC CCG GAG

                        260                                270                               280
      glu pro ala val his ala asp cys his arg ala ser leu asn ile ser phe gln glu leu gly trp asp arg trp ile val his pro pro
828 GAA CCC GCT GTG CAC GCC GAC TGC CAC AGA GCT TCC CTC AAC ATC TCC TTC CAG GAG CTG GGC TGG GAC CGG TGG ATC GTG CAC CCT CCC

                        290                                300                               310
      ser phe ile phe his tyr cys his gly gly cys gly leu pro thr leu pro asn leu pro leu ser val pro gly ala pro pro thr pro
918 AGT TTC ATC TTC CAC TAC TGT CAC GGG GGC TGC GGG CTG CCG ACC CTG CCC AAC CTG CCC CTG TCT GTC CCT GGG GCC CCC CCT ACC CCT

                        320                                330                               340
      val gln pro leu leu leu val pro gly ala gln pro cys cys ala ala leu pro gly thr met arg ser leu arg val arg thr thr ser
1008 GTC CAG CCC CTG TTG TTG GTG CCA GGG GCT CAG CCC TGC TGC GCT GCT CTC CCG GGG ACC ATG AGG TCC CTA CGC GTT CGC ACC ACC TCG

                        350                                360       364
      asp gly gly tyr ser phe lys tyr glu thr val pro asn leu leu thr gln his cys ala cys ile OC
1098 GAT GGA GGT TAC TCT TTC AAG TAC GAA ACG GTG CCC AAC CTT CTC ACC CAG CAC TGT GCC TGC ATC TAA GGGTGTCCCGCTGGTGGCCGAGCTCCC

1194 ACAGGCACCAGCCTGGAGGAAGGCAGAGTTCCCACCTCCCCTTTCCI TCCGCCTCTCCGCCTGGAGGCTCCCCTCCCTGTCCGCCCCTGTCCCATGGGTAATGTGACAATAAACAGCAT

1312 AGTGCAGATGACTCGGTGCGCAAAAAAAAAA
```

FIG. 6. Nucleotide and deduced protein sequences for the porcine inhibin α subunit precursor. Nucleotides are numbered at the left, and amino acids are numbered throughout. The amino acid sequence overlined was used to design a long synthetic DNA probe to screen a porcine ovarian cDNA library of approximately 6×10^6 clones in λgt10. The 364-amino acid precursor includes a hydrophobic signal sequence, a prosequence, and the mature α chain (amino acids 231–364). The proteolytic processing site Arg-Arg (black bar) immediately precedes the amino terminus of the α chain. Several other putative dibasic processing sites present in the proregion are indicated by open bars. Cysteine residues are shaded. The two potential N-linked glycosylation sites are shown by hatched bars. The polyadenylation signal AATAAA box close to the 3′ end of the mRNA is underlined.

sented by two main species of approximately 4.5 and 7.2 kb. The β_B precursor is encoded by a single mRNA of ~4.5 kb and is found at approximately half the level of the two β_A mRNAs. The relative abundance of the precursor mRNAs thus reflects the yields of inhibins A and B isolated from PFF: the amount of inhibin A isolated is at least 10-fold more than B.

This figure presents the nucleotide sequence and the deduced amino acid sequence of the coding region, with three-frame amino acid translations shown above/below the codons. Boxed residues and shaded cysteines indicate conserved features; arrows mark the start of the βA subunit and βB subunit.

```
        1                          10                              20
 1  AAAAGGGCCGTCACCACAACTTTGGCTGCCAGG  ATG CCC TTG CTT TGG CTG AGA GGA TTT TTG TTG GCG AGT TGC TGG ATT ATA GTG AGG AGT TCC
                                       met pro leu leu trp leu arg gly phe leu leu ala ser cys trp ile ile val arg ser ser

                         30                              40                            50
 97 CCC ACC CCA GGA TCC GGG GGG CAC AGC GCA GCC CCG GAC TGC CCG TCC TGT GCC ACC CTC CCA AAG GAT GTA CCC AAC TCT CAG
    pro thr pro gly ser gly gly his ser ala ala pro asp cys pro ser cys ala thr leu pro lys asp val pro asn ser gln
                                                                       CGG GCG GCG GGG GCG GAG GAG GAG CTG GGC CGG CTG GAC
                                                                       arg ala ala gly ala glu glu glu leu gly arg leu asp

                          70                             80
187 CCG GAG ATG GTG GAA GCA GTC AAG AAG CAC ATT TTA AAC ATG CTG CAC TTG AAG AAG AGA CCC GAT GTC ACC CAG CCG GTA AAG GCG
    pro glu met val glu ala val lys lys his ile leu asn met leu his leu lys lys arg pro asp val thr gln pro val lys ala
    GGC GAC TTC CTG GAG GCA GTG AAG CGC CAC ATC TTG AAC ATG CTG CAC TTG AAG AAG AGA CCC AAC CAT GAC GTC ACC CAG CCA GAC
    gly asp phe leu glu ala val lys arg his ile leu asn met leu his leu gln met arg gly arg pro asn ile thr his ala pro lys ala

                          90                            100
277 GCG CTT CTG AAC GCA ATC ATC AGA AAG CTT CAT GTG GGC GAC GAC ATC GGA GCG AGA
    ala leu leu asn ala ile arg lys leu his val gly asp asp ile gly ala arg
    GCC ATG GTC ACG GCC CTG CGC AAA CTA CAT GCG GAC AAG GTG CGC GAG GAC GGC CGG GTG GAG ATC CAC CTG GAC GGC GAC GCC AGC
    ala met val thr ala leu arg lys leu his ala gly lys val arg glu asp gly arg val glu ile his leu asp gly asp ala ser

                         120                            130
367 GAA ATG AAT GAA CTC ATC GAG CAG ACC TCG GAG ATC ATC ACC TTC GCG GAA GCA --- GGC ACC GCC --- --- AGG AAG ACG GTC CGC TTT
    glu met asn glu leu ile glu gln thr ser glu ile ile thr phe ala glu ala gly thr ala arg lys thr val arg phe
    CCT GGC GCC GAC CAA GAG GTC TCG GAG ATC ATC AGC TTC GCA GAG GCA GAT ggc leu ala ser arg arg val leu tyr phe

                  140                             150                              160
448 GAG ATC TCC AAG GAG GGT AGC GAT CTC TCC GTG GTG GAG CGC GCC GAG ATC TGG CTC TTC CTC TTC AAG GTC CCC AAG CGA ACC AGG
    glu ile ser lys glu gly ser asp leu ser val val glu arg ala glu ile trp leu phe leu phe lys val pro lys arg thr arg
    TTC ATC TCC AAC GAG GGT AAC CAG AAC CTG TTC GTG GTA CGC GCC AGT CTG TGG CTC TAC CTG AAG GTC CTG --- --- --- aac cgg acc agg
    phe ile ser asn glu gly asn gln asn leu phe val gln ala ser leu trp leu tyr leu lys val leu

                 170                                           190
538 ACC AAA GTC TCC ATC GGT CTC TTT CAA CAG CAG AGG CGC CCG CAA GGC GCG GAC GCA GGG GAG GCG GAG GAC GTG GGC TTC CCG
    thr lys val ser ile gly leu phe gln gln gln arg arg pro gln gly ala asp ala gly glu ala glu asp val gly phe pro
            CCT TAC GTT CTG GAG AAG GGC AGC AGG AGG aag gtt gac gtc gtc aag gtc tat cag gag glu pro
            pro tyr val leu glu lys gly ser arg arg                              lys val asp val val lys val tyr gln glu gln glu pro

                200                            210                              220
628 GAG GAG AAG TCG GAG GTG CTG ATT TCG GAG AAG GTG GTG GAT GAG AAG GTG AGC CGG CGT GTG CTG AAG CGC AGC AGC TGG CAC ATC ATC CAG
    glu glu lys ser glu val leu ile ser glu lys val val asp glu lys val ser arg arg val leu lys arg ser ser trp his ile ile gln
    GGC CAC GGC GAC CGC TGG GAC GTG GTG GAG GAG CGT GTG GAC CTG AAG CGC AGC AGC TGG CAC ATC ATC CAG
    gly his gly asp arg trp asp val val glu glu arg val asp leu lys arg ser ser gly trp his ile ile gln

                230                             240                             250
718 CGC TTG CTG GAC CAG GGC AAG AGC GCC CTG ACT GAC ACT GGG CAG CAG TGC CAC GAG GAC GCC AGC CTG GTC CTG CTG GGC
    arg leu leu asp gln gly lys ser ala leu thr asp thr gly gln gln cys his glu asp ala ser leu val leu leu gly
    GCC CTG TTT GAA CAG GGC AAG CGG GGC CTC AAC CTG AAC GTG CAG TGC cys cys gly gln gly leu val val pro val phe
    ala leu phe glu arg gly arg gly arg leu asn leu asn val gln cys cys

                                                                       280
808 AAG AAG AAG AAG GAG GAG GAG GCG GGG AGG AAG AGG GAC GGA TAC GGG GCG GTG GAG GAG AAG CAG gln ser his arg
    lys lys lys lys glu glu glu ala gly arg lys arg asp gly tyr gly ala val glu glu lys gln
                                                          GTG GCC GGC --- GAG GAG TCA CAC CGG
                                                          val ala gly glu glu ser his arg
                                                                       →βA subunit

                290                            300
898 CCT TTC CTC ATG CTG CAG GCC CGC CAG TCC GAA GAG CAC CCC CAC CGC AGG AGG cgg aggly gtc ggc ggc tgc gac ggc gtc aac atc
    pro phe leu met leu gln ala arg gln ser glu glu his pro his arg arg arg arg gly gly val gly gly cys asp gly val asn ile
    CCC TTC GTG GTG GTG CAG GCC CGA TCC GGT GAC AGC AGG --- CAC ATC CGC AGG AGG ggg ggc gtc gag tgt gac ggc cgg arg thr asn ile leu
    pro phe val val val gln ala arg leu gly asp ser arg his ile arg arg arg gly gly val glu cys asp gly arg
                                                                       →βB subunit

               320                            330
988 TGC TGT AAG CAG TTC TTT GTC AGT TTC CGC ATT GGC TGG AGT GAC TGG ATC ATC GCT CCC ACC GGC TAC TAT GGG TAC TAC TGT
    cys cys lys gln phe phe val ser phe arg ile gly trp asn asp trp ile ile ala pro thr gly tyr tyr gly tyr tyr cys
    cys cys arg gln gln phe phe ile asp phe leu ile ile gly trp asp trp ile ile ala pro leu gly tyr tyr asp tyr cys

               350                            360                            370
1078 GAG GGC GAG TGC CCC AGC CAC ATA GCG GGC ACG TCG GGC TCC TCG CTC TCG TTC CAC TCG ACG GTC ATC AAC CAC TAC CGC ATG CGG GGC
     glu gly glu cys pro ser his ile ala gly thr ser gly ser ser leu ser phe his ser thr val ile asn his tyr arg met arg gly
     gly gly ser cys pro tyr leu gln ser ala arg val pro arg gly leu ala tyr leu ser ser phe ser his thr val val asn his tyr arg met arg gly

             380                            390                            400
1168 CAC AGC CCG TTC GCC AAC CTG AAG TCG TGC TGC GTC CCC ACC AAG CTG AGG CCC ATG TCC ATG CTC TAC TTC GAT GAG GAG TAC AAC ATC
     his ser pro phe ala asn leu lys ser cys cys val pro thr lys leu arg pro met ser met leu tyr phe asp glu glu tyr asn ile
     leu asn pro --- gly thr val asn ser cys cys ile leu pro thr lys leu ser thr met ser met leu tyr phe asp asp glu glu tyr asn ile

            410                            420            424
1258 ATC AAG AAG GAC ATC CAG AAC ATG ATC GTG GAG GAG TGC GGG TGC TCC TAG  AGCGCCGGCCGGGGCCCGGGGCCCGGGGCCCGGGGACGGACGGCGGCCACGC
     ile lys lys asp ile gln asn met ile val glu glu cys gly cys ser AM
     val lys arg asp val glu ... asn met ile val glu val cys gly cys ala OP
     GTC AAG CGG GAC GTG CCC AAC ATG ATC GTG GAG TGT GGC TGT cys ala TGA  AAGCTAGGGCTCGGGACTGTCCCTGCGGGCACGGGGCACATGGCGGGGGGGG
     val lys arg asp val pro asn met ile val glu val cys gly cys

1360 GAAGACACGTTTACGGCCTCTGACCTAGGCGACCGCAAACATGGAAATGAACAAAAATAACCATAAACTAAAAACAAAACCTGAAACAGATGAAGGAAGACGTGGAAAAATTCCGTAGCC
     TGTGGTCTTGGTTGTTCCTTGTTCCTCCTCAGCAGTGCCAGGTGCCAGGTGGGAGGCCTGAGATACTTTCCTACTTCTTTATTGAGCAATCAGTCGAAACCAGAGGGCGGACCCTCCGTGGACACGAAAGA

1480 AGGGCTCGGCGATGACACCGTGAAGGAGACGGGACTCGGGGGGGAGGGAGGAGGCAGAACGTGGGGGGCGGGGCGGGGGGGGGACCCTTCCTTTCTTCCTCCAGCATCGGAGTGGGGAC
     CTTGAAAATGCACACGTAGATGCCCGCAGCAGACGCCTCCTGCCCCACACAGAGCCTCCGGGATACCAGCAAATGGCAGTGACAAATGGCAGCTTAGCTACAAACGCCTGTCAG

1600 AGCAGTTGCTCCAACGGGAATATTGTCCTCCTTTTCAGTTCCCTGCTGGAGCCTCGAAGTCAGCTTGTCTGGTCTGCAGCCATGTGGGCTGGCACAACCCAAATAGCGTCTAGA
     TCGGAGGAAAAGGGTGAGCAGCCACCATTCCCACCAGCTGGCCCGGCCACTCTGAATCGCTCCTTTCGAGCACACAGAAAAGCACAAAGACAGAGACACCGAGAGAGAGAGAGAGAGA

1720 AAGCCATGAGTTTGAAAGGGCCAGTTATAGGCACTTTCCCACCCAGTAACCCAGGCTGTAAGGTATGTCTGTGTGGACCCTCTCTCTGTGTATATCAGCCCATGCACACACCTACAAAGAC
     GAGACAGACAGACAGACAGAGAGAGAGACGAGAGAGAGACGAGAGAGAGGAGA

1840 ACACACACACACACACACACACACACACACACACACACACACACACACAACTTCCTCTGACTTTTCTGAGACAAAGAGGTGGGTATAAACTGACTCCAGGAAAACTCGAG
1960 TGGGAAAACGTGCCCTTTGGGTTGGGACAATTTAGATGGTGGAGCAAAGCAAAAAGGAGGCAACGGCAAGTATGTTCGTGATGGGCCTGTGCCCCTGAGGGAGGGGGTGAGGAAGTTCCCTA
2080 AGGGTGACCTTAGCCAGACAGTGACTCTAGAAGAAGGGGCTCGACAGGGTCATGTAAAGAGGAAGGAGCTAATTCAGTCAGAAGAACCCCTGGCACTCAAGAGAACCACCGTGGGAGTTCCCG
2200 TCGTGGCGCAGTGGTTAACGAATCCGACTAGGAACATGAGGTTGAGGGTTCGATCCCTGACCTGCAGTTAACGATCCGGCGTTGCGGTGAGCTGTGGCGTCAGCTACCAGCTCTCTTTCAG
2320 CGGCTCGGATCCTGCGTTGCTGTGGCTCTGGCGTAGGCGGGTGGCTACAGCTCCGATTCAACCCCTAGCCTGGGAACCTCCATATGCGCGGCCCAGAAGAATAGCAAAAAAAAAAAA
2440 AGAACCACCGTGGAGGCCCGTAGCAGAGCCGGTCCCTTTTAACCCAATGTAGGGAAAGGGGGAATGAGACTAACTAAGAAGTGAATTTTCTTGACAGTCGCAGGCAGAAGAGGCAGAGGGACGTC
2560 AGTGCCTCTTCCTGGGAAGGCCAGCCGCTCCGTAGGCTGCACAGGAGTTCGCTGAGGGGCCGGCGAGGAAAGGTGTGGACAGAGGTGGAGGCATGTATTCCACCTTTCGCTTTAGCAGTA
2680 TCTGAAGTCACGGCGAGACTAAGGGCTTCCATTCAGTCCCGTGTATTGCAAGAATCCATGAATTATCTGAATCATTTCGGCCACTTAATCAACCCTACAGTGTTTCACGTGATCTTGTT
2800 TGCTGGTTAAACCCTACACTATTTGAGAAACCAAAGCTGTGCTATTGCTCTAGCACCAGTTCCAAGGGCCACCTTCCTCCGGATAAGGCCTTGTCCAGACTGCTGCTTCCTCGGCCAGGTC
2920 ATTCCTCTCCTTCCTGCCCAGTCAACTCTTCCCAAGGAGATTCTGTCCCCTAAATATCTCTGGAAGCCACCTTAGTTTCTTCCATTCAGATTCTTCAGTGGCTTCCGTTGGCTTTTGAATAAAGTCCTA
3040 AATTCAAAGAGCTTTGCATAAGTTCAGCCTGTACCATGCATGTGTTCCCTAAGTTCCAGTCAAATTGACATGGTCTTCCCCATTCAGATTTCAGCCTTCCGGCACAGCAGACACGGAGTGTTC
3160 TCTCGGTTGTAAACATCCCATTTCCACCTTTTAATCCTAAATGTTTCTTCCTCGGGGAGACCTTTCTGATTTGTGATGTAGGTCAAGACTTTTAGTTAAATCTTCTCTTAGCACAA
3280 TGCGTGTTTCATAGCACTTATTACAATCATAATGTTACAGTAGACGTAATTGGCTGGCAGGCTGCTAGATGTTGAAGCTCATGAGGGCAGAAATACGTCCATCTTGTTCACTGCTGT
3420 ATTCCGAGTGTCGGGCACACAGTTGTTGTCAATAAATTTGACTTAATGAACTCAAAAAAAAAAAAAA
```

The structural organization of PFF inhibins shares some intriguing features with the pituitary and placental glycoprotein hormones. Thyroid-stimulating hormone, FSH, LH, and chorionic gonadotropin, like the molecules inhibins A and B, are high-molecular-weight glycoproteins composed of two subunits, one common to all four hormones within a single species, the other variable, and all encoded by different mRNA species (Pierce and Parsons, 1981; Fiddes and Talmadge, 1984). The mRNAs encoding the common α subunit for inhibins (Mason *et al.*, 1985) or for pituitary glycoprotein hormones (Counis *et al.*, 1982) occur in substantially greater abundance than the corresponding β subunit mRNAs, suggesting a similarity in the regulation of biosynthesis of each group of hormones. In the pituitary and placental glycoprotein hormones, the variable β subunit confers the different biological specificities of each molecule while the constant α subunit presumably has a crucial role in folding and overall conformation of the complex (Pierce and Parsons, 1981). At present, we have not found evidence for differences in biological properties of inhibins A and B. Unlike the case for known glycoprotein hormones, the subunits of each inhibin are linked by disulfide bridge(s), a situation more closely resembling the immunoglobulins.

Surprisingly, significant sequence similarity was found between the β subunit sequences of inhibin and the recently determined primary structure of human transforming growth factor-β (TGF-β) (Derynck *et al.*, 1985), as shown in Fig. 8. These peptides are of nearly equal length (inhibin β_A subunit, 116 residues; β_B subunit, 115; TGF-β, 112) and show a strikingly similar distribution of their nine cysteines. It is intriguing that members of these two related protein families should be involved in such seemingly unrelated activities as the control of reproduction and cellular growth. What determines the activity of each molecule? A clue may be found in the fact that TGF-β acts in a homodimeric form whereas inhibin acts as a heterodimer. However, more surprises were discovered by us and others when dimers of the β

FIG. 7. Nucleotide and deduced protein sequences for inhibin β subunit precursors. Nucleotide numbers at left refer to those of cloned β_A cDNA sequences. Amino acid numbers are for β_A precursor residues. The amino termini of the β subunits, which are preceded by basic processing sites (black bars), are indicated by arrows. The β_B sequence is shown underneath the β_A sequence and aligned with it for maximum similarity. Regions containing identical amino acid sequences are boxed. Cysteine residues are shaded, possible processing sites are indicated by open bars, and potential glycosylation sites are shown by hatched bars. A highly G+C-rich region 3' to the termination codon is underlined in one and overlined in the other sequence, and the AATAAA polyadenylation signal is underlined in the β_A subunit sequence.

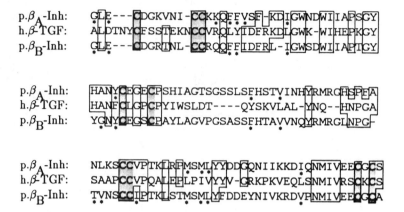

FIG. 8. Sequence similarities of inhibin β subunits and human TGF-β. Amino acids are represented by the one-letter code recommended by IUPAC–IUB. Identical residues are boxed and cysteine residues shaded. Asterisks denote conservative changes.

subunit of inhibin were found in PFF that have activities completely opposite to inhibin (see Section IV).

The distribution of the cysteine residues in the β subunits of inhibin are also similar to those located at the carboxy terminus of the newly characterized bovine Müllerian inhibiting substance (MIS) (Cate *et al.*, 1986). MIS is an M_r 140,000 glycoprotein comprised of two identical subunits. Its primary function is to cause regression of Müllerian ducts in male embryos, but this substance is also found to be present in BFF (Takahashi *et al.*, 1986).

B. Bovine, Human, and Murine Ovarian Inhibins

Using information from the amino-terminal amino acid sequence of the M_r 44,000 α subunit and the M_r 14,000 β subunit of the M_r 56,000 inhibin, Forage and colleagues deduced the amino acid sequence of the complete α subunit precursor as well as the partial sequence of the β subunit precursor from cDNA species derived from bovine granulosa cell mRNA (Forage *et al.*, 1986). As shown in Fig. 9, the overall structures of the bovine and porcine α subunit precursors are very similar. The bovine M_r 44,000 α subunit proper contains 300 amino acids (M_r 32,298) with two potential N-glycosylation sites. Glycosylation could thus account for the difference in molecular weight (M_r 44,000) observed in SDS–PAGE analysis versus that deduced from the amino acid sequence (M_r 32,298). In addition, the M_r 44,000 α subunit contains two potential proteolytic processing sites, the first located at

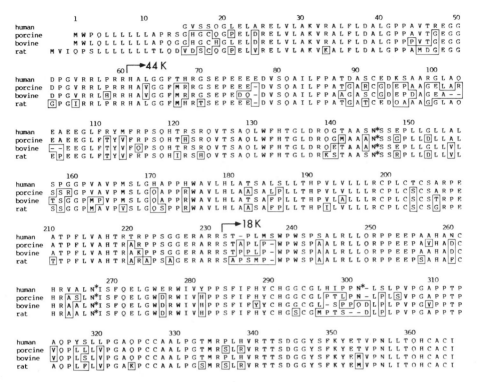

FIG. 9. Amino acid sequences of human (Mason *et al.*, 1986), porcine (Mason *et al.*, 1985), bovine (Forage *et al.*, 1986), and murine (Esch *et al.*, 1987) inhibin α subunit precursors. The numbers are aligned with the human sequence only. Amino acids differing from the human sequence are boxed. 18K and 44K denote the amino termini of the M_r 18,000 and 44,000 mature α subunits. Putative N-linked glycosylation sites are marked by asterisks.

eight residues from the amino terminus and the second at approximately the middle of the sequence. Processing at the second cleavage site would yield the corresponding bovine M_r 18,000 α subunit of the M_r 32,000 inhibin. The mature β subunit of the bovine M_r 56,000 inhibin is composed of 116 amino acids (M_r 12,977), and its sequence is completely identical to the β subunit of porcine inhibin A (Fig. 10).

Porcine inhibin α, $β_A$ and $β_B$ cDNAs have been used to deduce the complete amino acid sequences of the precursor forms of human (Mason *et al.*, 1986) and murine (Esch *et al.*, 1988) ovarian inhibins by nucleotide sequencing. With cDNAs coding for bovine inhibin A and B subunits, Stewart and co-workers have cloned the human inhibin genes (Stewart *et al.*, 1986). In addition, the complete α subunit precur-

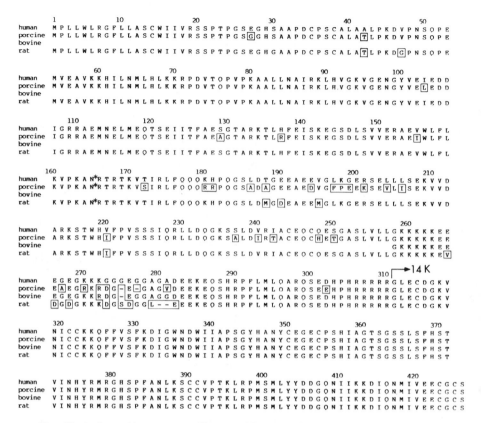

FIG. 10. Amino acid sequences of human (Mason *et al.*, 1986), porcine (Mason *et al.*, 1985), bovine (Forage *et al.*, 1986), and murine (Esch *et al.*, 1987) inhibin β_A subunit precursors. The numbers are aligned with the human sequence only. Amino acids differing from the human sequence are boxed. 14K denotes the amino termini of the M_r 14,700 mature β_A subunits. Putative N-linked glycosylation sites are marked by asterisks.

sor has been deduced from cDNAs obtained from a human placental genomic library (Mayo *et al.*, 1986). The predicted amino acid sequences of the α and β_A subunit precursors for human, porcine, bovine, and murine inhibins are presented in Figs. 9 and 10, respectively, and the precursors for the β_B subunit of human, porcine, and murine inhibins are shown in Fig. 11. Overall, the α subunits from the four species are very similar. The only notable difference is the presence, within the mature M_r 18,000 α subunit of human inhibin, of two potential N-glycosylation sites, whereas all the other species have only one.

To account for the production of two different sized α subunits, McLachlan and colleagues proposed that the inhibin released into follicular fluid from granulosa cells is predominantly of high-molecular-weight forms, such as the M_r 56,000 species with an M_r 44,000 α subunit (McLachlan *et al.*, 1986a). The high-molecular-weight forms are then processed to the M_r 32,000 active metabolite containing the M_r 18,000 α subunit in the follicular fluid or upon release into the circulation.

The similarities in the β subunits from the four species are even more striking. The mature β subunits of human, porcine, bovine, and murine inhibins are completely identical, whereas, within the mature $β_B$ subunits, the human, porcine, and murine species differ by only a few amino acids.

IV. Isolation and Characterization of Activins

In our original report on the isolation of the two inhibins from PFF (Ling *et al.*, 1985), we noted a side fraction, migrating after the M_r

```
         35      40          50            60          70          80
human    C T S C G G F R R P E E L G R V D G D F L E A V K R H I L S R L Q M R G R P N*I T H A V P K A A M V T A L
porcine          G G F R R P E E L G R L D G D F L E A V K R H I L N R L Q M R G R P N*I T H A V P K A A M V T A L
rat

             90          100         110         120         130         140
human    R K L H A G K V R E D G R V E I P H L D G H A S P G A D G Q E R V S E I I S P A E T D G L A S S R V R L Y
porcine  R K L H A G K V R E D G R V E I P H L D G H A S P G A D G Q E R V S E I I S P A E T D G L A S S R V R L Y
rat                                    H A S P G A D G Q E R V S E I I S P A E T D G L A S S R V R L Y

                     150         160         170         180         190
human    F F I S N E G N Q N L F V V Q A S L W L Y L K L L P Y V L E K G S R R K V R V K V Y F Q E Q G H G D R W N
porcine  F F I S N E G N Q N L F V V Q A S L W L Y L K L L P Y V L E K G S R R K V R V K V Y F Q E P G H G D R W D
rat      F F V S N E G N Q N L F V V Q A S L W L Y L K L L P Y V L E K G S R R K V R V K V Y F Q E Q G H G D R W N

             200         210         220         230         240
human    M V E K R V D L K R S G W H T F P L T E A I Q A L F E R G E R R L N L D V Q C D S C Q E L A V V P V F V D
porcine  V V E K R V D L K R S G W H T L P L T E A I Q A L F E R G E R R L N L D V Q C D G C Q E L A V V P V F V D
rat      V V E K K V D L K R S G W H T F P I T E A I Q A L F E R G E R R L N L D V Q C D S C Q E L A V V P V F V D

             250         260         270    ┌─►14K   280         290
human    P G E E S H R P F V V V Q A R L G D S R H R I R K R G L E C D G R T N L C C R Q Q F F I D F R L I G W N D
porcine  P G E E S H R P F V V V Q A R L G D S R H R I R K R G L E C D G R T N L C C R Q Q F F I D F R L I G W S D
rat      P G E E S H R P F V V V Q A R L G D S R H R I R K R G L E C D G R T S L C C R Q Q F F I D F R L I G W N D

         300         310         320         330         340         350
human    W I I A P T G Y Y G N Y C E G S C P A Y L A G V P G S A S S F H T A V V N Q Y R M R G L N P G T V N S C C
porcine  W I I A P T G Y Y G N Y C E G S C P A Y L A G V P G S A S S F H T A V V N Q Y R M R G L N P G T V N S C C
rat      W I I A P T G Y Y G N Y C E G S C P A Y L A G V P G S A S S F H T A V V N Q Y R M R G L N P G P V N S C C

             360         370         380
human    I P T K L S T M S M L Y F D D E Y N I V K R D V P N M I V E E C G C A
porcine  I P T K L S T M S M L Y F D D E Y N I V K R D V P N M I V E E C G C A
rat      I P T K L S S M S M L Y F D D E Y N I V K R D V P N M I V E E C G C A
```

FIG. 11. Amino acid sequences of human (Mason *et al.*, 1986), porcine (Mason *et al.*, 1985), and murine (Esch *et al.*, 1988) inhibin $β_B$ subunit precursors. The numbers are aligned with the human sequence only. Amino acids differing from the human sequence are boxed. 14K denotes the amino termini of the M_r 14,000 mature $β_B$ subunits. Putative N-linked glycosylation sites are marked by asterisks.

32,000 inhibins in the Sephacryl S-200 gel filtration step, which stimulates pituitary FSH secretion (fractions 41–43 in Fig. 2b). On further purification by RP-HPLC the FSH-releasing activity was resolved into two distinct forms in elution from the column. Both forms were purified to homogeneity by multiple HPLC steps (Ling *et al.*, 1986a,b).

A. Activin from Porcine Ovarian Follicular Fluid

Throughout the purification procedure, FSH-releasing activity was monitored by the same *in vitro* bioassay used for the isolation of inhibins (Ling *et al.*, 1985). In this assay the inhibin-containing fractions inhibit the basal release of FSH but not that of LH, as compared to release by control cells incubated with medium only. The FSH-releasing substance enhances release only of FSH in 48-hour incubations.

For purification (Ling *et al.*, 1986a), fractions containing the M_r 32,000 inhibins and FSH-releasing activity from the Sephacryl S-200 gel filtration of the heparin–Sepharose-adsorbed PFF proteins were pooled and lyophilized. The lyophilized material (~53 mg) was dissolved in 40 ml of 0.2 N acetic acid and filtered through a Millex-HA 0.45-μm filter. The filtrate was applied directly to a Vydac 5μ C_4 column (10 × 250 mm) as for the purification of the inhibins (Ling *et al.*, 1985). The column was washed with the aqueous solvent A until the UV absorption reached baseline levels. The inhibin and FSH-releasing activities were separated with a linear gradient of 24–36% acetonitrile in the Et₃NP solvent system in 120 min at a flow rate of 3 ml/min on a Beckman 322 gradient liquid chromatography system as above. Fractions of 9 ml were collected, monitored by UV absorption at 280 nm, and bioassayed. As shown in Fig. 12a, two zones of inhibin activity (designated A and B) were separated, as were two zones of FSH-releasing activity (denoted by the two solid bars). The FSH-releasing fractions denoted by the solid bar and eluting at 30% acetonitrile were pooled and, after mixing with an equal volume of 0.2 N acetic acid, pumped directly onto a Vydac 5μ C_4 column (10 × 250 mm) and eluted with a linear gradient of 25–34% acetonitrile in the TFA solvent system in 90 min at a flow rate of 3 ml/min. Fractions of 6 ml were collected, and measured by UV absorption at 210 nm, and bioassayed as shown in Fig. 12b.

The active material (denoted by the solid bar in Fig. 12b) was pooled and diluted to twice its original volume and rechromatographed on a Vydac 5μ phenyl column (10 × 250 mm) with a linear gradient of 25–34% acetonitrile in the Et₃NP system in 90 min at a flow rate of 1ml/min. Fractions of 2 ml were collected and monitored as shown in

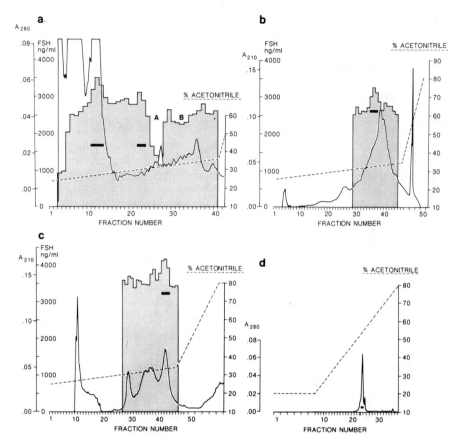

FIG. 12. Purification of the FSH-releasing substance, activin, from PFF. The Sephacryl S-200-purified material was processed through the following steps. (a) The material was chromatographed on a Vydac C_4 column and eluted with the indicated gradient of acetonitrile in the Et_3NP system. Two zones of inhibin activity, designated A and B, were separated, as were two zones of FSH-releasing activity, denoted by solid bars. (b) The FSH-releasing fractions denoted by the black bar and eluting at 30% acetonitrile in a were pooled and, after diluting with an equal volume of 0.2 N acetic acid, chromatographed directly on a Vydac C_4 column and eluted with the indicated gradient of acetonitrile in the TFA system. (c) The active fractions (denoted by solid bar in b) were pooled, diluted, and processed on a Vydac phenyl column with the indicated gradient of acetonitrile in the Et_3NP system. (d) The active material (solid bar in c) from four chromatographic runs was pooled and, after dilution, concentrated on an Aquapore RP-300 column using the indicated gradient of acetonitrile in the TFA system.

Fig. 12c. The active material (solid bar) from four chromatographic separations identical to those in Fig. 12c were pooled and, after dilution with 0.2 N acetic acid, concentrated by chromatography on an Aquapore 10μ RP-300 column (4.6 × 250 mm) using a linear gradient of 20–80% acetonitrile in the TFA system at a flow rate of 0.5 ml/min as shown in Fig. 12d. Fractions of 1 ml were collected and monitored by UV absorption only. The yield from 2 liters of PFF was ~32 μg of protein.

The purified protein caused half-maximal stimulation of FSH release at a concentration of 3.7 ± .05 ng/ml and maximal release at 16 ng/ml or higher (Ling *et al.*, 1986a). It did not affect secretion of LH. Manifestation of the FSH-releasing activity requires at least 24 hours; short-term incubation (4 hours) with this substance [the classic *in vitro* bioassay (Vale *et al.*, 1972) used to study the hypothalamic releasing hormones] will not release FSH. We suggest that the substance be called *activin* to signify that it shows biological effects opposite to those of inhibin and is different from the gonadotropin-releasing hormone.

The purified activin yielded a single band of apparent M_r 24,000 on SDS–PAGE analysis under nonreducing conditions (Fig. 13a). Microsequencing of the intact molecule revealed the first 32 amino-terminal residues as shown in Fig. 14a. These data are identical to those expected for simultaneous sequencing of the two β subunits of inhibins A and B together (see Fig. 14b). To determine the structure of the two subunits of activin, the molecule was compared with inhibins A and B using SDS–PAGE under reducing conditions. As shown in Fig. 13b, migration of the two reduced subunits of activin coincides with that of the reduced β subunits of inhibins A and B, respectively. Thus, based on the molecular weights of the reduced subunits and their amino-terminal sequences, we propose that activin, one of the FSH-releasing substances present in PFF, is a heterodimer comprised of the β subunits of inhibins A and B, linked by interchain disulfide bond(s).

B. Homoactivin A from Porcine Ovarian Follicular Fluid

Approximately 1 liter of frozen PFF was processed to isolate the second FSH-releasing substance (Ling *et al.*, 1986b). The first three steps of purification, consisting of heparin–Sepharose affinity chromatography, Sephacryl S-200 gel filtration, and RP-HPLC on a Vydac C_4 column with the Et_3NP solvent system, were the same as before (Ling *et al.*, 1986a). The FSH-releasing activity eluting at 30% acetonitrile from the first RP-HPLC step (Fig. 15a) had been previously purified to homogeneity and characterized as a heterodimer (activin) of

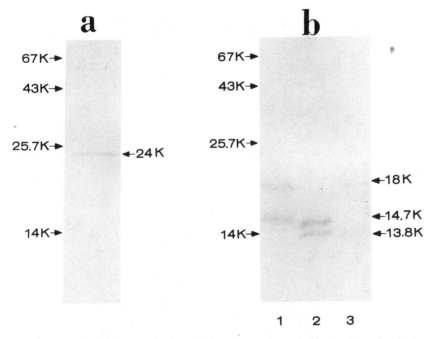

FIG. 13. SDS–PAGE analysis of purified activin under nonreducing (a) and reducing conditions (b). Lanes 1 and 3 in b denote purified porcine inhibins A and B, respectively, analyzed simultaneously with activin (lane 2). The high-molecular-weight band at 18K (M_r 18,000) is the common α subunit of the inhibins, and the low-molecular-weight bands at 14.7K and 13.8K correspond to the M_r 14,700 and 13,800 β subunits of inhibins A and B, respectively. Positions of molecular weight standards are indicated at left.

the β subunits of inhibins A and B linked by disulfide bond(s). The other FSH-releasing zone eluting at 27% acetonitrile was pooled (solid bar), further purified on a Vydac 5μ C$_4$ column (10 × 250 mm), and eluted with a linear gradient of 25–34% acetonitrile in the TFA system in 90 min at a flow rate of 3 ml/min. Fractions of 6 ml were collected and monitored by UV absorption at 210 nm and bioassayed as shown in Fig. 15b.

The FSH-releasing zone detected by bioassay was pooled (solid bar) and, after removing the acetonitrile in a Speed-Vac concentrator and adjusting the pH to 6.5 with 1 N ammonium hydroxide, pumped directly onto a Spherogel (Toyo Soda, Tokyo, Japan) 10μ IEX 535CM column (6 × 150 mm). The ion-exchange HPLC equipment consisted of a Beckman 332 gradient liquid chromatography unit equipped with a Spectroflow 770 UV detector (Kratos), a Linear 385 recorder (Linear, Irvine, CA), and a Redirac 2112 fraction collector. After loading, the column was washed with buffer A consisting of 10 mM Na$_2$HPO$_4$, pH

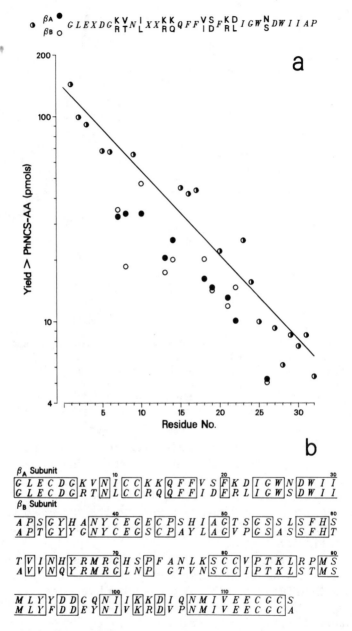

FIG. 14. (a) Amino-terminal sequence analysis of porcine activin. Residues that are common to both subunits are denoted by ◑. Unique residues present only in the β_A subunit are designated by ● and those present only in the β_B subunit by ○. X denotes an unidentified residue (cysteine?). (b) Primary structure of the β subunits of porcine

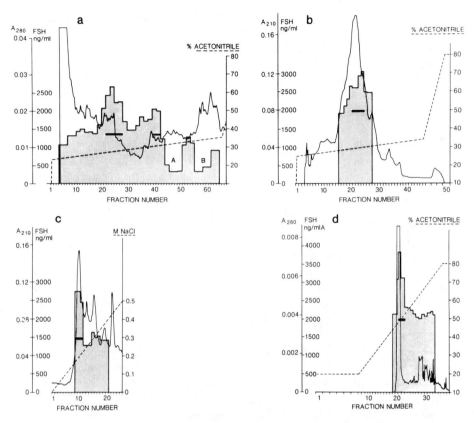

FIG. 15. Purification of the second FSH-releasing substance, homoactivin A, from PFF. The Sephacryl S-200-purified material was processed through the following steps. (a) The material was chromatographed on a Vydac C$_4$ column and eluted with the indicated gradient of acetonitrile in the Et$_3$NP system. Two zones of inhibin activity, A and B, were detected as were two zones of FSH-releasing activity. (b) The active fractions denoted by a black bar and eluting at 27% acetonitrile in a were pooled and, after being diluted to 2 times their original volume with 0.2 N acetic acid, applied directly onto a Vydac C$_4$ column and eluted with the indicated gradient of acetonitrile in the TFA system. (c) The active material (black bar in b) was pooled and further purified by ion-exchange HPLC on a TSK 535CM column and eluted with the indicated gradient of NaCl in 10 mM Na$_2$HPO$_4$, pH 6.5. (d) The ion-exchange HPLC-purified material (black bar in c) was concentrated on an Aquapore RP-300 column using the indicated gradient of acetonitrile in the TFA system.

inhibins A and B deduced from molecular cloning (Mason *et al.*, 1985). The regions containing identical residues are boxed. A gap is introduced at position 74 of β$_B$ to maximize sequence alignment with β$_A$.

6.5, until the UV absorption reached baseline levels. The FSH-releasing activity was eluted from the column with a linear gradient of 0–0.5 M NaCl in 10 mM Na_2HPO_4, pH 6.5, in 50 min at a flow rate of 1 ml/min. Fractions of 2 ml were collected and similarly assayed (Fig. 15c). The material recovered from the cation-exchange HPLC step (solid bar) was then concentrated by RP-HPLC on an Aquapore RP-300 column as before (Fig. 15d).

Analysis of the concentrated material using SDS–PAGE under nonreducing conditions revealed a major band migrating at apparent M_r 24,000 plus two minor bands at 32,000 and 34,000 (Fig. 16). Bioassay of the protein extracted from the gel revealed that only the M_r 24,000 band shows FSH-releasing activity. The remaining RP-HPLC-concentrated material was processed by preparative SDS–PAGE and subsequently purified to homogeneity by RP-HPLC using the same conditions as in Fig. 15d. Altogether, ~6 μg of the second FSH-releasing substance was purified from 1 liter of PFF.

The homogeneous material exhibited half-maximal stimulation of FSH release at a concentration of 3.7 ± 0.5 ng/ml and maximal release at 16 ng/ml or higher (Ling *et al.*, 1986b). The potency values are thus similar to those exhibited by activin.

Microsequencing from the amino terminus of the purified material revealed a single amino acid sequence, which is identical to the amino terminus of the β subunit of inhibin A (Fig. 17). In addition, the yield of the phenylthiohydantoin–amino acids was about twice the amount expected based on the quantity of proteins loaded on the sequencer, indicating that the protein being sequenced is composed of two identical chains of the β subunit of inhibin A. Thus, based on the M_r of the intact molecule and the deduced amino-terminal sequence, we propose that the second FSH-releasing substance found in PFF is a homodimer composed of two β subunits of inhibin A joined together by interchain disulfide bond(s). In keeping with the same terminology as above, we suggest the name *homoactivin A* to signify its origin from two β subunits of inhibin A and its relationship with activin.

The identical homodimeric FSH-releasing protein was independently purified and isolated by Vale and colleagues from PFF using a similar bioassay (Vale *et al.*, 1986). Their purification scheme consisted of ammonium sulfate precipitation, preparative RP-HPLC, and gel filtration on Sepharose CL6B, followed by cation-exchange FPLC, semipreparative RP-HPLC, gel permeation FPLC on Superose 12B, and multiple steps of analytical RP-HPLC. The purified material is effective in stimulating half-maximal FSH release and synthesis at ~25 pM. It has no effect on LH or any other pituitary hormone. Chem-

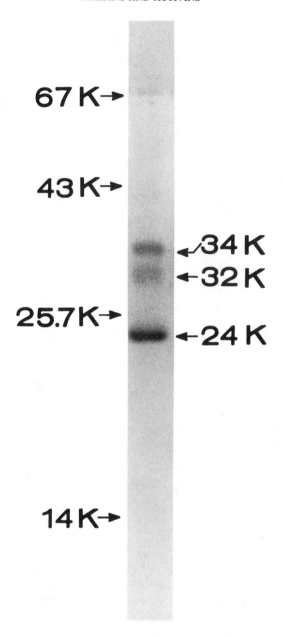

FIG. 16. SDS–PAGE analysis under nonreducing conditions of the FSH-releasing substance, homoactivin A, recovered from Fig. 15d. Only the 24K band (M_r 24,000) is biologically active. Positions of molecular weight standards are indicated at left.

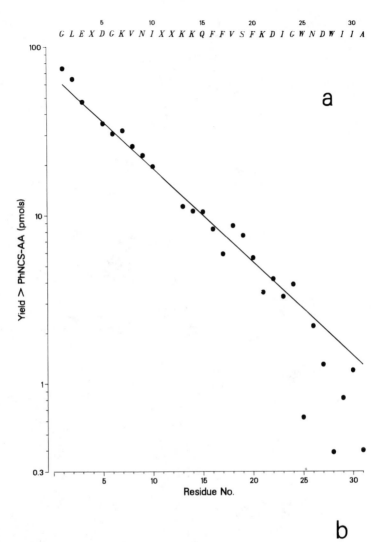

FIG. 17. (a) Amino-terminal sequence analysis of porcine homoactivin A. Fifty-four picomoles of protein were sequenced, and the yield of the released phenylthiohydantoin–amino acids indicated by ●. X denotes an unidentified residue (cysteine?) (b) Primary structure of the β subunit of porcine inhibin A deduced from molecular cloning (Mason *et al.*, 1985).

ical characterization revealed that it is a homodimer composed of two inhibin B_A subunits linked by disulfide bond(s). All these data are in agreement with ours.

In our original report on the structure of inhibins (Mason *et al.,* 1985), we noted the striking similarity between the β subunits of the two forms of inhibin and TGF-β (Fig. 8) and have recently shown that the homodimer TGF-β has intrinsic FSH-releasing activity (Ying *et al.,* 1986a). To observe FSH-releasing activity in a molecule consisting of the β subunits of inhibins A and B or two β subunits of inhibin A is thus in keeping with the TGF-β precedent. What is striking is that when each of the β subunits of the inhibins is combined with an α subunit the resulting molecule inhibits the release of FSH, whereas two β subunits ($β_Aβ_B$ and $β_Aβ_A$) joined together in a molecule release FSH (Fig. 18). It is conceivable that a homodimer composed of two β subunits of inhibin B could produce similar FSH-releasing activity. Such a precedent can be found in the case of platelet-derived growth factor (PDGF) (Waterfield *et al.,* 1983), a heterodimer of two closely related A and B subunits, the same PDGF-like biological activity

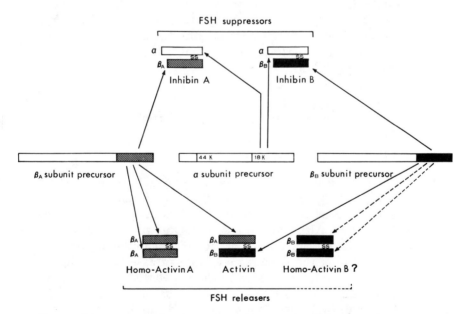

FIG. 18. Divergent arrangements of gene products from the α, $β_A$, and $β_B$ subunit precursors of inhibins A and B through disulfide bridging to yield FSH releasers and suppressors. 18K and 44K denote the M_r 18,000 and 44,000 mature α subunits, respectively. Dashed lines indicate a possible product which has not been isolated and characterized.

being exhibited by a homodimer of either the A or B subunits (Stroobant and Waterfield, 1984; Heldin *et al.*, 1986).

Our previous report on the structural characterization of inhibins A and B demonstrated that each subunit (α, β_A, β_B) is the product of a different mRNA rather than being processed from some unique, very large precursor, and we hypothesized the existence of multiple combinations of the inhibin subunits, including hybrids with the subunits of the ubiquitous TGF-β (Mason *et al.*. 1985). The characterization of activin as a heterodimer of the β subunits of inhibins A and B as well as homoactivin A as a homodimer of two β subunits of inhibin A reinforces that hypothesis. If such rearrangements of several gene products are the norm rather than the exception, this process clearly extends considerably the diversity of the final products (and of their biological activities) derived from a limited number of genes (Fig. 18).

At present, the physiological significance and anatomical distribution of activins are still unknown. Preliminary experiments have shown that the activity of activins is not mediated through the gonadotropin-releasing hormone receptors at the pituitary (Vale *et al.*, 1986). In addition, activins show local effects on the gonad to potentiate FSH-induced aromatase activity in granulosa cells (Ying *et al.*, 1986b), and the effects of activins are opposed by inhibins (Vale *et al.*, 1986; Ying *et al.*, 1986b). It is clear that more studies need to be done in order to elucidate the physiological functions of the β subunit dimers derived from the inhibins.

V. Biosynthesis, Secretion, and Distribution of Inhibin

A. Subunit Assembly of Inhibin

Molecular cloning of ovarian follicular fluid inhibin has revealed that the α, β_A, and β_B subunits are biosynthesized from separate precursors, each encoded by its own mRNA (Mason *et al.*, 1985, 1986; Forage *et al.*, 1986). Although little detail is known about the mechanism(s) regulating the translation of the mRNAs to the precursors as well as processing of the precursors and chain assembly of the subunits to the mature inhibin, it is well documented that in PFF and BFF the M_r 32,000 inhibin, consisting of an M_r 18,000–20,000 α subunit and an M_r 13,000–14,000 β subunit linked by disulfide bridge(s), is the smallest form with full intrinsic activity (Ling *et al.*, 1985; Miyamoto *et al.*, 1985; Rivier *et al.*, 1985; Fukuda *et al.*, 1986; Robertson *et al.*, 1986). The M_r 18,000–20,000 α subunit can be extended at its amino terminus, possibly all the way up to the first residue of the proregion, without loss of biological activity.

Miyamoto and colleagues have isolated from BFF, using immunoaffinity chromatography, six molecular forms of biologically active inhibin (120K, 108K, 88K, 65K, 55K, and 32K), five of which are larger than the M_r 32,000 species (Miyamoto *et al.*, 1986). Using two-dimensional SDS–PAGE to separate the individual subunits after reduction followed by immunoblotting with monoclonal antibodies specific for the α and β subunits, they showed that the 65K, 55K, and 32K inhibins are composed of a 13K β subunit linked by disulfide bridge(s) to a 57K, 44K, or 20K α subunit (Fig. 19a). The 57K α subunit presumably corresponds to the whole precursor minus the signal sequence, and the 44K species is derived from cleavage of the precursor at a processing site close to the amino terminus. The higher molecular weight forms, 120K, 108K, and 88K, were found to be comprised of three polypeptide subunits (Fig. 19b). In these forms, a polypeptide of 62K, immunologically related to the mature β subunit, is attached by disulfide bridge(s) as the third component to the respective 65K, 55K, and 32K inhibin forms. This three-component complex is an attractive model to explain the divergent formation of the inhibins and activins from a common precursor by restricted proteolytic processing and selective cleavage of the interchain disulfide bond(s).

At present, the detailed assignment of the disulfide bonds among the α and β subunits of inhibin is not known. Moreover, the relative

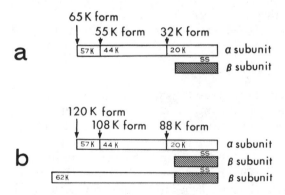

FIG. 19. Possible arrangements of subunits for the larger inhibins from BFF. (a) Arrangement of the 32K, 55K, and 65K forms representing inhibins of M_r 32,000, 55,000, and 65,000, respectively. (b) Arrangement of the 88K, 108K, and 120K forms representing inhibins of M_r 88,000, 108,000, and 120,000, respectively. 20K, 44K, and 57K correspond to the M_r 20,000, 44,000, and 57,000 mature α subunits. 62K is the complete β subunit precursor of M_r 62,000.

physiological significance of the different inhibin forms is still unclear.

B. SECRETION OF INHIBIN

Inhibin activity has been detected in the culture media of granulosa cells derived from rat (Erickson and Hsueh, 1978; Hermans et al., 1982), monkey (Channing et al., 1982), human (Channing et al., 1982), cow (de Jong et al., 1982; Henderson and Franchimont, 1983), and pig (Anderson and Hoover, 1982). The rate of inhibin production was stimulated by the addition of FSH. With the availability of specific antibodies, inhibin can now be measured by radioimmunoassay (Hasegawa et al., 1986; McLachlan et al., 1986a,b; Rivier et al., 1986; Ying et al., 1986c). In this regard, we as well as others we have found that immunoreactive inhibin in the culture media of rat granulosa cells is increased 24 hours after stimulation with FSH (Hasegawa et al., 1986; Ying et al., 1986c). Moreover, Hasegawa and co-workers have detected enhanced inhibin secretion from granulosa cells stimulated with low concentrations of LH; however, testosterone, estradiol, or progesterone alone had practically no effect (Hasegawa et al., 1986). In addition, Davis and colleagues found that treatment of rats with pregnant mare serum gonadotropin (PMSG) increased the level of inhibin mRNA in the ovaries, suggesting modulation of ovarian inhibin synthesis by PMSG at the transcription level (Davis et al., 1986). All these findings support the concept of a negative feedback mechanism such that increased pituitary FSH secretion will elevate the inhibin level in the gonad, which, in turn, attenuates FSH production.

C. DISTRIBUTION OF INHIBIN

Availability of the protein sequence for the inhibin subunits has enabled us to generate antibodies against synthetic peptide fragments that recognize the parent molecule (Ying et al., 1986c). Specifically, we have produced a polyclonal antibody in rabbit, using a synthetic [Tyr^{30}]α-subunit(1–30) fragment of porcine inhibin coupled to bovine serum albumin. This antiserum recognizes native inhibins A and B.

To ascertain what cell types in the gonad produce inhibin, we have used immunohistochemistry and this antiserum to localize inhibin-like immunoreactivity in male and female gonads (Cuevas et al., 1987). Intense staining was observed in rat follicular granulosa cells but not in the theca layers outside the basement membrane (Fig. 20a). This observation is in agreement with the finding of Erickson and

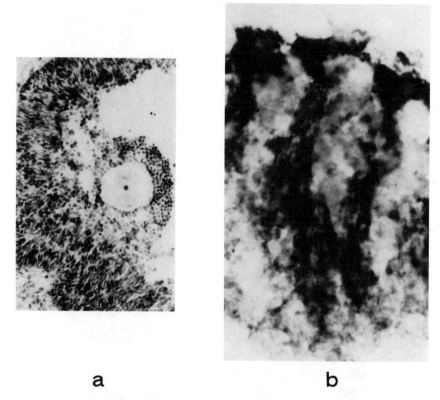

a   b

FIG. 20. Immunohistochemical detection of inhibin in (a) granulosa cells on the follicular wall and the cumulus oophus of a rat ovarian follicle and in (b) Sertoli cells of rat testis.

Hsueh, who first showed that inhibin was produced by granulosa cells in the ovary (Erickson and Hsueh, 1978). In addition, the intensity of the staining correlates with the stages of maturity of the follicles: more intense immunostaining was detected in the larger follicles. Again, this result is in accord with observations that correlated inhibin production with follicle size (Chappel et al., 1980). In rat testes, only the Sertoli cells revealed immunoreactivity with the inhibin antiserum (Fig. 20b). This observation is in agreement with the work of Steinberger and Steinberger (1976), who first demonstrated inhibin production by cultures of Sertoli cells. The positive staining in the gonadal tissues could be blocked completely by preadsorbing the serum with either the synthetic peptide or native inhibin. Immunostaining was not detected in brain, pituitary, thymus, stomach, pancreas,

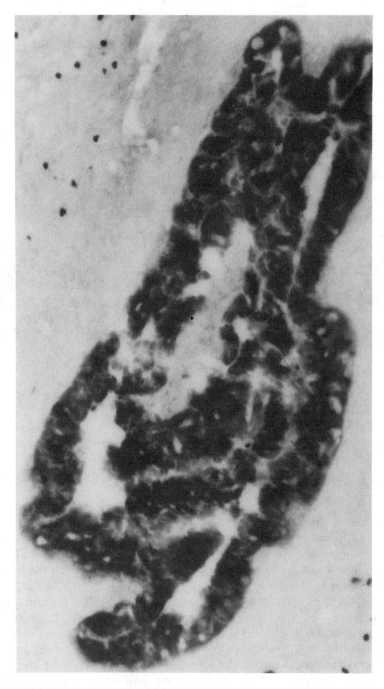

FIG. 21. Immunohistochemical detection of inhibin in rat corpus luteum.

kidney. or adrenal sections, thus confirming that inhibin originates only from specific cells of the gonad.

Unexpectedly, luteal cells in the corpus luteum were also stained by the inhibin antiserum (Fig. 21), but this observation is in accord with a recent publication which reported the detection of a substantial level of mRNA encoding the α subunit precursor in rat corpus luteum (Davis *et al.*, 1986). Recently, McLachlan and colleagues reported the detection of inhibin activity in human placenta extract (McLachlan *et al.*, 1986c). This finding corroborated the results of Mayo and co-workers, who cloned and sequenced the mRNA encoding the inhibin α subunit precursor from a human placental cDNA library (Mayo *et al.*, 1986).

VI. Biological Studies with Inhibin

At present, very few reports on biological studies with purified inhibin have appeared in the literature. The lack of data is due to the paucity of inhibin which at present can only be obtained by tedious purification from ovarian follicular fluid. Most recent biological studies with inhibin concerned measurement of plasma inhibin levels in various physiological states. In one report (McLachlan *et al.*, 1986b), the plasma levels of inhibin were measured in 26 women undergoing treatment to induce follicle growth and maturation for *in vitro* fertilization procedures. These women were treated with clomiphene citrate and human menopausal gonadotropin. Levels of plasma inhibin rose progressively in parallel with estradiol during the treatment with gonadotropin. Peak plasma inhibin levels correlated with the number of developing follicles as assessed by ultrasonography and by the number of oocytes recovered at laparoscopy. The increased inhibin production by the ovaries induced by exogenous FSH is in keeping with its proposed role as a negative feedback regulator of FSH.

Similar animal studies with inhibin antisera have been reported by Rivier and colleagues, who showed that plasma inhibin levels in immature female rats could be increased by administration of PMSG whereas ovariectomy caused an abrupt decrease in plasma inhibin which could not be prevented by PMSG treatment (Rivier *et al.*, 1986). When antibody to inhibin was injected into rats in proestrus as well as diestrus, plasma FSH levels rose but the level of LH was not affected. This finding may explain to some extent the incomplete synchrony of FSH and LH secretion during the estrus cycle (Elias and Blake, 1980; Hasegawa *et al.*, 1981).

VII. Summary

Physiological studies carried out 50 years ago led to the concept that the gonad secretes a polypeptide hormone, inhibin, which acts as a feedback regulator to suppress secretion of pituitary FSH. In 1985, inhibin was finally isolated and purified from porcine and bovine ovarian follicular fluid by four independent research groups. Two forms of M_r 32,000 inhibin, A and B, were isolated from the porcine fluid, each comprised of a common α subunit of M_r 18,000 linked by disulfide bridge(s) to a distinct but related β subunit of M_r 14,000–14,700. From the bovine fluid, a similar M_r 32,000 form of inhibin as well as a M_r 56,000 form, comprised of a M_r 44,000 α subunit joined to a M_r 14,000 β subunit by disulfide bond(s), were identified.

The message encoding each of the subunits (α, $β_A$, $β_B$) of the inhibins has been cloned from porcine and bovine ovarian cDNA libraries. DNA sequence analysis showed that the inhibin α subunit is initially synthesized as a large precursor protein with potential N-linked glycosylation sites. Proteolytic processing at arginine pair sites yields the mature M_r 18,000 or 44,000 α subunit at the carboxy terminus of the precursor. The two β subunits were also found to be derived from large polypeptide precursors and cleavage at the processing sites to yield the mature β subunits at the carboxy termini of the precursors. In addition, the mature β subunits of inhibin were found to be related to a newly characterized homodimeric protein, TGF-β.

Using the porcine cDNAs as hybridization probes, the human and murine inhibin subunit precursors have also been cloned and sequenced. Overall, the amino acid and nucleotide sequences of these inhibin subunits are highly conserved among the four species. These data, all obtained since 1985, end the past confusion regarding the existence and molecular structure of inhibin.

In addition to the inhibins, two FSH-releasing proteins, named activin and homoactivin A, were also isolated from porcine follicular fluid. The former was characterized as a heterodimer, comprised of the β subunits of inhibins A and B, linked by disulfide bridge(s), while the latter was identified as a homodimer of two β subunits of inhibin A. Preliminary studies showed that the biological effects of the activins are opposed to those of the inhibins and vice versa. Now that the activins have been discovered, all the early physiological studies on inhibin, carried out with partially purified porcine follicular fluid, must be viewed with caution.

With the availability of specific antibodies, immunohistochemical localization of inhibin in the granulosa and Sertoli cells of the gonad has been completed. In addition, inhibin has been determined in human and rat plasma; a negative correlation between plasma FSH and inhibin has been established, lending credence to the hypothesis that inhibin is a negative feedback regulator of FSH release. Undoubtedly, more physiological data will be forthcoming in the near future to ascertain the role of inhibin as a new gonadal hormone.

ACKNOWLEDGMENTS

We would like to thank F. Castillo, R. Schroeder, M. Regno, T.-C. Chiang, R. Hu, M. Mercado, K. Cooksey, A. Becker, J. Czvik, and D. Angeles for technical assistance; Bernice Gayer and D. Higgins for preparing the manuscript. This work was supported by NIH Program Project Grants HD-09690 and AM-18811, and NICHD contract NO1-HD-6-2944. Additional financial support was provided by the Robert J. Kleberg, Jr., and Helen C. Kleberg Foundation.

REFERENCES

Aebersold, R. H., Teplow, D. B., Hood, L. E., and Kent, S. B. H. (1986). Electroblotting onto activated glass. High efficiency preparation of proteins from analytical sodium dodecyl sulfate polyacrylamide gels for direct sequence analysis. *J. Biol. Chem.* **261,** 4229–4238.

Akiyama, K., Yoshioka, Y., Schmid, K., Offner, G. D., Troxler, R. F., Tsuda, R., and Hara, M. (1985). The amino acid sequence of human β-microseminoprotein. *Biochim. Biophys. Acta* **829,** 288–294.

Anderson, L. D., and Hoover, D. J. (1982). Hormonal control of inhibin secretion. *In* "Intraovarian Control Mechanisms" (C. P. Channing and S. J. Segal, eds.), pp. 53–78. Plenum, New York.

Baker, H. W. G., Bremner, W. J., Burger. H. G., de Krester, D. M., Dulmanis, A., Eddie, L. W., Hudson, B., Keogh, E. J., Lee, V. W. K., and Rennie, G. C. (1976). Testicular control of follicle-stimulating hormone secretion. *Recent Prog. Horm. Res.* **32,** 429–469.

Baker, H. W. G., Eddie, L. W., Higginson, R. E., Hudson, B., Keogh, E. J., and Niall, H. D. (1981). Assays of inhibin. *In* "Intragonadal Regulation of Reproduction" (P. Franchimont and C. P. Channing, eds.), pp. 193–228. Academic Press, New York.

Beksac, M. S., Khan, S. A., Eliasson, R., Skakkebaek, N. E., Sheth, A. R., and Diczfalusy, (1984). Evidence for the prostatic origin of immunoreactive inhibin-like material in human seminal plasma. *Int. J. Androl.* **7,** 389–397.

Böhlen, P., and Schroeder, R. (1982). High-sensitivity amino acid analysis: Methodology for the determination of amino acid compositions with less than 100 picomoles of peptides. *Anal. Biochem.* **126,** 144–152.

Cahoreau, C., Blank, M. R., Dacheux, J. L., Pisselet, I., and Courot, M. (1979). Inhibin activity in ram rete testis fluid: Depression of plasma FSH and LH in the castrated cryptorchid ram. *J. Reprod. Fertil. Suppl.* **26,** 97–116.

Cate, R. L., Mattaliano, R. J., Hession, C., Tizard, R., Farber, N. M., Cheung, A., Ninfa, E. G., Frey, A. Z., Gash, D. J., Chow, E. P., Fisher, R. A., Bertonis, J. M., Torres, G., Wallner, B. P., Ramachandran, K. L., Ragin, R. C., Manganaro, T. F., MacLaughlin, D. T., and Donahoe, P. K. (1986). Isolation of the bovine and human genes for Müllerian inhibiting substance and expression of the human gene in animal cells. *Cell* **45,** 685–698.

Channing, C. P., Anderson, L. D., Hoover. D., Kolena, J., Osteen, K., Pomerantz, S. H., and Tanable, K. (1982). The role of nonsteroidal regulators in control of oocyte and follicular maturation. *Recent Prog. Horm. Res.* **38**, 331–408.

Channing, C. P., Gordon, W. L., Liu, W.-K., and Ward, D. N. (1985). Physiology and biochemistry of ovarian inhibin. *Proc. Soc. Exp. Biol. Med.* **178**, 339–361.

Chappel, S. C., Holt, J. A.. and Spies, H. G. (1980). Inhibin: Differences in bioactivity within human follicular fluid in the follicular and luteal stages of the menstrual cycle. *Proc. Soc. Exp. Biol. Med.* **163**, 310–314.

Chari, S., Duraiswami, S., and Franchimont, P. (1978). Isolation and characterization of inhibin from bull seminal plasma. *Acta Endocrinol.* **87**, 434–448.

Chari, S., Hopkinson, C. R. N., Duame, E., and Strum, G. (1979). Purification of "inhibin" from human ovarian follicular fluid. *Acta Endocrinol.* **90**, 157–166.

Counis, R., Corbani, M., Poissonnier, M., and Jutisz, M. (1982). Characterization of the precursors of α and β subunits of follitropin following cell-free translation of rat ovine pituitary mRNAs. *Biochem. Biophys. Res. Commun.* **107**, 998–1005.

Cuevas, P., Ying, S.-Y., Ling, N., Ueno, N., Esch, F., and Guillemin, R. (1987). Immunohistochemical detection of inhibin in the gonad. *Biochem. Biophys. Res. Commun.* **142**, 23–30.

Davies, R. V., Main, S. J., and Setchell, B. P. (1978). Inhibin: Evidence for its existence, methods of bioassay and nature of the active material. *Int. J. Androl. Suppl.* **2**, 102–104.

Davis, S. R., Dench, F., Nikolaidis, I., Clements, J. A., Forage, R. G., Krozowski, Z., and Burger, H. G. (1986). Inhibin A-subunit gene expression in the ovaries of immature female rats is stimulated by pregnant mare serum gonadotrophin. *Biochem. Biophys. Res. Commun.* **138**, 119–1195.

de Jong, F. H. (1979). Inhibin: Fact or artifact. *Mol. Cell. Endocrinol.* **13**, 1–10.

de Jong, F. H., and Robertson, D. M. (1985). Inhibin: 1985 update on action and purification. *Mol. Cell. Endocrinol.* **42**, 95–103.

de Jong, F. H., and Sharpe, R. M. (1976). Evidence for inhibin-like activity in bovine follicular fluid. *Nature (London)* **263**, 71–72.

de Jong, F. H., Jansen, E. H. J. M., and van der Molen, H. J. (1981). Purification and characterization of inhibin. *In* "Intragonadal Regulation of Reproduction" (P. Franchimont and C. P. Channing, eds.), pp. 229–250. Academic Press, New York.

de Jong, F. H., Jansen, E. H. J. M., Hermans, W. P., and van der Molen, H. J. (1982). Purification, characterization and physiological significance of inhibin from ovarian follicular fluid. *Adv. Biosci.* **34**, 73–84.

Derynck, R., Jarrett, J. A., Chen, E. Y., Eaton, D. H., Bell, J. R., Assoian, R. K., Roberts, A. B., Sporn, M. B., and Goeddel, D. V. (1985). Human transforming growth factor-β complementary DNA sequence and expression in normal and transformed cells. *Nature (London)* **316**, 701–705.

Dobos, M., Burger, H. G., Hearn, M. T. W.. and Morgan, F. J. (1983). Isolation of inhibin from ovine follicular fluid using reversed-phase liquid chromatography. *Mol. Cell. Endocrinol.* **31**, 187–198.

Elias, K. A., and Blake, C. A. (1980). A change in basal FSH release accompanies the onset of the second or selective phase of increased serum FSH in the cyclic rat. *Life Sci.* **26**, 749–755.

Erickson, G. F., and Hsueh, A. J. W. (1978). Secretion of "inhibin" by rat granulosa cells *in vitro*. *Endocrinology* **103**, 1960–1963.

Esch, F. S. (1984). Polypeptide microsequence analysis with the commercially available gas-phase sequencer. *Anal. Biochem.* **136**, 39–47.

Esch, F. S., Shimasaki, S., Cooksey, K., Mercado, M., Mason, A. J., Ying, S.-Y., Ueno, N., and Ling, N. (1987). Complementary deoxyribonucleic acid (cDNA) cloning and DNA sequence analysis of rat ovarian inhibins. *Mol. Endocrinol.* **1,** 388–396.

Fevold, H. L., Hisaw, F. L., and Leonard, S. L. (1931). The gonad-stimulating and luteinizing hormones of the anterior lobe of the hypophysis. *Am. J. Physiol.* **97,** 291–301.

Fiddes, J. C., and Talmadge, K. (1984). Structure, expression, and evolution of the genes for the human glycoprotein hormones. *Recent Prog. Horm. Res.* **40,** 43–78.

Forage, R. G., Ring, J. M., Brown, R. W., McInerney, B. V., Cobon, G. S., Gregson, R. P., Robertson, D. M., Morgan, F. J., Hearn, M. T. W., Findlay, J. K., Wettenhall, R. E. H., Burger, H. G., and de Kretser, D. M. (1986). Cloning and sequence analysis of cDNA species coding for the two subunits of inhibin from bovine follicular fluid. *Proc. Natl. Acad. Sci. U.S.A.* **83,** 3091–3095.

Franchimont, P. (1985). Inhibin and gonadal parahormones: Possible contraceptive agents. *In* "Male Contraception: Advances and Future Prospects" (G. I. Zatuchni, A. Goldsmith, J. M. Spieler, and J. J. Sciarra, eds.), pp. 408–418. Harper & Row, Philadelphia.

Franchimont, P., Chari, S., and Demoulin, A. (1975a). Hypothalamus–pituitary–testis interaction. *J. Reprod. Fertil.* **44,** 335–350.

Franchimont, P., Chari. S., Hagelstein, M. T., and Duraiswami, S. (1975b). Existence of a follicle-stimulating hormone inhibiting factor "inhibin" in bull seminal plasma. *Nature (London)* **257,** 402–404.

Franchimont, P., Demoulin, A., Verstraelen-Proyard, J., Hazee-Hagelstein, M. T., and Tunbridge, W. M. G. (1979a). Identification in human seminal fluid of an inhibin-like factor which selectively regulates FSH secretion. *J. Reprod. Fertil. Suppl.* **26,** 123–133.

Franchimont, P., Verstraelen-Proyard, J., Hazee-Hagelstein, M. T., Renard, Ch., Demoulin, A., Bourguignon, J. P., and Hustin, J. (1979b). Inhibin: From concept to reality. *Vitam. Horm.* **37,** 243–302.

Fukuda, M., Miyamoto, K., Hasegawa, Y., Nomura, M., Igarashi, M., Kangawa, K., and Matsuo, H. (1986). Isolation of bovine follicular fluid inhibin of about 32 kDa. *Mol. Cell. Endocrinol.* **44,** 55–60.

Hasegawa, Y., Miyamoto, K., Yazaki, C., and Igarashi, M., (1981). Regulation of the second surge of follicle-stimulating hormone; effects of antiluteinizing hormone-releasing hormone, serum, and pentobarbital. *Endocrinology* **109,** 130–135.

Hasegawa, Y., Suzuki, T., Ui, M., Rokukawa, S., and Igarashi, M. (1986). Measurement of inhibin production from porcine granulosa cells by a specific radioimmunoassay. *Annu. Meet. Endocrine Society, 68th, Anaheim, CA,* Abstr. No. 168.

Heldin, C.-H., Johnsson, A., Wennergren, S., Wernstedt, C., Betsholtz, C., and Westermark, B. (1986). A human osteosarcoma cell line secretes a growth factor structurally related to a homodimer of PDGF A-chains. *Nature (London)* **319,** 511–514.

Henderson, K. M., and Franchimont, P. (1983). Inhibin production by bovine ovarian tissues *in vitro* and its regulation by androgens. *J. Reprod. Fertil.* **67,** 291–298.

Hermans, W. P., Van Leeuwen, E. C. M., Debets, H. T. H., Sander, H. J., and de Jong, F. H. (1982). Estimation of inhibin-like activity in spent medium from rat ovarian granulosa cells during long-term culture. *Mol. Cell. Endocrinol.* **27,** 277–290.

Jansen, E. H. J. M., Steenbergen, J., de Jong, F. H., and van der Molen, H. J. (1981). The use of affinity matrices in the purification of inhibin from bovine follicular fluid. *Mol. Cell. Endocrinol.* **21,** 109–117.

Johansson, J., Sheth, A., Cederlund, E., and Jörnvall, H. (1984). Analysis of an inhibin preparation reveals apparent identity between a peptide with inhibin-like activity and a sperm-coating antigen. *FEBS Lett.* **176**, 21–26.

Keogh, E. J., Lee, V. W., Rennie, G. C., Burger, H. G., Hudson, B., and de Kretser, D. M. (1976). Selective suppression of FSH by testicular extract. *Endocrinology* **98**, 997–1004.

Klinefelter, H. F., Reifenstein, E. C., and Albright, F. (1942). Syndrome characterized by gynecomastia, aspermatogenesis without A-Leydigism, and increased excretion of follicle-stimulating hormone. *J. Clin. Endocrinol.* **2**, 615–627.

Kohan, S., Fröysa, B., Cederlund, E., Fairwell, T., Lerner, R., Johansson, J., Khan, S., Ritzen, M., Jörnvall, H., Cekan, S., and Diczfalusy, E. (1986). Peptides of postulated inhibin activity. Lack of *in vitro* inhibin activity of a 94-residue peptide isolated from human seminal plasma, and of a synthetic replicate of its C-terminal 28-residue segment. *FEBS Lett.* **199**, 242–248.

Laemmli, U. (1970). Cleavage of structural proteins during the assembly of the head of bacteriophage T4. *Nature (London)* **227**, 1677–1685.

Li, C. H., Hammonds, R. G., Jr., Ramasharma, K., and Chung, D. (1985). Human seminal α inhibins: Isolation, characterization, and structure. *Proc. Natl. Acad. Sci. U.S.A.* **82**, 4041–4044.

Lilja, H., and Jeppsson, J. O. (1985). Amino acid sequence of the predominant basic protein in human seminal plasma. *FEBS Lett.* **182**, 181–184.

Ling, N., Ying, S.-Y., Ueno, N., Esch, F., Denoroy, L., and Guillemin, R. (1985). Isolation and partial characterization of a M_r 32,000 protein with inhibin activity from porcine follicular fluid. *Proc. Natl. Acad. Sci. U.S.A.* **82**, 7217–7221.

Ling, N., Ying, S.-Y., Ueno, N., Shimasaki, S., Esch, F., Hotta, M., and Guillemin, R. (1986a). Pituitary FSH is released by a heterodimer of the β subunits from the two forms of inhibin. *Nature (London)* **321**, 779–782.

Ling, N., Ying, S.-Y., Ueno, N., Shimasaki, S.. Esch, F., Hotta, M., and Guillemin, R. (1986b). A homodimer of the β subunits of inhibin A stimulates the secretion of pituitary follicle stimulating hormone. *Biochem. Biophys. Res. Commun.* **138**, 1129–1137.

Lorenzen, J. R., Channing, C. P., and Schwartz, N. B. (1978). Partial characterization of FSH suppressing activity (Folliculostatin) in porcine follicular fluid using the metestrous rat as an *in vivo* bioassay model. *Biol. Reprod.* **19**, 635–640.

Lugaro, G., Casellato, M. M., Mazzola, G., Fachini, G., and Carrea, G. (1974). Evidence for the existence in spermatozoa of a factor inhibiting the follicle stimulating hormone releasing hormone synthesis. *Neuroendocrinology* **15**, 62–68.

McCullagh, D. R. (1932). Dual endocrine activity of the testes. *Science* **76**, 19–20.

McLachlan, R. I., Robertson, D. M., Burger, H. G., and de Kretser, D. M. (1986a). The radioimmunoassay of bovine and human follicular fluid and serum inhibin. *Mol. Cell. Endocrinol.* **46**, 175–185.

McLachlan, R. I., Robertson, D. M., Healy, D. L., de Kretser, D. M., and Burger, H. G. (1986b). Plasma inhibin levels during gonadotropin-induced ovarian hyperstimulation for IVF: A new index of follicular function? *Lancet* **1**, 1233–1234.

McLachlan, R. I., Healy, D. L., Robertson, D. M., Burger, H. G.. and de Kretser, D. M. (1986c). The human placenta: A novel source of inhibin. *Biochem. Biophys. Res. Commun.* **140**, 485–490.

Main, S. J., Davies, R. V., and Setchell, B. P. (1979). The evidence that inhibin must exist. *J. Reprod. Fertil. Suppl.* **26**, 3–14.

Mason, A. J., Hayflick, J. S., Ling, N., Esch, F., Ueno, N., Ying, S.-Y., Guillemin, R., Niall, H., and Seeburg, P. H. (1985). Complementary DNA sequences of ovarian follicular fluid inhibin show precursor structure and homology with transforming growth factor-β. *Nature (London)* **318,** 659–663.

Mason, A. J., Niall, H. D., and Seeburg, P. H. (1986). Structure of two human ovarian inhibins. *Biochem. Biophys. Res. Commun.* **135,** 957–964.

Mayo, K. E., Cerelli, G. M., Spiess, J., Rivier, J., Rosenfeld, M. G., Evans, R. M., and Vale, W. (1986). Inhibin A-subunit cDNAs from porcine ovary and human placenta. *Proc. Natl. Acad. Sci. U.S.A.* **83,** 5849–5853.

Midgley, A. R., Jr. (1966). Radioimmunoassay: A method for human chorionic gonadotropin and human luteinizing hormone. *Endocrinology* **79,** 10–18.

Midgley, A. R., Jr. (1967). Radioimmunoassay for human follicle-stimulating hormone. *J. Clin. Endocrinol. Metab.* **27,** 295–299.

Miyamoto, K., Hasegawa, Y., Fukuda, M., Nomura, M., Igarashi, M., Kangawa, K., and Matsuo, H. (1985). Isolation of porcine follicular fluid inhibin of 32K daltons. *Biochem. Biophys Res. Commun.* **129,** 396–403.

Miyamoto, K., Hasegawa, Y., Fukuda, M., and Igarashi, M. (1986). Demonstration of high molecular weight forms of inhibin in bovine follicular fluid (bFF) by using monoclonal antibodies to bFF 32K inhibin. *Biochem. Biophys. Res. Commun.* **136,** 1103–1109.

Mottram, J. C., and Cramer, W. (1923). On the general effects of exposure to radium on metabolism and tumour growth in the rat and the special effects on testis and pituitary. *Q. J. Exp. Physiol.* **13,** 209–229.

Pierce, J. G., and Parsons, T. F. (1981). Glycoprotein hormones: Structure and function. *Annu. Rev. Biochem.* **50,** 465–495.

Ramasharma, K., Sairam, M. R., Seidah, N. G., Chrétien, M., Manjunath, P., Schiller, P. W., Yamashiro, D. and Li, C. H. (1984). Isolation, structure, and synthesis of a human seminal plasma peptide with inhibin-like activity. *Science* **223,** 1199–1202.

Rivier, C., Rivier, J., and Vale, W. (1986). Inhibin mediated feedback control of follicle-stimulating hormone secretion in the female rat. *Science* **234,** 205–208.

Rivier, J., Spiess, J., McClintock, R., Vaughan, J., and Vale, W. (1985). Purification and partial characterization of inhibin from porcine follicular fluid. *Biochem. Biophys. Res. Commun.* **133,** 120–127.

Robertson, D. M., Foulds, L. M., Leversha, L., Morgan, F. J., Hearn, M. T. W., Burger, H. G., Wettenhall, R. E. H., and de Kretser, D. M. (1985). Isolation of inhibin from bovine follicular fluid. *Biochem. Biophys. Res. Commun.* **126,** 220–226.

Robertson, D. M., de Vos, F. L., Foulds, L. M., McLachlan, R. I., Burger, H. G., Morgan, F. J., Hearn, M. T. W., and de Kretser, D. M. (1986). Isolation of a 31 kDa form of inhibin from bovine follicular fluid. *Mol. Cell. Endocrinol.* **44,** 271–277.

Sairam, M. R., and Papkoff, H. (1974). Chemistry of pituitary gonadotropins. *Handb. Physiol.* **4,** 111–131.

Schwartz, N. B., and Channing, C. P. (1977). Evidence for ovarian "inhibin": Suppression of the secondary rise in serum follicle stimulating hormone levels in proestrous rats by injection of porcine follicular fluid. *Proc. Natl. Acad. Sci. U.S.A.* **74,** 5721–5724.

Seidah, N. G., Arbatti, N. J., Rochemont, J., Sheth, A. R., and Chrétien, M. (1984). Complete amino acid sequence of human seminal plasma β-inhibin. *FEBS Lett.* **175,** 349–355.

Setchell, B. P., and Jacks, F. (1974). Inhibin-like activity in rete testis fluid. *Endocrinology* **62,** 675–676.

Setchell, B. M., Davies, R. V., and Main, S. J. (1977). Inhibin. *In* "The Testis" (A. D. Johnson and W. R. Gomes, eds.), Vol. 4, pp. 198–238. Academic Press, New York.

Sherman, B. M., and Korenman, S. G. (1975). Hormonal characteristics of the human menstrual cycle throughout reproductive life. *J. Clin. Invest.* **55,** 699–706.

Steinberger, A., and Steinberger, E. (1976). Secretion of an FSH-inhibiting factor by cultured Sertoli cells. *Endocrinology* **99,** 918–921.

Stewart, A. G., Milborrow, H. M., Ring, J. M., Crowther, C. E., and Forage, R. G. (1986). Human inhibin genes. *FEBS Lett.* **206,** 329–334.

Stroobant, P., and Waterfield, M. D. (1984). Purification and properties of porcine platelet-derived growth factor. *EMBO J.* **4,** 1945–1949.

Takahashi, M., Hayashi, M., Manganaro, T. F., and Donahoe, P. K. (1986). The ontogeny of Müllerian inhibiting substance in granulosa cells of bovine ovarian follicle. *Biol. Reprod.* **35,** 447–453.

Vale, W., Grant, G., Amoss, M., Blackwell, R., and Guillemin, R. (1972). Culture of enzymatically dispersed anterior pituitary cells: Functional validation of a method. *Endocrinology* **91,** 562–572.

Vale, W., Rivier, J., Vaughan, J., McClintock, R., Corrigan, A., Woo, W., Karr, D., and Spiess, J. (1986). Purification and characterization of an FSH releasing protein from porcine ovarian follicular fluid. *Nature (London)* **321,** 776–779.

Ward, D. N. (1981). In pursuit of physiological inhibitors of and from the ovary. *In* "Regulators of Reproduction" (G. Jagiello and H. Vogel, eds.), pp. 371–387. Academic Press, New York.

Waterfield, M. D., Scrace, G. T., Whittle, N., Stroobant, P., Johnsson, A., Wasteson, A., Westermark, B., Heldin, C.-H., Huang, J. S., and Deuel, T. F. (1983). Platelet-derived growth factor is structurally related to the putative transforming protein p28^{sis} of simian sarcoma virus. *Nature (London)* **304,** 35–39.

Williams, A. T., Rush, M. E., and Lipner, H. (1979). Isolation and preliminary characterization of inhibin-f. *In* "Ovarian Follicular and Corpus Luteum Function" (C. P. Channing, J. M. Marsh, and W. A. Sadler, eds.), pp. 429–435. Plenum, New York.

Yamashiro, D., Li, C. H., Ramasharma, K., and Sairam, M. R. (1984). Synthesis and biological activity of human inhibin-like peptide-(1–31). *Proc. Natl. Acad. Sci. U.S.A.* **81,** 5399–5402.

Ying, S.-Y., Becker, A., Baird, A., Ling, N., Ueno, N., Esch, F., and Guillemin, R. (1986a). Type beta transforming growth factor (TGF-β) is a potent stimulator of the basal secretion of follicle stimulating hormone (FSH) in a pituitary monolayer system. *Biochem. Biophys. Res. Commun.* **135,** 950–956.

Ying, S.-Y., Becker, A., Ling, N., Ueno, N., and Guillemin, R. (1986b). Inhibin and beta type transforming growth factor (TGF-β) have opposite modulating effects on the follicle stimulating hormone (FSH)-induced aromatase activity of cultured rat granulosa cells. *Biochem. Biophys. Res. Commun.* **136,** 969–975.

Ying, S.-Y., Ling, N., Ueno, N., Esch, F., and Guillemin, R. (1986c). Immunoneutralization and radioimmunoassay of inhibin isolated from porcine follicular fluid. *Annu. Meet. Endocrine Society, 68th, Anaheim, CA,* Abstr. No. 766.

VITAMINS AND HORMONES, VOL. 44

Guanine Nucleotide Binding Proteins and Signal Transduction

ALLEN M. SPIEGEL

Molecular Pathophysiology Section, Metabolic Diseases Branch
National Institute of Diabetes, Digestive, and Kidney Diseases
National Institutes of Health
Bethesda, Maryland 20892

I. Introduction

Rodbell and co-workers (1980) provided the first evidence for involvement of guanine nucleotides in transmembrane signal transduction. Their experiments indicated that GTP is essential for hormonal stimulation of adenylate cyclase but that, under certain conditions,

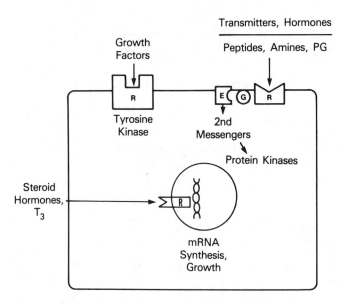

FIG. 1. Three major transmembrane signaling pathways. Steroid and thyroid hormones cross the cell membrane and bind to intracellular receptors (R) that are DNA-binding proteins. Ligand-activated receptors alter transcription of specific gene sequences. Many growth factors bind to cell surface receptors that act as tyrosine kinases. Thus, a major action of such factors is stimulation of phosphorylation of key protein substrates on tyrosine residues. A third class of agonists also binds to cell surface receptors, but these apparently are devoid of kinase activity. Instead, such receptors are coupled to separate effector (E) molecules by G-proteins (G). Effectors may be enzymes that produce second messengers that in turn can activate distinct protein (generally serine/threonine) kinases.

guanine nucleotides could also inhibit adenylate cyclase. They also found that GTP modulates the affinity of agonists in binding to receptors. These observations led first to the discovery of the guanine nucleotide binding protein (G-protein) associated with stimulation of adenylate cyclase, G_s, then to the discovery of the distinct G-protein, G_i, associated with inhibition of adenylate cyclase, and ultimately to the realization that there is a sizeable family of structurally distinct G-proteins involved in coupling diverse receptors to diverse effectors. G-proteins are components of one of three major pathways for transmembrane signaling (Fig. 1).

In contrast to other guanine nucleotide binding proteins such as elongation and initiation factors, involved in protein synthesis, and tubulin, involved in cytoskeletal function (Hughes, 1983), the members of the G-protein family are membrane-bound signal transducers.

In addition to G_s and G_i, known G-proteins include two forms of transducin, involved in photoreceptor function, and G_o, a G-protein of unknown function abundant in brain. Receptor-stimulated phosphoinositide (PI) breakdown is also a G-protein-coupled event, but the identity of the G-protein(s) involved is not yet known. The products of *ras* protooncogenes are presumed to act as signal transducers by analogy to the G-proteins, but this has not yet been rigorously proved.

Many aspects of the structure and function of known G-proteins have recently been elucidated. New G-proteins of unknown function and new G-protein-mediated functions have also been uncovered by recent work. Recent progress in this field is summarized in this article, and the likely direction of future research is indicated.

II. General Aspects of G-Protein Structure and Function

A. Receptor–Effector Coupling and the GTPase Cycle

Members of the G-protein family share certain common features. G-proteins act to couple receptors and effectors. In general, receptors with which G-proteins interact appear to be transmembrane glycoproteins capable of being activated by specific extracellular signals or "first messengers." These signals are diverse and include peptide and glycoprotein hormones, neurotransmitter amines, prostaglandins, chemical odorants, photons of light, and perhaps others. Activation of the receptor involves more than specific binding. Pure antagonists bind to the receptor, often with high affinity, but do not elicit some critical change in receptor structure responsible for signal transmission. The nature of the change elicited by an agonist is unknown, but the result of agonist binding is to convey a signal from the receptor to a G-protein capable of interacting with that receptor. G-proteins in the inactive state contain tightly bound GDP (Ferguson *et al.,* 1986; Poe *et al.,* 1985). Agonist activation of receptor leads to displacement of tightly bound GDP from the receptor-associated G-protein. This enables the G-protein to bind GTP, which is present in the cell in much higher concentration (about 10-fold) than GDP. GTP binding to G-protein has two major consequences: dissociation of G-protein from receptor and activation of effector by the GTP-bound G-protein. The former effect is responsible for the reduction in agonist affinity noted on addition of GTP to plasma membranes; agonists bind to receptors with higher affinity when receptors are associated with G-proteins rather than free.

Known effectors interacting with G-proteins are membrane-bound enzymes, often involved in second messenger metabolism. These include adenylate cyclase, responsible for cAMP formation, and phospholipase C, responsible for diacylglycerol and inositol trisphosphate formation. Effectors interacting with G-proteins may not be limited to enzymes. Preliminary evidence suggests that ion channels may be directly coupled to receptors by one or more G-proteins.

G-protein–effector interaction is transient under physiologic conditions and is terminated by a GTPase activity intrinsic to the G-protein. GTP hydrolysis leads to release of inorganic phosphate and a return of the G-protein to its GDP-bound, inactive state. In this form, the G-protein is again dependent on interaction with agonist-activated receptor to begin another found of the GTPase cycle. The high affinity (submicromolar) of guanine nucleotide binding to G-proteins reflects the relatively slow dissociation rate of bound GDP. This prevents spontaneous activation of G-proteins despite a ratio of GTP/GDP concentration in the cell of about 10. Instead, interaction of G-protein with agonist-activated receptor is needed for release of GDP. Another important feature of G-protein function is that the intrinsic GTPase rate is relatively slow. This is necessary to permit the GTP-bound form of G-protein to survive long enough for effector interaction. Conversely, a further reduction in rate of GTPase activity would lead to prolonged and potentially inappropriate effector activation (see Fig. 2).

Agonist stimulation of effector function involves a series of interactions among receptor, G-protein, and effector. each of which can be measured in crude membrane preparations as well as in phospholipid vesicle systems reconstituted with purified components. Reduction in agonist affinity for receptors by added guanine nucleotides is one measure of receptor–G-protein interaction. This effect reflects the dissociation of G-protein from receptor by added guanine nucleotide. This action of guanine nucleotides may be the first indication that a given receptor is coupled to a G-protein (Glossman et al., 1974; Hinkle and Phillips, 1984).

The interaction between agonist-activated receptor and G-protein can also be monitored by measuring agonist stimulation of guanine nucleotide binding and of GTPase activity. The latter effect is not due to direct stimulation of G-protein enzymatic activity but instead reflects agonist-promoted guanine nucleotide binding. Since GTPase activity is dependent on binding of substrate after each round of hydrolysis, agonist-promoted GTP binding results in apparent stimulation of overall GTPase activity. These parameters of receptor–G-protein interaction are conveniently measured in artificial phospholipid vesi-

Active
Receptor

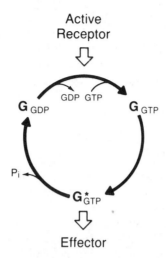

Effector

FIG. 2. The G-protein GTPase cycle. Activated receptor enables G-protein to release tightly bound GDP and to bind GTP. GTP-bound G-protein is the activated form that interacts with and in turn activates effector. Effector and G-protein activation is terminated by the intrinsic GTPase activity of G-protein that hydrolyzes bound GTP and releases free inorganic phosphate. The inactive, GDP-bound form of G-protein must recycle to receptor to undergo activation.

cle systems (Pedersen and Ross, 1982; Cerione *et al.*, 1985), but they can also be measured in crude membrane preparations (Cassel and Selinger, 1977) if appropriate conditions (submicromolar GTP concentration, millimolar concentration of ATP analogs) are used to block nonspecific nucleotide triphosphatases.

Agonist stimulation of effector activity reflects the interaction of all three components: receptor, G-protein, and effector. In appropriate preparations, e.g., highly purified plasma membranes, agonist stimulation of effector activity can be shown to be entirely dependent on added guanine nucleolides. This reflects the participation of a G-protein in signal transduction and its requirement for GTP to displace bound GDP. Use of nonhydrolyzable analogs of GTP, e.g., guanosine 5'-*O*-(3-thiotriphosphate) (GTPγS), leads to stimulation of effector activity by agonist that is quasi-irreversible, as predicted by the GTPase model.

G-proteins may be activated directly, i.e.. without first activating receptor, using nonhydrolyzable GTP analogs or fluoride. Agonist-activated receptor permits release of bound GDP to proceed relatively rapidly even at low $[Mg^{2+}]$ (<5 mM). Increased $[Mg^{2+}]$ facilitates receptor-independent release of bound GDP and activation by newly bound GTP. Fluoride in the millimolar range is a general activator of G-proteins. It appears to interact as a complex, AlF_4^-, with GDP bound to the G-protein (Sternweis and Gilman, 1982; Bigay et al., 1985). The AlF_4^- complex mah mimic the γ phosphate of GTP, thereby converting GDP-bound, inactive G-protein to an activated form. Both fluoride and nonhydrolyzable GTP analogs can activate effectors by directly activating G-proteins.

B. Subunit Structure

Purified G-proteins in solution behave as monomers of approximately 100 kDa. Each G-protein is composed of three distinct subunits (Fig. 3A): α, β, and γ. These are readily separated and visualized after sodium dodecyl sulfate–polyacrylamide gel electrophoresis (SDS–PAGE) (Fig. 3B). Under nondenaturing conditions, however, the β and γ subunits remain tightly, but not covalently, linked. α subunits bind guanine nucleotide, contain GTPase activity, and are substrates for covalent modification by bacterial toxins (see below). The α subunit of each G-protein is distinct and appears to confer specificity for receptor and effector interactions. α subunits range in size on SDS–PAGE from 39 to 52 kDa. The *ras* oncogene products, as discussed below, may be functionally analogous to the G-protein α subunit but are substantially smaller (about 21 kDa).

β subunits migrate as 36-kDa proteins on SDS–PAGE. The β subunits of several G-proteins appear highly similar on peptide mapping (Manning and Gilman, 1983) and immunochemical studies (Gierschik et al., 1985; Fig. 3B). Amino acid sequences predicted by cDNA sequencing show complete identity among several of the β subunits (Codina et al., 1986). A more rapidly migrating (35-kDa) form of β subunit is observed in some tissues (Sternweis and Robishaw, 1984). γ subunits are low-molecular-weight components (8,000–11,000). Although γ subunits of different G-proteins are similar in size, structure (Fig. 3B), and possibly function (Cerione et al., 1987), differences are present.

The holoprotein appears necessary for effective receptor interaction (Fung, 1983; Florio and Sternweis, 1985). Activation of G-protein in solution by nonhydrolyzable guanine nucleotide analogs or by fluoride leads to dissociation of α from β/γ subunits. Mg^{2+} facilitates activation (Iyengar and Birnbaumer, 1982; Katada et al., 1984b), and at high $[Mg^{2+}]$ (50 mM) α subunits dissociate without addition of GTP (Deterre et al., 1984). Resolved, activated α subunits are capable of in-

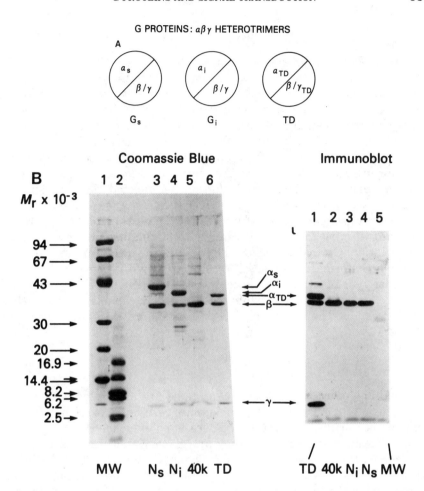

FIG. 3. (A) G-proteins consist of distinct α, β, and γ subunits. The α subunits of G_s, G_i, and transducin (TD) are each unique, while β subunits appear to be identical. TD-γ differs in structure from G_s- and G_i-γ. On G-protein activation in solution, the α subunit dissociates from the β/γ complex. β and γ remain tightly associated under all but denaturing conditions. (B) SDS–PAGE and immunoblot analysis of G_s and G_i (here labeled N_s and N_i) and of transducin (TD). α subunits of differing size (G_s 42, G_i 41, TD 39 kDa) and identical size β (36 kDa) and γ (~8 kDa) subunits are seen on the protein-stained gel (left). Immunoblot with the first antibody directed against holotransducin shows staining of TD α, β, and γ; only β subunits of G_s and G_i cross-react with antibody (right). 40k refers to the β/γ complex of G_s and G_i. (Reproduced, with permission, from Gierschik *et al.*, 1985.)

teracting with and activating effectors (May *et al.*, 1985; Shinozowa *et al.*, 1980; Stryer, 1986).

Since β/γ subunits are not required for effector–G-protein interaction, and since it may be necessary for β/γ subunits to dissociate from α subunits to be activated, the β/γ complex has been viewed as an inhibitor of G-protein activation (Gilman, 1984). It is still not clear, however, whether subunit dissociation is necessary or even occurs during G-protein activation by GTP. Subunits can be readily dissociated in solution, but it has not been proved that such occurs normally in the membrane-bound state *in vivo*. Activation of G-proteins causes important changes in α subunit conformation, as reflected in altered susceptibility to trypsin (Hurley *et al.*, 1984b), and changes in exposure of sulfhydryl groups (Ho and Fung, 1984). These changes may portend reduced affinity for the β/γ complex and thereby promote subunit dissociation. On hydrolysis of GTP to GDP, the α subunit should reassume a conformation favoring reassociation with β/γ. This is necessary for reassociation with receptor since, as mentioned earlier, isolated α subunits are incapable or only poorly capable of interacting with receptor. The properties of G-protein subunits are summarized in Table I.

C. Subcellular Localization

Available data suggest that G-proteins are associated with either the plasma membrane or, for the special case of transducin, with rod photoreceptor disk membranes. There is no evidence that G-proteins span the membrane or that they are glycosylated. Instead they are presumed to be bound to the inner (cytoplasmic) surface of the membrane. The nature and extent of G-protein membrane insertion has not been well defined. With the exception of transducin, G-proteins require detergent to remove them from the membrane. Nonionic detergents such as Lubrol 12A9 are less effective than ionic detergents, particularly cholate (Sternweis *et al.*, 1981). Transducin can be released from rod outer segment membranes in aqueous, hypotonic buffers without detergent (Kuhn, 1980). G-protein α subunits appear to be relatively hydrophilic and behave as monodisperse species in buffers without detergent (Neer *et al.*, 1984; Sternweis, 1986). β/γ subunits (except for that of transducin), in contrast, require detergent for solubility. Thus, it has been suggested that β/γ subunits may serve to anchor G-proteins in the membrane (Sternweis, 1986). The difference in behavior of the transducin β/γ complex almost certainly is due to its unique γ subunit. The latter is relatively hydrophilic (Hurley *et al.*,

TABLE I
SELECTED FEATURES OF G-PROTEIN
SUBUNIT STRUCTURE
AND FUNCTION

α subunits
    Unique for each G-protein
    Approximately 39–52 kDa
    Bind guanine nucleotides; act as GTPase
    Substrate for bacterial toxin ADP ribosylation
    Bind to receptors, effectors, and β/γ complex
β/γ complex
    Binds to α subunit; may function as inhibitor of G-protein activation
    Probably required for G-protein–receptor interaction but not for effector interaction
β subunits
    May be identical for all G-proteins
    36 kDa (an additional 35-kDa form, structurally distinct from the 36-kDa form, also copurifies with some G-proteins)
    Binds tightly, but not covalently, to γ subunit (β/γ complex dissociates only under denaturing conditions)
γ subunit
    That of transducin differs from those of other G-proteins
    Structure of other G-protein γ subunits not yet known
    All are low molecular weight (about 8,000–11,000)
    May be involved in G-protein membrane attachment

1984a; Ovchinnikov *et al.*, 1985); the greater hydrophobicity of other G-protein γ subunits could explain their stronger membrane attachment.

Similarities between the primary sequences of G-protein subunits and those of certain other proteins lead to speculations concerning posttranslational modifications relevant to membrane insertion. G-protein α subunits (with the exception of that of G_s) contain cysteine as the fourth residue from the carboxy terminus. This is similar to the structure of *ras* p21 proteins which are palmitylated in this position. The latter modification is critical for *ras* p21 memrane attachment (Willumsen *et al.*, 1984). It seems unlikely, however, that this cysteine is acylated in the G-α subunit and is accessible to pertussis toxin for ADP ribosylation (see Section II,D). G_s-α is devoid of this cysteine (see Fig. 7C). Interestingly, transducin-γ contains a cysteine in the identical position (see Fig. 7C), and its flanking sequence shows even greater similarity to that of *ras* p21 than does that of G-protein α subunits (Hurley *et al.*, 1984a). This could suggest that the γ subunit of transducin (and perhaps the γ subunits of other G-proteins whose primary sequence is not yet known) could be palmitylated by analogy to *ras* p21.

The amino terminus of all known G-protein α subunits begins with the amino acids Met and Gly. The first 10–15 amino acids show weak similarity to the corresponding region of the *src* oncogene. The latter is known to undergo myristylation on the Gly at the amino terminus (persumably after the Met–Gly bond is cleaved) (Pellman *et al.*, 1985). This acylation is distinct from the palmitylation discussed earlier but is functionally similar in being absolutely required for *src* membrane attachment. The weak homology between G-protein α subunits and *src* in this region provides a tenuous basis for speculation, but certain observations are consistent with the notion that G-protein α subunits may undergo myristylation at the amino terminus. The amino terminus of the α subunits is known to be blocked (Hurley *et al.*, 1984b). In addition, tryptic digestion of membranes containing G_s-α (42 kDa) radioactively labeled with ^{32}P-labeled ADP–ribose release a 41-kDa fragment (Hudson *et al.*, 1981). We (B. Eide and A. M. Spiegel, unpublished observations) have made similar observations for G_o-α in brain membranes. In the latter instance, tryptic cleavage of an amino-terminal 1 to 2-kDa fragment releases the remainder (37 kDa) of the protein from the membrane.

It is worth emphasizing that hypotheses concerning fatty acid acylation of any G-protein subunits must await confirmation with direct evidence for (or against) these or other posttranslational modifications.

The possibility that G-protein α subunits may be released from the membrane under normal physiologic conditions is another interesting speculation (Rodbell, 1985). In certain cell types, G-proteins may be found partially (neutrophils; Okajima *et al.*, 1984) or completely (mast cells; Nakamura and Ui, 1985) in the cytosol. What is not clear is whether this reflects native conditions or merely some artifact of cell disruption. Even if it were the latter, the observation could indicate an important difference in tightness of membrane attachment. If α subunits indeed dissociate from β/γ on activation by GTP in the lipid membrane milieu, and if β/γ is the sole anchor for α subunits in the membrane, one might well expect α subunits to be released from the membrane during the course of normal activation cycles. Such released G-protein α subunits might interact with effectors at points remote from the plasma membrane itself (Rodbell, 1985). Much further work will be necessary to define the nature and extent of G-protein and membrane attachment. The possibility that G-proteins may exist and function as signal transducers in other membrane compartments of the cell also deserves consideration.

D. Effects of Bacterial Toxins

Diphtheria toxin transfers ADP–ribose from NAD to a highly modified form of histidine (trivial name, diphthamide) found in the soluble guanine nucleotide binding protein, elongation factor 2 (EF-2) (Kohno *et al.*, 1986). The diphtheria toxin-dependent ADP ribosylation of EF-2 reduces its interaction with ribosomes and its GTPase activity and thereby inhibits peptide chain elongation. An analogous reaction involving signal-transducing G-proteins is catalyzed by cholera and pertussis toxins (Gill and Meren, 1978; Cassel and Pfeuffer, 1978; Ui, 1984). The toxins bind to cell surface receptors. After binding, one class of subunit, an ADP-ribosyltransferase enzyme, penetrates the cell and uses endogenous NAD to ADP ribosylate a G-protein bound to the inner surface of the cell membrane. In broken cell preparations, the enzymatically active toxin subunit must be generated by reducing disulfide bonds with thiol-containing compounds, and NAD must be added to the reaction mixture.

The α subunit (Fig. 4) is the substrate for toxin-catalyzed ADP ribosylation. Cholera toxin transfers ADP–ribose to an arginine in G_s and TD (see Fig. 7B). This covalent modification appears to reduce the intrinsic GTPase activity of the substrate (Cassel and Selinger, 1977; Abood *et al.*, 1982). This prolongs the half-life of the G-α–GTP complex and permits longer-lived activation of effector. Guanine nucleotide is required for efficient cholera toxin-catalyzed ADP ribosylation of G_s. This requirement appears to reflect the participation of an additional guanine nucleotide binding protein termed ARF (ADP ribosylation

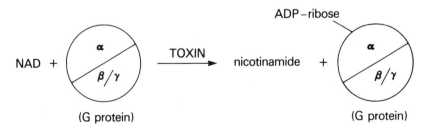

Fig. 4. Bacterial toxins ADP ribosylate G-proteins. Using NAD as cofactor, bacterial toxins such as those of cholera and pertussis transfer ADP–ribose to specific amino acids (see text and Fig. 7) on the G-protein α subunit. The functional consequences vary with the toxin.

factor) in the cholera toxin catalyzed reaction (Kahn and Gilman, 1986). The precise role of ARF remains to be determined. Under certain conditions (no added guanine nucleotide), substrates for cholera toxin-catalyzed ADP ribosylation (other than G_s) are found in cell membranes from fat cells (Owens et al., 1985) or neutrophils (Verghese et al., 1986). These substrates comigrate with those ADP ribosylated by pertussis toxin and could represent G_i and/or G_o. The amino acid target for these substrates has not been identified, but an arginine residue is found in all G-α subunits studied to date in a position identical to that of G_s (see Fig. 7B). Differences in the sequence flanking this arginine residue as well as other differences in secondary and tertiary structure could explain the apparent preferential ADP ribosylation of G_s by cholera toxin. The functional consequences of cholera toxin-catalyzed modification of substrates other than G_s and transducin (TD) have not been well defined, but there is some evidence (Aksamit et al., 1985; Imboden et al., 1986) that rather than activation, as for G_s, other substrates may be inactivated.

Pertussis toxin transfers ADP–ribose to a cysteine near the carboxy terminus of TD, G_i, and G_o-α (West et al., 1985). G_s-α, lacking a cysteine residue in this position, is not a substrate for pertussis toxin. Interestingly, TD-γ as well as the p21 ras gene products contain a cysteine in the same position, but these proteins have not been shown to be ADP ribosylated by pertussis toxin (see Fig. 7C). ADP ribosylation by pertussis toxin appears to cause uncoupling of G-protein from receptor (Ui, 1984; Van Dop et al., 1984b). This leads to reduced agonist-stimulated GTPase activity that reflects the uncoupling of G-protein from receptor rather than a change in the intrinsic GTPase activity of the G-protein. Pertussis toxin may in addition impair G_i activation by nonhydrolyzable GTP analogs (Jakobs et al., 1984). The effect of pertussis toxin is to interfere with signal transduction through the pathway coupled by the relevant G-protein substrate.

The holoprotein rather than isolated G-α is the preferred pertussis toxin substrate. Agents such as fluoride and nonhydrolyzable GTP analogs that promote subunit dissociation inhibit pertussis toxin-catalyzed ADP ribosylation (Neer et al., 1984; Tsai et al., 1984). The molecular basis for the holoprotein requirement is not clear. It could reflect an interaction between the toxin and the β/γ complex or a specific conformation of the α subunit induced by the β/γ complex. The stoichiometry and affinity of α to β/γ subunits are important factors in considering the susceptibility of G-protein to pertussis toxin modification. Unlike the action of cholera toxin, pertussis toxin appears to catalyze ADP ribosylation of substrate without participation of additional proteins such as ARF.

Bacterial toxins have been extremely useful probes of G-protein structure and function. With radioactively labeled NAD as cofactor, toxin-catalyzed ADP ribosylation has been used to identify G-α subunits in membranes. Toxin-catalyzed reactions have been monitored in intact cells by studying receptor–G-protein–effector interaction.

III. Specific G-Proteins and Their Functions

A. G_s

G_s was the first signal-transducing G-protein to be identified. G_s couples receptors for agonists that stimulate cAMP formation to the catalyst, adenylate cyclase. Numerous receptors, including those for β-adrenergic catecholamines, prostaglandins, and many peptide hormones, mediate stimulation of adenylate cyclase. Such receptors can be transferred by cell fusion techniques (Orly and Schramm, 1976) from one cell type to another with resultant acquisition of adenylate cyclase stimulation by ligand for the newly acquired receptor. This implied that receptors and catalyst are distinct and modular.

GTP-affinity chromatography (Pfeuffer, 1977; Spiegel et al., 1979) and complementation studies with mutant S49 mouse lymphoma cells termed CYC$^-$ (Ross et al., 1978) showed that a GTP-binding protein is a distinct component interposed between receptor and adenylate cyclase. Reconstitution studies initially performed with relatively crude detergent extracts and membranes showed that interaction of G_s with receptor leads to increased affinity of receptor for agonist (Sternweis and Gilman, 1979), that interaction of G_s with catalyst is required for guanine nucleotide and fluoride stimulation of catalyst (Ross et al., 1978; Nielsen et al., 1980), and that G_s is the substrate for cholera toxin (Johnson et al., 1978). With the purification of receptors (Dixon et al.. 1986), G_s (Sternweis et al., 1981), and cyclase catalyst (Pfeuffer et al., 1985), reconstitution of receptor–G-protein–effector interaction in artificial phospholipid vesicles has been accomplished (Cerione et al., 1984; May et al., 1985).

G_s is found in all vertebrate cell types, reflecting the ubiquitous distribution of the cAMP transduction pathway. The latter is also found in lower eukaryotes and in prokaryotes. It is not yet clear whether a G_s-like protein performs a similar function in invertebrate systems. Cholera toxin-catalyzed ADP ribosylation identifies at least two G_s-α substrates in most but not all cell types (Johnson et al., 1978; Gilman, 1984). Purification of G_s confirms this heterogeneity and shows that each form of α subunit is associated as a heterotrimer with β and γ subunits (Sternweis et al., 1981; Hildebrandt et al., 1985).

Cholera toxin stimulates cAMP formation directly and also increases the sensitivity of adenylate cyclase to stimulation by agonists. The toxin also augments plasma membrane adenylate cyclase activity in response to GTP. These effects reflect the decrease in G_s GTPase activity discussed earlier.

Forskolin, a diterpene, can activate adenylate cyclase without G_s (Seamon et al., 1984). Forskolin may bind directly to a site on the catalyst, a glycoprotein of approximately 130 kDa (Pfeuffer et al., 1985). Forskolin binding to this site is potentiated by interaction of catalyst with activated G_s, and, in turn, forskolin-bound adenylate cyclase shows enhanced stimulation by G_s (Seamon et al., 1984; Darfler et al., 1982). The relevant sites for G_s-α and forskolin interaction with adenylate cyclase have not yet been defined, but they appear to be distinct, as reflected by differential susceptibility to inhibition by chymotrypsin (Gierschik and Spiegel, 1985).

B. G_i

Guanine nucleotide-dependent inhibition of adenylate cyclase was recognized at the same time as guanine nucleotide-dependent stimulation. Kinetic and other indirect evidence suggested that GTP-mediated inhibition of adenylate cyclase involved a binding site distinct from that mediating stimulation (Rodbell, 1980). With the availability of pertussis toxin [islet-activating protein (Ui, 1984)], G_i was identified and ultimately purified as a distinct G-protein mediating inhibition of adenylate cyclase (Codina et al., 1983; Katada et al., 1984a). Pertussis toxin ADP ribosylates G_i, thereby inactivating it and blocking agonist inhibition of adenylate cyclase. In CYC$^-$ cells, genetically lacking G_s, agonist (somatostatin)- and guanine nucleotide-mediated inhibition of adenylate cyclase is still observed, implicating a distinct G-protein in adenylate cyclase inhibition. In CYC$^-$ as in other cells, this protein was found to be a pertussis toxin substrate, G_i (Hildebrandt et al., 1982).

Based on pertussis toxin-catalyzed ADP ribosylation and on inhibition of adenylate cyclase, G_i appears to be as ubiquitous as G_s. G_i may be about 10-fold more abundant than G_s in plasma membranes (Gilman, 1984). Recent evidence (reviewed in Section V,A) suggests that there are multiple forms of G_i. Differences in tissue distribution and in function between these subtypes have not yet been defined. A central question concerns the mechanism of inhibition of adenylate cyclase.

The general model for G-protein function described earlier would suggest that G_i is activated to bind GTP by agonist-activated receptor, and that receptor bound to G_i will display high affinity for agonists. Substantial evidence confirms this supposition and indicates that pertussis toxin interferes with these interactions (Hsia et al., 1984; Ui, 1984). The model then suggests that activated G_i (α subunit?) should interact directly with adenylate cyclase and decrease activity of the catalyst. Evidence in support of this step is not definitive. On resolution of α and β/γ subunits of purified G_i, potent cyclase-inhibitory activity comigrates with β/γ rather than α subunits (Katada et al., 1984b). Since β/γ subunits of G_s and G_i may be identical, this has led to the suggestion (Gilman, 1984) that inhibition of adenylate cyclase may in fact reflect the action of β/γ subunits on dissociation of G_s. Thus, activation of G_i would lead to dissociation of G_i-α and -β/γ subunits. The latter, given the $10:1$ ratio of Gi to Gs, could block G_s dissociation and activation by a mass action effect.

β/γ subunits are clearly potent inhibitors of adenylate cyclase, and, although one report suggested a direct action on the cyclase catalyst (Katada et al., 1986), it seems more likely that β/γ subunits act by blocking G_s activation. Both TD-β/γ and G-β/γ from brain, the latter more potently, inhibit G_s activation of adenylate cyclase in artificial phospholipid vesicles, but neither inhibits cyclase catalyst directly (Cerione et al., 1986b, 1987). Nonetheless, this action of β/γ may not accurately reflect the mechanism of cyclase inhibition in cell membranes. The dissociation of G_s subunits in the membrane, particularly with the natural activator, GTP, has not yet been demonstrated. Thus, it is not clear whether β/γ inhibition, which assumes the need for G_s-α dissociation, is relevant to the intact cell. Also, the β/γ action on dissociation of G_s cannot explain cyclase inhibition in CYC$^-$ cells. Although the latter are obviously mutant cells, a direct role for G_i-α subunits (much less likely an action of β/γ subunits) on the catalyst is evident.

Further work will be necessary to clarify the basis for adenylate cyclase inhibition. One immediate implication of the uncertainty surrounding the mechanism of inhibition is the difficulty in assigning a specific function to G_i-like proteins. The latter are defined by similarity in structure of their α subunits (see Section V,A), but, if the α subunit is not required for cyclase inhibition, the designation "G_i" is meaningless. If β/γ subunits, moreover, account for cyclase inhibition, and if β/γ subunits are all structurally (or, for TD, functionally) equivalent, then any G-protein with β/γ subunits is a potential "G_i."

C. TRANSDUCIN

In retinal photoreceptor cells, a G-protein (Shinozawa et al.. 1980) termed transducin (Stryer, 1986) couples photon receptors to cGMP phosphodiesterase. In rod cells, the photon receptor is rhodopsin; in cones, related but distinct proteins serve as photon receptors (Nathans et al., 1986). Each of the opsins contains retinal which isomerizes on photoactivation by light of the appropriate wavelength. Photoactivation of opsin is equivalent to agonist binding to hormone or neurotransmitter receptors. Activated opsin permits release of GDP from TD; subsequent binding of GTP activates TD which in turn activates cGMP phosphodiesterase. Indirect evidence suggests that TD-α dissociates from β/γ on activation by GTP (Fung, 1983). The GTP-bound α subunit binds to and apparently displaces an inhibitory γ subunit from the cGMP phosphodiesterase complex (Yamazaki et al., 1983). Effector activation is terminated by GTP hydrolysis on TD-α, although other mechanisms may also be involved. A "48K" protein (Wistow et al., 1986) may compete with TD for binding to rhodopsin.

Light alters photoreceptor synaptic transmission by changing membrane potential. In rods, the photon receptor is an intrinsic membrane protein contained in disks stacked in a specialized outer segment. Rod outer segment disk membranes are not contiguous with the plasma membrane. Thus, a diffusible messenger must transmit the light impulse from rhodopsin in the disk membranes to the plasma membrane, where a change in potential occurs. TD and the cGMP phosphodiesterase are peripheral proteins associated with the disk membranes. Recent electrophysiologic studies (reviewed by Stryer, 1986) suggest that cGMP itself is the diffusible messenger. cGMP apparently holds open a cation channel in the rod outer segment plasma membrane. Light-activated hydrolysis of cGMP reduces the concentration of the latter sufficiently to permit channel closing and altered membrane potential.

In cones, photopigments are present in the plasma membrane itself, obviating the need for a diffusible messenger. Nonetheless, cGMP appears to serve a similar function in cones as in rods. A form of cGMP phosphodiesterase related to but perhaps not identical to that in rods is found in cone cells (Hurwitz et al., 1985). Immunohistochemical studies showed that a putative cone TD must differ from rod TD (Grunwald *et al.*, 1986). A cDNA coding for a G-α subunit closely related to but distinct from that for rod TD-α was cloned from a retinal library (Lochrie *et al.*, 1985). Antibodies raised against synthetic peptides from unique regions of the two forms of TD localized the proteins to either rods or cones (Lerea *et al.*, 1986).

Unlike G_s and G_i, TD shows a highly restricted distribution; it is limited to photoreceptor cells in the retina and perhaps to photorecep-tor-like cells in nonmammalian vertebrate pineal gland (Van Veen *et al.*, 1986). TD (the rod form for which there is direct evidence, but presumably the cone form as well) serves as both a pertussis and cholera toxin substrate. The sites of ADP ribosylation by the two tox-ins are distinct (see Section II,D), and the functional consequences are opposite (cholera, activation; pertussis, inactivation).

D. G_o

A G-protein of unknown function (hence termed G_o for other) was discovered in the course of purification of G-proteins from brain (Sternweis and Robishaw, 1984; Neer *et al.*, 1984). The common G-protein β subunit is present in higher concentration in brain than in any tissue with the exception of rod outer segment membranes, the site of highly abundant TD (Gierschik *et al.*, 1985). The high β subunit concentration reflects the presence of high concentrations of G_o (roughly 1% of total membrane protein) in addition to G_i (one-fifth to one-tenth the concentration of G_o) and G_s (Gierschik *et al.*, 1986b). G_o-α is a district protein as shown by immunochemical comparisons with other G-proteins (Huff *et al.*, 1985; Mumby *et al.*, 1986; Gierschik *et al.*, 1986b; Fig. 5) and by differential susceptibility to proteolysis (Sternweis and Robishaw, 1984; Winslow *et al.*, 1986). cDNA cloning confirms that G_o is a distinct member of the G-protein family (see Section V,A).

G_o is, like G_i and TD, a pertussis toxin substrate. G_o shows certain unique features including relatively lower affinity of its α for β/γ subunits, even when the former are in the GDP-bound form, higher "basal" GTPase activity, and more rapid exchange of bound guanine nucleotide, particularly at low Mg^{2+} concentration (Sternweis and Robishaw, 1984; Neer *et al.*, 1984). G_o appears to be less widely dis-tributed than G_s and G_i but more widely than TD. In addition to marking brain, specific antibodies localize G_o immunoreactivity in heart (Huff *et al.*, 1985) and in 3T3-L1 fibroblasts and adipocytes (Gierschik *et al.*, 1986c). Relatively little if any G_o is present in liver (Huff *et al.*, 1985) or in neutrophils (Gierschik *et al.*, 1986a).

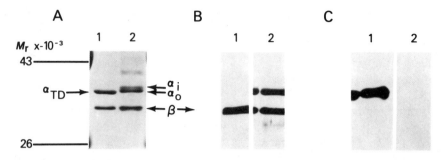

FIG. 5. SDS–PAGE and immunoblot analysis of purified transducin and brain G_i/G_o. (A) Protein stain shows a doublet of brain α subunits (41-kDa G_i and 39-kDa G_o) and a doublet of brain β subunits (predominant 36-kDa form and slight 35-kDa form). TD-α (39 kDa) and -β (36 kDa) appear as single bands. (B) Antibodies directed against brain, G-proteins react with brain G_o-α and -β and cross-react with TD-β but not TD-α. (C) Antibody directed against TD-α fails to react with brain G_i/G_o α subunits.

G_o is assumed to be a signal transducer on the basis of its association with the inner surface of the plasma membrane and its heterotrimeric structure, analogous to that of other G-proteins whose signal transduction function has been identified. The specific function of G_o, however, has not been identified. Purified G_o has been found capable of coupling to muscarinic cholinergic (Florio and Sternweis, 1985), α_2-adrenergic (Cerione et al., 1986a), and fMet-Leu-Phe (Kikuchi et al., 1986) receptors as efficiently as G_i; however, none of these studies proves that G_o is actually coupled to any of these receptors in the cell.

With respect to effector interactions, activated G_o-α will not substitute for TD in stimulating cGMP phosphodiesterase, for G_s-α in stimulating adenylate cyclase, nor for G_i-α in inhibiting cyclase activity in CYC$^-$ cells (Roof et al., 1985). Speculation concerning effector interaction of G_o centers on phosphoinositide (PI) breakdown and on ion channels. One or more G-proteins, some pertussis toxin sensitive, appear to be involved in these effector pathways (see Section IV,A). Immunohistochemical localization of G_o in brain corresponds more closely to the distribution of protein kinase C than to that of adenylate cyclase (Worley et al., 1986). This has been interpreted to suggest G_o involvement in PI breakdown. In pertussis toxin-treated HL-60 cells, purified brain G_o was found to restore agonist-stimulated PI breakdown. Purified brain G_i was equally effective, raising questions of specificity in this response (Kikuchi et al., 1986). Ultimately, reconstitution of receptor–G-protein–effector interactions with purified components as well as more precise methods for probing specific

TABLE II

FUNCTION AND DISTRIBUTION OF KNOWN AND PUTATIVE G-PROTEINS

G-protein	Function	Distribution
Transducin$_1$	Couples rhodopsin to cGMP phosphodiesterase	Rod photoreceptors
Transducin$_2$	Couples cone opsins to cGMP phosphodiesterase	Cone photoreceptors
G_s	Couples many receptors to stimulation of adenylate cyclase	Ubiquitous
G_i	Couples many receptors to inhibition of adenylate cyclase; may have other functions	Several forms; tissue-specific expression likely
G_o	Unknown; probably couples neurotransmitter receptors to one or more effectors (?ion channels)	Most abundant in brain; present in some (e.g., heart) but not all other tissues
G_{pi}	Couples many receptors to stimulation of phosphoinositide breakdown	In neutrophils and some other cells, G_{pi} is pertussis toxin sensitive and may be related to G_i; in most cells G_{pi} is insensitive to pertussis toxin and may be a different G-protein
$G_{\text{"ionchannel"}}$	Couples neurotransmiter receptors directly (?) to ion channels	Pertussis toxin-sensitive form identified in heart and neurons

functions within the cell will be necessary to elucidate functions of G_o and other novel G-proteins. Table II summarizes properties of known and putative G-proteins.

IV. OTHER POSSIBLE G-PROTEINS AND G-PROTEIN-MEDIATED FUNCTIONS

A. G-PROTEIN(S) LINKED TO PHOSPHOINOSITIDE BREAKDOWN (G_{pi})

Agonists for many different cell surface receptors cause breakdown of PI and generation of second messengers inositol trisphosphate (IP$_3$) (calcium mobilization) and diacylglycerol (activation of protein kinase C) (reviewed in Berridge and Irvine, 1984). Much recent evidence suggests that a G-protein couples such receptors to the effector enzyme, phospholipase C. Aluminum floride, a universal G-protein activator, can stimulate PI breakdown directly, as can nonhydrolyzable GTP analogs. Agonist stimulation of PI breakdown in plasma membranes can also be shown to be guanine nucleotide dependent (Litosch *et al.,* 1985; Cockroft and Gomperts, 1985). Agonists shown to act by stimulating PI breakdown, moreover, have been found to stimulate high affinity GTPase and to display altered affinity for receptors after addition of guanine nucleotides, both clues to receptor–G-protein interaction (e.g., for TRH, Hinkle and Phillips, 1984).

In certain cell types the G-protein coupling receptor to phospholipase C appears to be a pertussis toxin substrate. This has been best shown in neutrophils (Okajima *et al.,* 1984; Smith *et al.,* 1985). The identity of the relevant G-protein is not yet clear, since several pertussis toxin substrates, including G_i, G_o, and TD, exist. Immunochemical studies (Gierschik *et al.,* 1986a; Falloon *et al.,* 1986) suggest that the protein is neither TD nor G_o. Immunochemical differences, moreover, were noted between a form of G_i detected in brain and the pertussis toxin substrate of neutrophils (Fig. 6). These data suggest that novel forms of pertussis toxin substrate exist and are consistent with the cloning of cDNAs (see Section V,A) for multiple forms of "G_i." As yet it is unclear which if any of these forms of G_i corresponds to the pertussis toxin-sensitive G-protein linked to phospholipase C in neutrophils. The relevant G-protein may also be unique in its susceptibility to ADP ribosylation (Aksamit *et al.,* 1985; Verghese *et al.,* 1986) and inactivation (Imboden *et al.,* 1986) by cholera toxin. This, or a related protein, may also be found in other cell types including mast cells (Nakamura and Ui, 1984), lymphocytes (Jakway and DeFranco, 1986), and macrophages (Johnson and Davies, 1986).

In numberous other cell types, including pancreatic acinar cells, pituitary cells, and liver (reviewed in Williamson, 1986), a G-protein coupling receptors to phospholipase C appears to be pertussis toxin insensitive. This could reflect altered accessibility to toxin, variations in ratio of α to β/γ subunits, or other factors. A simpler explanation would be that this is an entirely different G-protein. If so, its identity is yet to be discovered. Pertussis toxin differentiates this "G_{pi}" from "G_i." Thus, in kidney, the toxin uncouples α_2-adrenergic receptors linked to cyclase inhibition from G-protein, but not α_1 receptors linked to PI breakdown (Boyer *et al.,* 1984). Similar observations have been made for muscarinic cholinergic receptors (Master *et al.,* 1985), although the receptor subtypes are not as clearly defined. Limited data (Enjalbert *et al..* 1986) also suggest that a G-protein, perhaps linked to the D_2-dopamine receptor, may couple receptors to inhibition of PI breakdown. Such dual regulation would parallel that for adenylate cyclase.

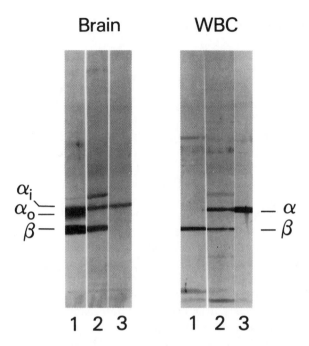

FIG. 6. Immunochemical identification of brain and neutrophil pertussis toxin substrates. In human brain membranes abundant G_o is detected with specific antibodies (1), whereas in human neutrophil membranes (WBC) G_o is undetectable. A polyclonal antiserum raised against transducin but reactive with G_i and an antiserum raised against a synthetic peptide related to G_i-α detect equal amounts of G_i-α in brain membranes (2 and 3, respectively); in neutrophil membranes, the peptide antiserum (3) detects substantially more immunoreactive material than does transducin antiserum (2). β subunits are detected by appropriate antisera in each case. The data suggest that neutrophils contain a pertussis toxin substrate immunochemically distinct from those in brain (see text). (Reproduced from Falloon *et al.*, 1986, with permission.)

Three independent reports of guanine nucleotide stimulation of a soluble form of phospholipase C have appeared (Baldassare and Fisher, 1986; Deckmyn *et al.*, 1986; Banno *et al.*, 1986). These raise the possibility that a soluble G-protein max interact with a soluble form of phospholipase C in platelets, and perhaps elsewhere. Agonist modulation of this activity was not observed, and further work will be needed to define its significance. Enzymes of the PI metabolic pathway other than phospholipase C may also be subject to regulation by guanine nucleotides and perhaps by G-proteins. Stimulation of phosphorylation of PI 4-phosphate by GTPγS in placental membranes has been reported (Urumow and Wieland, 1986). If confirmed, this would mean that synthesis of the precursor for IP_3 formation is also regulated by guanine nucleotides.

B. *ras* AND *ras*-LIKE G-PROTEINS

ras gene products, like G-protein α subunits, bind guanine nucleotides, show GTPase activity, and are associated with the cytoplasmic surface of the cell membrane (Gibbs *et al.*, 1984). Palmitylation of a cysteine near the carboxy terminus is critical for membrane insertion and *ras* function (Willumsen *et al.*, 1984). Unlike G-protein α subunits, there is no evidence that *ras* gene products associate with G-protein β/γ subunits or analogous structures (Broek *et al.*, 1985). Indirect evidence suggests that *ras* gene products, like G-proteins, are signal transducers, but this has not been rigorously proved.

Three mammalian *ras* genes code for three closely related proteins of 188 or 189 amino acids (apparent M_r on SDS–PAGE is 21,000, hence p21), (Taparowsky *et al.*, 1983). The three forms of p21 are identical except for a variable region just before the carboxy terminus (amino acids 165–185). The significance of this heterogeneity is not clear, but, if *ras* gene products are indeed signal transducers, the variable region could confer specificity to receptor or effector interaction. Amino acid sequence similarities between portions of *ras* p21 and G-protein α subunits (see Section V,A) likely reflect a common evolutionary origin. Such regions relate primarily to sites involved in binding guanine nucleotides. Thus, these similarities alone do not constitute evidence that *ras* p21 is a signal transducer.

Evidence for this notion comes from analysis of mutant, oncogenic forms of p21. These occur within retroviral genomes (e.g., Kirsten or Harvey sarcoma viruses), and have also been isolated from several human tumors by transfection assays. Substitutions, generally involving amino acids 13, 59, 61, and, in particular, glycine 12 (see Fig. 7A), lead to forms of p21 capable of transforming NIH 3T3 cells. Most (McGrath *et al.*, 1984; Sweet *et al.*, 1984; Gibbs *et al.*, 1984), but not all (Lowy and Willumsen, 1986), forms of p21 causing malignant transformation also show reduced GTPase activity. The latter, by analogy with the GTPase cycle of G-proteins, could lead to constitutive activation of *ras* p21 and a putative effector protein with which it interacts. If, as has been postulated, growth factors and growth factor receptors (Kamata and Feramisco, 1984), are the physiologic activators of *ras* p21, oncogenic forms of p21, with reduced GTPase activity, would be active independent of receptor interaction.

The receptors and effectors for *ras* p21 have not been directly identified. Indirect evidence links *ras* p21 to stimulation of PI breakdown

(Fleischman *et al.*, 1986; Preiss *et al.*, 1986). Experiments involving overexpression of the protooncogenic form of *N-ras* suggest that this form of p21 may couple bombesin receptors to PI breakdown (Wakelam *et al.*, 1986). Interestingly, pertussis toxin has been reported to block the effects of bombesin on *myc* expression and DNA synthesis in Swiss 3T3 cells (Letterio *et al.*, 1986). The latter effects, it is believed, result from stimulation of PI breakdown. Since *ras* p21 is not known to be pertussis toxin sensitive, toxin blockade of bombesin mitogenic effects would appear inconsistent with a role for p21 in coupling the bombesin receptor to PI breakdown. Further work is needed to identify the nature and precise function of the pertussis toxin-sensitive G-protein.

ras gene products are found, and are highly conserved, throughout nature. In yeast, *Saccharomyces cerevisiae*, 2 *ras* gene products code for proteins closer in size to G-protein α subunits (about 39 kDa). These are nearly identical to mammalian *ras* p21 in the amino-terminal half of the molecule, but the yeast forms diverge from mammalian p21, and from each other, in a large carboxy-terminal segment (DeFeo-Jones *et al.*, 1983). Both *S. cerevisiae ras* genes code for proteins linked to regulation of adenylate cyclase (Kataoka *et al.*, 1985). Interestingly, although mammalian *ras* p21 can substitute for yeast *ras* products in reconstituting adenylate cyclase activity in deficient mutants, there is no evidence that *ras* p21 regulates adenylate cyclase positively or negatively in mammals (Beckner *et al.*, 1985) or even in other yeasts, such as *Schizosaccharomyces pombe* (Fukui *et al.*, 1986). Additional evidence suggests that *ras* gene products may also regulate glucose-induced PI breakdown in *S. cerevisiae* (Kaibuchi *et al.*, 1986).

Although much evidence connects *ras* gene products to control of cell division, studies on neurons implicate *ras* gene products in other functions. Paradoxically, microinjection of oncogenic p21 into PC12 cells induces differentiation into sympathetic neurons (Bar-Sagi and Feramisco, 1985). Abundant expression of *ras* proteins in *Aplysia* neurons (Swanson *et al.*, 1986) also suggests that *ras* gene products may subserve functions unrelated to control of cell division.

cDNAs coding for *ras*-related proteins have recently been identified. The *rho* gene (similar to *ras;* Madaule and Axel, 1985) was first identified in *Aplysia* but is present and highly conserved in mammals. *rho* gene products show strong similarity to *ras* in regions involved in guanine nucleotide binding but diverge in other regions that may specify target protein interactions. The *YPT* gene product in *S. cerevisiae* codes for a guanine nucleotide binding protein distinct from that encoded by the two *ras* genes; it may be involved in microtubule function (Schmitt *et al.*, 1986).

ARF, a 21-kDa protein originally identified as a cofactor for cholera toxin-catalyzed ADP ribosylation of G_s, is itself a guanine nucleotide binding protein (Kahn and Gilman, 1986). It seems likely that it serves an endogenous function unrelated to cholera toxin. Despite similar M_r, ARF and ras p21 are apparently distinct proteins. Another guanine nucleotide binding protein smaller than G-protein α subunits and closer to ras p21 in size has been isolated from placental membranes and termed "G_p" (Evans et al., 1986). The function of this protein is at present unknown. It seems clear, though, that in addition to the expanding family of G-proteins with α subunits in the 40-kDa range there is a related family of guanine nucleotide binding proteins of approximately 20 kDa. Much more work will be necessary to elucidate the function of the latter.

C. Olfaction

Olfactory transduction involves conversion of extracellular signals (a vast array of chemical odorants) into altered synaptic transmission by chemosensitive neurons. The latter are functionally and anatomically analogous to the photoreceptor cells of the retina. Although chemical odorants rather than photons of light are the "first messengers," specialized olfactory cilia similar to photoreceptor outer segments (themselves modified cilia) are the site of transduction.

Recent evidence implicates G-proteins in olfactory transduction. Olfactory cilia are extraordinarily rich in both adenylate cyclase activity and a cholera toxin substrate that is either G_s or a closely related protein (Pace et al., 1985). Slight differences in size and nucleotide binding specificity between olfactory cilia and liver G_s (Pace and Lancet, 1986) may relate to G_s-α heterogeneity (see Section V,A) or may indicate that the olfactory protein is unique. Adenylate cyclase activity in olfactory cilia membranes is stimulated by odorants in a guanine nucleotide-dependent manner. This suggests that G_s may couple odorant receptors to adenylate cyclase in a manner analogous to the hormone- and neutrotransmitter-sensitive adenylate cyclase of other tissues (Pace et al.. 1985). Olfactory dysfunction in humans with deficient G_s (see Section VII,A) is consistent with this model (Weinstock et al., 1986).

Another study of olfactory epithelial adenylate cyclase activity confirms odorant and guanine nucleotide sensitivity (Sklar et al., 1986). Putrid (as opposed to fruity and herbaceous) odorants, however, did not stimulate the enzyme. This suggests that certain odorants utilize signal transduction pathways other than G_s-coupled stimulation of adenylate cyclase. Indeed, certain odorants may stimulate PI break-down in olfactory cilia, again in a guanine nucleotide-dependent man-ner (Huque and Bruch, 1986). The nature of the G-protein involved is not yet clear.

D. Ion Channels and Exocytosis

Ion channels, pores in the plasma and other cell membranes that permit the passage of certain ions, are subject to complex regulation. One of the best studied systems, the nicotinic cholinergic receptor, combines ligand recognition and channel function in one molecule. The function of several other types of channel may be modified indi-rectly by cell surface receptors. Thus, ligands that stimulate cAMP formation may lead to phosphorylation of channel proteins by cAMP-dependent protein kinase. As discussed earlier, ligands that stimulate PI breakdown and IP_3 formation raise intracellular calcium through the action of IP_3 on a calcium-gating mechanism in endoplasmic re-ticulum. In rod and cone photoreceptor cells, a second messenger, cGMP, directly modifies channel function by acting to keep open a cation channel. G-proteins, by coupling cell surface receptors to ef-fector enzymes that catalyze second messenger formation, are indi-rectly involved in regulation of ion channel function. G-proteins may also regulate certain ion channels directly.

A pertussis toxin-sensitive G-protein appears to link a muscarinic cholinergic receptor to an inwardly rectifying potassium channel in chick (Pfaffinger *et al.*, 1985) and frog heart (Breitweiser and Szabo, 1985). Similar results have been reported for a potassium channel activated by serotonin and γ-aminobutyric acid B receptors in rat hip-pocampus (Andrade *et al.*, 1986). In studies of excised patches from guinea pig atrial cells, Yatani *et al.* (1987) found that exogenous pu-rified human erythrocyte "G_i" restores potassium channel activation by muscarinic cholinergic agonists to cells treated with pertussis toxin. The identity of the relevant G-protein (which the authors termed "G_k") is not known, since purified erythrocyte "G_i" may consist of several G-proteins. G_o, purified from bovine brain, showed much less activity (5% of equivalent amounts of erythrocyte "G_i"). This low activity may be due to small amounts of other G-proteins contaminating the G_o preparation. Although not explicitly stated, the study of Yatani *et al.* (1987) implies that the activated α subunit of "G_k" directly activates the potassium channel. This finding, is apparently contradicted by the work of Logothetis *et al.* (1987), who showed that isolated β/γ subunits from brain (and not α subunits of G_i or G_o) directly activate a potassium channel in chick embryonic atrial cells. This finding raises important questions concerning specificity of effector activation by G-proteins. Since G-protein β/γ subunits had been assumed to be functionally equivalent, and since β/γ subunits might be released by activation of any G-protein, it is not clear why only certain agonists activate a potassium channel. Further studies are needed to answer this question and to resolve the apparent contradiction between the results of Yatani et al. (1987) and Logothetis et al. (1987).

Intracellular calcium concentration may be raised by release of calcium from intracellular stores (in particular, the endoplasmic reticulum) and by activation of voltage-sensitive (and perhaps other) calcium channels in the plasma membrane. The latter permit transmembrane flux of calcium from outside the cell and may be responsible for the sustained response of cells to calcium-mobilizing agents. Introduction of nohydrolyzable analogs of GTP into permeabilized cells provided the first evidence for a cyclic nucleotide-independent action of G-proteins in the regulation of intracellular calcium concentration (Gomperts, 1983). The initial observations have been confirmed in several cell types, but the evidence suggests that guanine nucleotides may affect calcium transport at several distinct sites. In dorsal root ganglion cells, α_2-adrenergic and γ-aminobutyric acid B receptors are coupled to inhibition of voltage-sensitive calcium channels by a pertussis toxin-sensitive G-protein (Holz et al., 1986). A similar G-protein appears to couple somatostatin receptors to voltage-sensitive calcium channels in a cultured pituitary cell line (Koch et al., 1985; Schlegel et al., 1985; Lewis et al., 1986). In neither instance can the effects of the G-protein be linked to alterations in cyclic nucleotide synthesis, since direct application of cyclic nucleotides does not mimic the effect of G-protein activation or inactivation. These data suggest that receptors may communicate with ion channels directly through a G-protein without involvement of intervening, second messengers.

Certain calcium-mobilizing agonists, e.g., angiotensin II in adrenal glomerulosa cells, increase intracellular calcium in at least two ways. Angiotensin stimulates PI breakdown, which leads to IP_3-mediated release of intracellular calcium, and angiotensin also stimulates calcium influx from outside the cell. The latter action, but not stimulation of PI breakdown, is inhibited by pertussis toxin in adrenal glomerulosa cells (Kojima et al., 1986). Similar observations have been made in cultured vascular smooth muscle cells (Kanaide et al., 1986). In neutrophils, both PI breakdown and influx of extracellular calcium are inhibited by pertussis toxin (Okajima and Ui, 1984).

Parathyroid cells provide an interesting system in which to study regulation of calcium transport. Considerable evidence suggests that increased ionized extracellular calcium per se inhibits parathyroid hormone secretion. The mechanism of this inhibition is still unknown. Studies with calcium channel agonists suggest that calcium entry via calcium channels is required for extracellular calcium inhibition of hormone secretion (Fitzpatrick et al., 1986). Interestingly, pertussis toxin was reported to block inhibition of hormone secretion by calcium channel agonists. This suggests that a putative G-protein may link a calcium channel to an as yet unidentified effector involved in hormone secretion. Note that in this case the G-protein would be "distal" to rather than "proximal" to the calcium channel, as in the earlier examples. Also, although activation of this G-protein should inhibit hormone secretion, nonhydrolyzable guanine nucleotides introduced into permeabilized parathyroid cells are potent secretagogues (Oetting et al., 1986). The latter effect, however, could reflect the sum total of GTP analog activation of distinct G-proteins.

In most cells, increased intracellular calcium stimulates exocytosis. Guanine nucleotides may regulate exocytosis in several ways (Gomperts, 1986). One site, the G-protein linked to stimulation of IP_3 formation and subsequent release of calcium, has been discussed. Several studies (Henne and Soling, 1986; Chueh and Gill, 1986; Knight and Baker, 1985) point to direct effects of guanine nucleotides on release of calcium from endoplasmic reticulum and on calcium-dependent exocytosis. Guanine nucleotides appear to act by a mechanism distinct from that of IP_3. Nonhydrolyzable guanine nucleotides, in contrast to their effects on other G-protein-mediated actions, are ineffective in releasing calcium from endoplasmic reticulum. The mechanism of guanine nucleotide action, its physiologic relevance, and the nature of a putative G-protein mediating this action require further study.

E. G-Proteins in Invertebrates

As discussed earlier, highly conserved ras gene products are found in invertebrate (e.g., Drosophila, slime molds, yeast) as well as vertebrate cells. Less clearly established is the existence, and function, of invertebrate homologs of the vertebrate, heterotrimeric G-proteins. Phototransduction by invertebrate photoreceptors appears to involve coupling by a G-protein of opsinlike receptors to stimulation of PI breakdown (Fein, 1986). A 41-kDa pertussis toxin substrate has been identified in octopus photoreceptors, as has a 36-kDa protein reactive with antisera prepared against bovine TD-β (Tsuda et al., 1986). A recent study (Johnson et al., 1986) suggests that cGMP, rather than PI breakdown products, may be the relevant second messenger in *Limulus* photoreceptors.

Microinjection studies of sea urchin eggs suggest that a G-protein mediates the effect of sperm on IP_3 formation and calcium dependent exocytosis (Turner *et al.*, 1986). A 39-kDa pertussis toxin substrate has been purified from sea urchin egg membranes (Oinuma *et al.*, 1986). The protein copurified with a 37-kDa protein cross-reactive with β subunit antisera. The relationship between this invertebrate G-protein and those of vertebrates extends to dissociation of the 39- from the 37-kDa protein by nonhydrolyzable GTP analogs. A γ subunit equivalent was not identified (Oinuma *et al.*, 1986). Similar observations have been reported for sea urchin sperm membranes (Bentley *et al.*, 1986). These studies support the notion that not only *ras* gene products, but heterotrimer G-proteins as well, find counterparts among invertebrate species. Elucidation of the structure and function of these proteins should provide useful information on the evolution of G-proteins.

V. MOLECULAR BIOLOGY OF G-PROTEINS

A. α SUBUNITS

TD-α and G_o-α have been purified in sufficient quantity to permit amino acid sequencing (Hurley *et al.*, 1984b). The amino terminus of these and other (e.g., G_i) G-α subunits is blocked by an as yet unidentified group. Sequencing of several tryptic peptides, however, revealed regions of sequence identity between G_o and TD as well as divergent regions. One highly conserved region also shows strong similarity to the sequences of *ras* p21 (Hurley *et al.*, 1984b). This region (see Fig. 7A) includes the glycine 12 position of *ras* p21, a known site of oncogenic mutation. Oligodeoxynucleotide probes based on this region have been used by several groups to screen cDNA libraries for G-α subunits.

Two distinct cDNA clones coding for TD related α subunits were obtained with antibody probes (Tanabe *et al.*, 1985; Medynski *et al.*, 1985; Yatsunami and Khorana, 1985) or with oligodeoxynucleotide probes (Lochrie *et al.*, 1985). The cDNAs encode proteins 350 and 354 amino acids long, respectively, and these have about 80% sequence similarity. On Northern blots, each cDNA hybridizes to retinal mRNA only (consistent with the highly restricted distribution of TD). Antibodies directed against synthetic peptides based on the cDNA-pre-

A

$G_{S\alpha}$: 42-59   R L L L L G A G E S G K S T I V K Q

$G_{i\alpha}$: 35-52   K L L L L G A G E S G K S T I V K Q

$G_{o\alpha}$: —   K L L L L G A G E S G K S T I V K Q

T_{α}: 31-48   K L L L L G A G E S G K S T I V K Q

ras: 5-22   K L V V V G A G G V G K S A L T I Q

B

$G_{S\alpha}$: 192-207   P S D Q D L L R C R V L T S G I

$G_{i\alpha}$: 170-185   P T Q Q D V L R T R V K T T G I

$G_{o\alpha}$: —   P T E Q D I L R T R V K T T G I

T_{α}: 165-180   P T E Q D V L R S R V K T T G I

C

$G_{S\alpha}$: 384-395   Q R M H L R Q Y E L L

$G_{i\alpha}$: 345-355   I K N N L K D C G L F

$G_{o\alpha}$: —   I A N N L R G C G L Y

T_{α}: 340-350   I K E N L K D C G L F

48K: R Q N L K D A G E Y

T_{γ}:   K E L K G G C V I S

ras_H: C K C V L S

ras_N: L P C V V M

ras_K: K K C I I M

FIG. 7. Selected regions of similarity in primary sequence of G-protein α subunits. Sequences shown are based on either direct amino acid sequencing or predictions from cDNA clones (references cited in text). (Numbering, where shown, refers to amino acid residue number.) The single-letter amino acid code is used. (A) A highly conserved region near the amino terminus also showing sequence similarity to *ras* p21 proteins and other guanine nucleotide binding proteins. The *ras* sequence shown is identical for all three forms of mammalian *ras* (*N, K,* and *H*). The indicated lysine (asterisk) corresponds to a lysine residue conserved in all guanine nucleotide binding proteins and shown for EF-Tu to interact with the phosphate groups of GDP. Mutations leading to substitution of the indicated glycine caused reduced GTPase activity in *ras* p21, and such mutant forms cause malignant transformation. (B) Site of cholera toxin ADP ribosylation (arginine, asterisk). Note the relative conservation of sequence in this region among G_s, G_i, G_o, and transducin, and in particular note that all contain arginine in a position identical to that of G_s. G_s is the preferred cholera toxin substrate. This may relate to unique features of its sequence flanking the substituted arginine and/or to other aspects of its secondary and tertiary structure. (C) Carboxy terminus of G-protein α subunits and of related proteins. The indicated cysteine (asterisk) is the site of pertussis toxin ADP ribosylation in transducin, G_i and G_o α subunits. G_s, lacking this cysteine, is not a pertussis toxin substrate. The retinal "48K" protein (see text) shows similarity of a portion (not at the carboxy terminus) of its sequence to this region of G-protein α subunits. Transducin-γ and the *ras* p21 proteins (all three forms are shown) contain a cysteine in the identical position relative to G-α subunits (fourth from the carboxy terminus). In *ras* p21 proteins, this cysteine is the site of palmitylation required for insertion in the plasma membrane.

```
CAG CGC AAC GAG GAG AAG GCG CAG CGT GAG GCC AAC AAA AAG ATC GAG AAG CAG CTG CAG   60
Gln Arg Asn Glu Glu Lys Ala Gln Arg Glu Ala Asn Lys Lys Ile Glu Lys Gln Leu Gln   20

AAG GAC AAG CAG GTC TAC CGG GCC ACG CAC CGC CTG CTG CTG CTG GGT GCT GGA GAA TCT  120
Lys Asp Lys Gln Val Tyr Arg Ala Thr His Arg Leu Leu Leu Leu Gly Ala Gly Glu Ser   40

GGT AAA AGC ACC ATT GTG AAG CAG ATG AGG ATC CTG CAT GTT AAT GGG TTT AAT GGA GAG  180
Gly Lys Ser Thr Ile Val Lys Gln Met Arg Ile Leu His Val Asn Gly Phe Asn Gly Glu   60

GGC GGC GAA GAG GAC CCG CAG GCT GCA AGG AGC AAC AGC GAT GGC AGT GAG AAG GCA ACC  240
Gly Gly Glu Glu Asp Pro Gln Ala Ala Arg Ser Asn Ser Asp Gly Ser Glu Lys Ala Thr   80

AAA GTG CAG GAC ATC AAA AAC AAC CTG AAA GAG GCG ATT GAA ACC ATT GTG GCC GCC ATG  300
Lys Val Gln Asp Ile Lys Asn Asn Leu Lys Glu Ala Ile Glu Thr Ile Val Ala Ala Met  100

AGC AAC CTG GTG CCC CCC GTG GAG CTG GCC AAC CCC GAG AAC CAG TTC AGA GTG GAC TAC  360
Ser Asn Leu Val Pro Pro Val Glu Leu Ala Asn Pro Glu Asn Gln Phe Arg Val Asp Tyr  120

ATT CTG AGT GTG ATG AAC GTG CCT GAC TTT GAC TTC CCT CCC GAA TTC TAT GAG CAT GCC  420
Ile Leu Ser Val Met Asn Val Pro Asp Phe Asp Phe Pro Pro Glu Phe Tyr Glu His Ala  140

AAG GCT CTG TGG GAG GAT GAA GGA GTG CGT GCC TGC TAC GAA CGC TCC AAC GAG TAC CAG  480
Lys Ala Leu Trp Glu Asp Glu Gly Val Arg Ala Cys Tyr Glu Arg Ser Asn Glu Tyr Gln  160

CTG ATT GAC TGT GCC CAG TAC TTC CTG GAC AAG ATC GAC GTG ATC AAG CAG GCT GAC TAT  540
Leu Ile Asp Cys Ala Gln Tyr Phe Leu Asp Lys Ile Asp Val Ile Lys Gln Ala Asp Tyr  180

GTG CCG AGC GAT CAG GAC CTG CTT CGC TGC CGT GTC CTG ACT TCT GGA ATC TTT GAG ACC  600
Val Pro Ser Asp Gln Asp Leu Leu Arg Cys Arg Val Leu Thr Ser Gly Ile Phe Glu Thr  200

AAG TTC CAG GTG GAC AAA GTC AAC TTC CAC ATG TTT GAC GTG GGT GGC CAG CGC GAT CAA  660
Lys Phe Gln Val Asp Lys Val Asn Phe His Met Phe Asp Val Gly Gly Gln Arg Asp Glu  220

CGC CGC AAG TGG ATC CAG TGC TTC AAC GAT GTG ACT GCC ATC ATC TTC GTG GTG GCC AGC  720
Arg Arg Lys Trp Ile Gln Cys Phe Asn Asp Val Thr Ala Ile Ile Phe Val Val Ala Ser  240

AGC AGC TAC AAC ATG GTC ATC CGG GAG GAC AAC CAG ACC AAC CGC CTG CAG GAG GCT CTG  780
Ser Ser Tyr Asn Met Val Ile Arg Glu Asp Asn Gln Thr Asn Arg Leu Gln Glu Ala Leu  260

AAC CTC TTC AAG AGC ATC TGG AAC AAC AGA TGG CTG CGC ACC ATC TCT GTG ATC CTG TTC  840
Asn Leu Phe Lys Ser Ile Trp Asn Asn Arg Trp Leu Arg Thr Ile Ser Val Ile Leu Phe  280

CTC AAC AAG CAA GAT CTG CTC GCT GAG AAA GTC CTT GCT GGG AAA TCG AAG ATT GAG GAC  900
Leu Asn Lys Gln Asp Leu Leu Ala Glu Lys Val Leu Ala Gly Lys Ser Lys Ile Glu Asp  300

TAC TTT CCA GAA TTT GCT CGC TAC ACT ACT CCT GAG GAT GCT ACT CCC GAG CCC GGA GAG  960
Tyr Phe Pro Glu Phe Ala Arg Tyr Thr Thr Pro Glu Asp Ala Thr Pro Glu Pro Gly Glu  320

GAC CCA CGC GTG ACC CGG GCC AAG TAC TTC ATT CGA GAT GAG TTT CTG AGG ATC AGC ACT 1020
Asp Pro Arg Val Thr Arg Ala Lys Tyr Phe Ile Arg Asp Glu Phe Leu Arg Ile Ser Thr  340

GCC AGT GGA GAT GGG CGT CAC TAC TGC TAC CCT CAT TTC ACC TGC GCT GTG GAC ACT GAG 1080
Ala Ser Gly Asp Gly Arg His Tyr Cys Tyr Pro His Phe Thr Cys Ala Val Asp Thr Glu  360

AAC ATC CGC CGT GTG TTC AAC GAC TGC CGT GAC ATC ATT CAG CGC ATG CAC CTT CGT CAG 1140
Asn Ile Arg Arg Val Phe Asn Asp Cys Arg Asp Ile Ile Gln Arg Met His Leu Arg Gln  380

TAC GAG CTG CTC TAA  GAAGGGAACCCCCAAATTTAATTAAAGCCTTAAGCACAATTAATTAAAAGTGAAACGT 1213
Tyr Glu Leu Leu Term                                                             384

AATTGTACAAGCAGTTAATCACCCACCATAGGGCATGATTAACAAAGCAACCTTTCCCTTCCC                  1276
```

FIG. 8. Nucleotide and amino acid sequences of a cDNA clone from a human brain library encoding the α subunit of G_s. The first amino acid residue corresponds to amino acid 12 of the complete sequence. The underlined nucleotides represent the sites of hybridization of probes used to screen the library. Amino acids 60–76 in the sequence shown (71–87 in the complete sequence) correspond to a variable region in which four

dicted amino acid sequence localize the 350-amino acid protein to rod photoreceptor cells and the 354-amino acid protein to cones (Lerea *et al.*, 1986). The rod TD cDNA hybridizes to an approximately 2.3-kb mRNA in retina, while the cone cDNA hybridizes to less abundant transcripts of 5.5 and 6 kb.

Multiple cDNAs encoding G_s-α have been obtained from bovine (Harris *et al.*, 1985; Nukada *et al.*, 1986a), rat (Itoh *et al.*, 1986), mouse (Sullivan *et al.*, 1986), and human (Mattera *et al.*, 1986; Bray *et al.*, 1986) cDNA libraries. Several of these were obtained by screening brain cDNA libraries with oligodeoxynucleotide probes corresponding to highly conserved regions of G-α subunits. This is somewhat surprising, given the low abundance of G_s in brain and other tissues relative to G_o and G_i. This suggests the possibility that G-α subunit mRNA and protein abundance may be inversely correlated.

Since the amino acid sequence of G_s-α protein is unavailable, indirect methods were necessary to identify the putative Gs-α cDNA. These included absence of hybridizing mRNA on Northern blots of mutant CYC$^-$ cells, known to lack G_s-α protein, and specific reactivity of cDNA-predicted peptide antibodies with purified G_s-α (Harris *et al.*, 1985). The cDNA hybridizes to an approximately 1.9-kB mRNA in all tissues tested, consistent with the ubiquitous distribution of G_s. G_s-α shows extraordinarily high conservation among species (human, cow, rat, mouse) at both the amino acid (>99%) and nucleotide levels (~94% in the coding region). Interestingly, both 5'-untranslated and 3'-untranslated regions of G_s-α mRNA are highly conserved (~90%) between species. This suggests that these noncoding regions could serve some important function.

G_s-α cDNAs obtained from bovine (Robishaw *et al.*, 1986a; Nukada *et al.*, 1986a), rat (Itoh *et al.*, 1986), and human (Fig. 8) (Bray *et al.*, 1986) brain libraries encode a 394-amino acid protein. Additional cDNAs obtained from bovine adrenal (Robishaw *et al.*, 1986b), human brain (Bray *et al.*, 1986), human liver (Mattera *et al.*, 1986), and mouse macrophage libraries (Sullivan *et al.*, 1986) encode G_s-α cDNAs which vary in a limited region (amino acids 71–87 of the 394-amino acid form). These variations involve substitution of an aspartic for a glutamic acid residue (position 71), deletion of the 15-amino acid peptide

---

forms of mRNA have been distinguished (see text and Fig. 9). The cDNA sequence shown is of that type designated α_s-2 in Fig. 9. Overall, the G_s-α amino acid sequence shows about 40% sequence similarity to other G-α subunits. The regions between amino acids 60–190 and 290–384 (as numbered here) show much greater variability in sequence among G-α subunits than the rest of the protein and may correspond to regions of effector and receptor interaction, respectively.

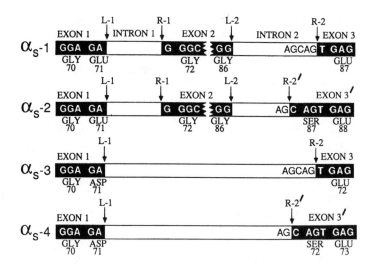

Fig. 9. Proposed alternative splicing mechanism leading to production of four forms of G_s-α mRNA. A 45-base exon (arbitrarily labeled exon 2) may (G_s-α types 1 and 2) or may not (G_s-α types 3 and 4) be included in the final mRNA. In addition, the postulated splice junction between exons 1 or 2 and exon 3 may occur before (G_s-α types 2 and 4) or after (G_s-α types 1 and 3) the indicated CAG. The consequences in terms of amino acid sequence are shown and discussed in the text. (Reproduced from Bray *et al.*, 1986, with permission.)

following position 71, and insertion of a serine at position 87. Four types of cDNA corresponding to various combinations of these changes were obtained from the same human brain library (Bray *et al.*, 1986). A plausible but unproved model for generation of these four forms of G_s-α mRNA by alternative splicing is illustrated in Fig. 9. Two of these forms of G_s-α have been independently cloned from human (Mattera *et al.*, 1986) and bovine (Robishaw *et al.*, 1986b) cDNA libraries, and a third form has been obtained from a mouse cDNA library (Sullivan *et al.*, 1986). Thus, multiple forms of G_s-α mRNA occur in several mammalian species.

S1 nuclease analysis (Robishaw *et al.*, 1986b; Bray *et al.*, 1986) provides direct evidence for the existence of at least three of these forms of G_s-α mRNA in several tissues. Because the different forms differ by at most 48 bases, heterogeneity of mRNA size on Northern blots is not apparent. While it is likely that all four forms arise by alternative splicing of a common transcript from a single gene, the possibility that there are multiple G_s-α genes has not been totally excluded.

G_s-α protein is known to exist in at least two forms of approximately 45 and 52 kDa (due to variability in molecular size standards these have also been referred to as 42 and 47 kDa). Proteolytic peptide mapping indicates that these two proteins are identical but for a single peptide, and both are absent in the G_s-deficient CYC$^-$ mutant (Johnson et al., 1978). This originally led to the suggestion that these two forms arise from a posttranslational modification. Recent evidence suggests instead that heterogeneity of G_s-α protein reflects directly heterogeneity of G_s-α mRNA. An antibody directed against a synthetic peptide corresponding to the region deleted in "short" forms of G_s-α mRNA reacts with the 52- but not the 45-kDa form of G_s-α (Robishaw et al., 1986b). Expression of "short" and "long" forms of G_s-α mRNA in cos cells, moreover, leads to synthesis of 45- and 52-kDa forms of G_s-α, respectively (Robishaw et al., 1986b). Based on the multiplicity of G_s-α mRNAs, it is likely, but not yet proven, that the 45- and 52-kDa forms of protein are themselves heterogeneous.

Interestingly, the cDNA predicted M_r and the apparent M_r on SDS–PAGE of G_s-α subunit forms are discrepant. "Short" forms of mRNA encode a 43,000 protein which migrates as 45,000, and "long" forms of mRNA encode a 44,000–45,000 protein which migrates as 52,000. This is likely due to anomalous behavior on SDS–PAGE. The region of variability between forms of G_s-α corresponds to a segment showing very little similarity to other G-α subunits. This segment could relate to effector interaction. There is some evidence that the 52-kDa form of G_s-α interacts more efficiently with adenylate cyclase than does the 45-kDa form (Sternweis et al., 1981). Thus the variability in forms of G_s-α could have functional significance. Also, three serines, potential sites for phosphorylation, occur in this variable region. Differences in the proportion of forms of G_s-α occur, but the mechanism underlying tissue-specific differences has not yet been defined.

Partial cDNA clones encoding G_o-α have been obtained from rat (Itoh et al., 1986) and bovine libraries (Angus et al., 1986). The identity of the cDNAs was established by comparison of predicted and tryptic peptide-derived amino acid sequences. The protein shows high overall sequence similarity (60–70%) to TD and G_i. Size and distribution of mRNA were not reported.

cDNAs encoding proteins related to G_i have been obtained from bovine brain, rat brain, human brain, and mouse macrophage libraries. The bovine brain cDNA encodes a 354-amino acid protein whose sequence corresponds exactly to that of multiple tryptic peptides derived from the 41-kDa form of G_i in both bovine and rat brain (Nukada et al., 1986b). The human brain cDNA encodes a protein identical to the bovine form (Bray et al., 1987). The rat brain cDNA (Itoh et al., 1986) encodes a 355-amino acid protein virtually identical to the mouse macrophage cDNA (Sullivan *et al.,* 1986) but clearly different from the bovine and human brain cDNAs. It is unlikely that these differences are due solely to species difference. Instead, several lines of evidence suggest that there are many genes encoding multiple forms of "G_i-α" (note that because of the difficulty in assigning a specific function of G_i, this designation is not very meaningful). At least three distinct forms of G_i-α cDNA have been obtained within the same species (rat) from an olfactory mucosa library (R. Reed and D. Jones, personal communication). Also, there is high conservation in the 3'-untranslated region (~90%) between the human and bovine brain G_i-α cDNAs but very low conservation between the comparable region of bovine and rat or mouse G_i-α cDNA. A comparison of the untranslated regions of mRNA for different G-α subunits among various species suggests that, as in the actin gene family, nucleotide sequences are highly conserved among species for a given "isotype" (form of G-α) and are very poorly conserved within a single species between isotypes (Bray *et al.,* 1987).

Two forms of "G_i-α" cDNA were cloned from a bovine pituitary library (Michel *et al.,* 1986). One form is nearly identical to the bovine brain cDNA (Nukada *et al.,* 1986b), but the other form is similar to but distinct from both the bovine and rat brain forms of G_i-α cDNA. Southern blot analysis of bovine genomic DNA using the two pituitary cDNAs as probes showed that each probe recognized distinct fragments, consistent with the existence of multiple distinct genes. The mRNA size of the bovine brain-related form of G_i (~3.3 kb) also differs from that of the rat brain and mouse macrophage form (~2.2 kb).

In summary, there appear to be multiple forms of "G_i-α" mRNA that are likely to be products of distinct genes. The significance of this heterogeneity in terms of function and tissue distribution is not yet apparent. This heterogeneity is consistent with immunochemical evidence for G_i heterogeneity (Gierschik *et al.,* 1986a).

Comparison of the nucleotide sequences of G-α subunit cDNAs leads to several interesting conclusions. These proteins constitute a gene family likely to be related to a common evolutionary precursor. The multiple forms of TD, G_i, and G_o show 60–70% sequence similarity at the amino acid level. G_s-α is more distantly related (~40% similarity with the others). Signal-transducing G-α subunits, in turn, are part of a super-gene family which includes the *ras*-related proteins as well as other guanine nucleotide binding proteins such as those involved in protein synthesis. Four regions conserved within the G-α subunit family also show sequence similarity to regions within other guanine nucleotide binding proteins and are likely related to nucleotide binding

(Halliday, 1984). The X-ray crystal structure of EF-Tu (Jurnak, 1985) has revealed amino acids directly related to guanine nucleotide binding. A lysine (see Fig. 7A) is believed to interact with the phosphate group of bound nucleotide. This lysine is conserved in all known guanine nucleotide binding proteins, as are an aspartate and asparagine residue thought to interact with the guanine ring. Note that the glycine substituted in oncogenic forms of *ras* p21 (with attendant reduction in GTPase activity) neighbors the lysine involved in phosphate group binding (see Fig. 7A).

The site of cholera toxin-catalyzed ADP ribosylation is the arginine shown in Fig. 7B. Although not in a region directly linked to GTP binding, this arginine is close to a site whose susceptibility to proteolytic cleavage is affected by bound guanine nucleotide. This may help explain why covalent modification of this arginine alters GTPase activity.

The site of pertussis toxin-catalyzed ADP ribosylation is the cysteine shown in Fig. 7C. Since this modification uncouples pertussis toxin substrates from receptors, the carboxy-terminal region may be part of a receptor recognition domain. This region also shows sequence similarity to a retinal 48K protein (Wistow *et al.*, 1986) which may compete with transducin for binding to rhodopsin (see Fig. 7C).

Substantial diversity in amino acid sequence between different forms of G-α subunits is limited to small regions of the molecule. Such regions could confer specificity in receptor and effector interaction. One such region (roughly between amino acids 100 and 140) could be involved in effector interaction. Interestingly, the amino-terminal 1 to 2-kDa piece is rather divergent in sequence. This is superficially inconsistent with a postulated role in interacting with the common G-β/γ subunit (Medynski *et al.*, 1985). Future studies, employing expression, site-directed mutagenesis, and other techniques, will undoubtedly help define the key functional domains of G-α subunits.

B. β Subunits

On SDS–PAGE, the β subunit of TD appears to be a single protein of approximately 36 kDa. In other tissues, a doublet is apparent (Sternweis and Robishaw, 1984). In brain, a minor, more rapidly migrating species (about 35 kDa) is seen in addition to the dominant 36-kDa form, whereas in liver the two forms are about equal in abundance. Immunochemical studies (Mumby *et al.*, 1985) suggest that these two forms of β subunit are distinct, and that the 35-kDa form is not merely a proteolytic product of the 36-kDa protein. The structural basis for this heterogeneity and its functional significance (if any) have not yet been defined.

The amino terminus of the TD-β subunit and of G-β from other tissues is blocked. Tryptic digestion of soluble, purified β/γ subunits of TD, or of brain plasma membranes (Pines *et al.*, 1985), yields 15- and 26-kDa fragments of the β subunit. Amino acid sequencing indicates that the 15-kDa fragment is the amino-terminal portion of β. The tryptic cleavage site is apparently accessible in β/γ subunits that are membrane bound. This region presumably is not involved in α or γ subunit interaction, or in membrane attachment.

The amino acid sequence from the amino terminus of the 26-kDa tryptic fragment (Fong *et al.*, 1986), or from other proteolytic fragments (Sugimoto *et al.*, 1985), was used to synthesize oligodeoxynucleotide probes. The latter were used to screen bovine retinal cDNA libraries, and cDNAs encoding TD-β were obtained. The identity of these cDNAs is based on their correspondence to the amino acid sequence obtained from fragments of 36-kDa TD-β. The cDNA encodes a protein of 340 amino acids (calculated M_r 37,375). The cDNA hybridizes to mRNAs of about 1.8 and 3.2 kb in Northern blots of retina as well as other tissues. Heterogeneity in mRNA size may relate to two possible sites for polyadenylation. When a cDNA probe consisting of a 5' fragment of TD-β (untranslated region) was used in Northern analysis, specific hybridization was limited to retinal mRNA (Sugimoto *et al.*, 1985). Subsequently, cDNA encoding the β subunit from human liver has been cloned (Codina *et al.*, 1986). The amino acid sequence predicted by the human liver β cDNA is identical to that for bovine TD-β.

These findings are consistent with peptide mapping studies (Manning and Gilman, 1983) and immunochemical studies (Gierschik *et al.*, 1985) that show similarity if not identity in the β subunits of TD and of other G-proteins. The cDNAs presumably correspond to the 36-kDa form of the β subunit, since this is the only form known for TD. Although the coding regions are identical, TD-β and the β subunit of other G-proteins may be products of separate genes, since clear differences are present in the untranslated portion of the mRNA. Such differences could relate to specialized mechanisms for regulating synthesis in photoreceptor cells (for TD-β) as opposed to other tissues.

C. γ SUBUNITS

γ subunits are low-molecular-weight (~10,000) proteins, tightly associated with β subunits. β/γ association is noncovalent (e.g., does not involve disulfide bonds), since the subunits are resolved by SDS–

PAGE without disulfide reduction. It is not clear whether specific domains of γ are linked to β subunits, nor is it clear whether γ directly interacts with other components such as the α subunit or receptors.

The γ subunit of TD is similar in size to those of G_s and G_i but is immunochemically distinct (Gierschik et al., 1985). Peptide mapping studies confirm this difference, and suggest that the γ subunits of G_s, G_i, and G_o are similar or identical (Hildebrandt et al., 1985). The entire amino acid sequence of TD-γ has been determined (Ovchinnikov et al., 1985), and cDNA clones have been obtained (Hurley et al., 1984a; Yatsunami et al., 1985). The protein consists of 73 amino acids and is relatively hydrophilic and acidic. The similarity in sequence of the carboxy terminus to ras p21 (see Fig. 7C) has prompted speculation concerning a role for TD-γ (and other γ subunits?) in membrane anchoring. On Northern analysis, TD-γ cDNA hybridizes to an approximately 0.6-kB mRNA in retina but not in other tissues (Van Dop et al., 1984a). This result is consistent with the notion that TD-γ differs substantially from other G-γ subunits.

VI. SPECIFICITY OF RECEPTOR–G-PROTEIN–EFFECTOR INTERACTIONS

Since G-proteins differ primarily in terms of α subunit structure, this subunit likely confers specificity in receptor and effector interactions. Domains of G-α subunits that diverge in amino acid sequence may directly interact with receptors and effectors, but as yet such domains have not been definitively identified. Receptor interaction is presumed to alter the guanine nucleotide binding site and permit exchange of GDP for GTP. GTP binding in turn is presumed to alter G-α subunit conformation. This may lead to β/γ subunit dissociation and permit interaction of G-α with effector.

Recently, the primary structures of several receptors that interact with G-proteins have been defined. Rhodopsin and the cone opsins (Nathans et al., 1986), the $β_2$- (Dixon et al., 1986) and $β_1$-adrenergic receptors (Yarden et al., 1986), and the muscarinic cholinergic receptor (Kubo et al., 1986) all show some degree (~25%) of amino acid sequence similarity, and, more importantly, all show a similar putative transmembrane structure. Based on hydrophobicity plots, these receptors are believed to span the plasma membrane seven times. This may emerge as a unique feature of receptors coupled to G-proteins. Three peptide loops and the carboxy terminus are presumably exposed on the cytoplasmic surface of the cell membrane. Regions responsible for G-protein interaction may well be localzed to one or more of these loops.

Receptor–G-protein coupling shows relative rather than absolute

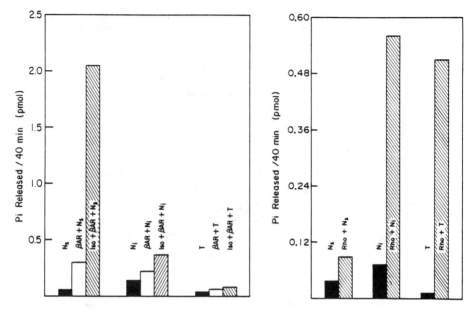

FIG. 10. Specificity in receptor–G-protein coupling. Purified hamster lung β-adrenergic receptors (BAR, left) or bovine rhodopsin (Rho, right) were inserted in artificial phospholipid vesicles with purified G_s (N_s) and G_i (N_i) from human erythrocytes and with transducin (T) purified from bovine retina. GTPase was measured for G-protein alone (solid black bars), for BAR + G-protein (open bars), and for either agonist-stimulated (iso) BAR + G-protein or light-activated rhodopsin + G-protein (hatched bars). (Reproduced from Cerione et al., 1985, with permission.)

specificity. In artificial phospholipid vesicles reconstituted with purified receptors and G-proteins, agonist stimulation of GTPase activity is a good measure of receptor–G-protein coupling. Such studies indicate that rhodopsin and the β-adrenergic receptor couple poorly with G_s and TD, respectively (see Fig. 10). G_i, surprisingly, interacts with the β-adrenergic receptor, but significantly less well than G_s (Cerione et al., 1985). Studies with the purified α_2-adrenergic receptor (Cerione et al., 1986b) show that G_s interacts poorly with this receptor but that G_o and G_i (purified from brain) interact equally well and somewhat better than TD. Other studies comparing G_i and G_o interaction, e.g.. with the muscarinic cholinergic receptor (Florio and Sternweis, 1985), similarly show no differences among the two in receptor interaction. These data may reflect the closer amino acid sequence similarity (~65%) among G_i, G_o, and TD compared to that between any of these and G_s (~40%). It is also possible that artificial reconstitution obscures subtle but relevant aspects of specificity of receptor–G-protein coupling.

Effector–G-protein coupling may show greater specificity. Only TD activated cGMP phosphodiesterase, only G_s activated adenylate cyclase, and only G_i inhibited CYC⁻ membrane adenylate cyclase (Roof et al., 1985). G_o was ineffective in all these assays. G-protein stimulation of purified phospholipase C has not been reported. In HL-60 cell membranes treated with pertussis toxin, either G_i or G_o (purified from brain) substituted for endogenous G-protein in activating phospholipase C (Kikuchi et al., 1986). The possibility that this effect is due to yet another G-protein in both the G_i and G_o preparations has not been completely excluded.

VII. QUALITATIVE AND QUANTITATIVE CHANGES IN G-PROTEINS: EFFECT ON SIGNAL TRANSDUCTION

Changes in G-proteins can profoundly alter signal transduction. Several examples of genetic changes in G-protein structure and of covalent modifications of G-proteins have already been defined; others undoubtedly exist.

A. GENETIC AND DEVELOPMENTAL CHANGES

One of the best studied systems is the S49 mouse lymphoma cell line (Salomon and Bourne, 1981). Since increased levels of cAMP are lethal in this cell line, mutants in the cAMP transduction system are readily selected. Several of these show abnormalities in G_s. The CYC⁻ mutant lacks G_s activity in functional assays (no cAMP stimulation by receptor agonists or by fluoride, cholera toxin, and guanine nucleotides) and lacks cholera toxin substrate (Johnson et al., 1978). Apparently, no G_s-α is synthesized, as the corresponding mRNA is totally undetectable (Harris et al., 1985). The UNC mutant (Haga et al., 1977) does not respond to receptor agonists with increased cAMP formation and shows only low affinity binding of agonists to receptor. cAMP stimulation by agents acting directly on G_s is intact. Cholera toxin substrate is detectable but subtly altered in p*I* on two-dimensional PAGE (Schleifer et al., 1981). UNC is presumed to result from a G_s lesion that impairs receptor–G_s but not G_s–cyclase interaction. Another mutant, H21A, shows the opposite defect, i.e., normal receptor–G_s interaction but defective G_s–cyclase interaction (Bourne et al., 1982). The molecular basis for these mutations has not yet been defined.

A form of the human genetic disease, pseudohypoparathyroidism (PHP), may also reflect a G_s-α abnormality (Spiegel et al., 1985). Affected individuals are resistant to diverse agents acting via stimulation of adenylate cyclase. Plasma membranes from several cell types of affected individuals show an approximately 50% reduction in G_s measured by functional assay and by cholera toxin-catalyzed labeling. Recent studies (Carter et al., 1988) show reduced G_s-α mRNA in affected subjects. These findings indicate that reduction, as opposed to complete absence, of G_s-α may also impair signal transduction. Reduced agonist stimulation of cAMP in a S49 mutant with partial reduction in G_s is also consistent with this conclusion (Salomon and Bourne, 1981).

As yet, genetic lesions in other G-α subunits, or in β or γ subunits, have not been described. By analogy with PHP, certain forms of rod photoreceptor dysfunction, retinitis pigmentosa, could result from TD-α defects. Genetic receptor defects have been defined for some forms of color blindness (Nathans et al., 1986), but defective cone TD-α is another theoretical possibility. Mutations in ras p21 coding genes have been discussed earlier. Several oncogenic mutants show reduced GTPase activity and presumably constitutive effector activation. Similar mutants of other G-α subunits could lead to a receptor-independent activated phenotype.

Development and differentiation of G-proteins also may vary. Such changes (together with, or rather than, receptor and effector changes) could explain developmental differences in signal transduction. Examples include ontogenetic changes in retinal transducin (Grunwald et al., 1986), and in brain G_i and G_o (Milligan et al., 1987). Adenylate cyclase responsiveness to hormones changes during differentiation of 3T3-L1 cells from fibroblasts to adipocytes. These may reflect variations in G_s (Lai et al., 1981) and/or inhibitory G-proteins (Gierschik et al., 1986c).

Muscarinic cholinergic receptors as well as G-proteins may be modified in development of embryonic chick heart (Halvorsen and Nathanson, 1984; Liang et al., 1986), leading to altered response to cholinergic agonists. Innervation of rat cardiocytes in culture and maturation in vivo are accompanied by an altered α_1-adrenergic response and an altered response to pertussis toxin (Steinberg et al., 1985). The latter may reflect the appearance of a new G-protein, pertussis toxin substrate. These few examples serve to indicate that developmental differences in G-protein synthesis may be an important cause of altered signal transduction. One can speculate that agents altering mRNA expression, e.g., steroids and thyroid hormone, may also alter G-protein synthesis. Further work is needed to explore this hypothesis.

B. Covalent Modifications

In discussing G-protein structure, posttranslational modifications, including amino-terminal blockade of α and β subunits, and possible fatty acid acylation of α and γ subunits have been discussed. Other, reversible covalent modifications could represent an important mechanism for regulating G-protein function and thereby signal transduction. The most obvious example is ADP ribosylation catalyzed by bacterial toxins, discussed in detail earlier. Although "nonphysiologic," toxin-catalyzed ADP ribosylation is relevant to the pathophysiology of cholera and pertussis infections and also provides an example of the potential functional significance of covalent modification of G-proteins. The possibility that endogenous ADP-ribosyltransferases alter G-proteins deserves careful consideration. A preliminary report concerning endogenous ADP ribosylation of G_s in fat cells requires confirmation (Jacquemin et al., 1986).

Protein phosphorylation is one of the most common and most important covalent modifications. At least one member of the extended guanine nucleotide binding protein family, eukaryotic initiation factor 2, is regulated by a reversible phosphorylation. Preliminary data suggest that signal-transducing G-proteins may also be regulated by phosphorylation. Much of the data relates to the effects of phorbol esters, activators of protein kinase C. Phorbol ester treatment of intact cells of diverse types may lead to potentiation or inhibition of agonist-stimulated cAMP formation. Inhibitory effects may be found on prolonged incubation with phorbol esters and may relate to receptor phosphorylation and uncoupling (see, for example, Sibley et al., 1984).

Brief exposure (<30 minutes) to phorbol esters generally potentiates the cellular cAMP response to agonists. Indirect evidence suggests that this effect is due to protein kinase C-catalyzed phosphorylation of one or more components of the receptor–G-protein–cyclase complex. In platelets and S49 mouse lymphoma cells, phorbol esters were reported to reduce G_i-mediated inhibition of cyclase (Katada et al., 1985; Bell and Brunton, 1986). In contrast, phorbol esters enhance the cAMP response to GRF in anterior pituitary cells without reducing inhibition by somatostatin (Cronin et al., 1986). In this and another study (Pines et al., 1986), moreover, phorbol ester effects were additive to those of pertussis toxin.

No simple interpretation of these data is possible. *In vitro* studies with purified G_i and protein kinase C (Katada *et al.*, 1985) show that G_i-α is a substrate for C-kinase phosphorylation. If G_i-α phosphorylation impairs function, e.g., by increasing affinity for β subunits, the effects of phorbol esters could be explained. Other targets for C-kinase phosphorylation, such as adenylate cyclase catalyst (Naghshineh *et al.*, 1986), must also be considered and could explain certain phorbol ester effects, e.g., additivity in some systems with the effects of pertussis toxin.

A report concerning phosphorylation of the G-protein β subunit by EGF-receptor-associated tyrosine kinase (Valentine-Braun *et al.*, 1986) has not been confirmed. A protein of similar molecular weight, lipocortin, rather than G-β, is likely to be the relevant tyrosine kinase substrate (Huang *et al.*, 1986). G-protein α subunits may be substrates for tyrosine phosphorylation. Purified TD-α is phosphorylated by the insulin receptor kinase and by protein kinase C on tyrosine and serine residues, respectively (Zick *et al.*, 1986). The preferred substrate, as was found for C-kinase phosphorylation of G_i (Katada *et al.*, 1985), is the free TD-α subunit in the GDP-bound form.

The physiologic relevance of any of these phosphorylations remains to be seen. In particular, G-proteins have not yet been identified as phosphorylation substrates for any kinase in intact cells. Nonetheless, the hypothesis that G-protein function is regulated by one or more kinases is attractive. It provides for "cross-talk" between parallel transduction pathways, e.g., activation of tyrosine kinase leading to phosphorylation of cyclase-coupled G-protein, and for feedback regulation, e.g., C-kinase phosphorylation of G-protein coupled to PI breakdown and C-kinase stimulation.

VIII. Conclusions and Future Prospects

There has been rapid progress in defining the function and structure of members of the signal-transducing G-protein family. This progress has led to an appreciation of the fundamental similarity in the mechanism of transduction of signals as diverse as neurotransmitters, hormones, odorants, and photons of light. Alterations in G-proteins have been recognized as the basis for several human diseases.

The results of ongoing and future studies should provide answers to several key questions. The function of several identified G-proteins, e.g., G_o and the multiple forms of "G_i," will be defined. The function of *ras* and *ras*-related gene products likewise should be elucidated. The

G-protein(s) linked to stimulation of PI breakdown should be identified. New G-proteins, and new functions for G-proteins, will likely be discovered. Rapid progress in defining G-protein, receptor, and effector structures is likely. From this should emerge a clearer idea of the structural basis for receptor–G-protein–effector interactions and the specificity of these interactions. Novel therapeutic approaches could result from an appreciation of these structural and functional details.

Much remains to be learned about G-protein subcellular localization and membrane attachment. Covalent modifications related to the latter should be defined. Other covalent modifications that may regulate G-protein function should be sought. Regulation of G-protein subunit synthesis also needs study. Coordination of synthesis of components of the heterotrimer and the basis for tissue-specific expression are among the interesting topics to be explored.

REFERENCES

Abood, M. E., Hurley, J. B., Pappone, M.-C., Bourne, H. R., and Stryer, L. (1982). Functional homology between signal-coupling proteins: Cholera toxin inactivates the GTPase activity of transducin. *J. Biol. Chem.* **257**, 10540–10543.

Aksamit, R. R., Backlund, P. S., Jr., and Cantoni, G. L. (1985). Cholera toxin inhibits chemotaxis by a cAMP-independent mechanism. *Proc. Natl. Acad. Sci. U.S.A.* **82**, 7475–7479.

Andrade, R., Malenka, R. C., and Nicoll, R. A. (1986). A G protein couples serotonin and GABA$_B$ receptors to the same channels in hippocampus. *Science* **234**, 1261–1265.

Angus, C. W., Van Meurs, K. P., Tasi, S.-C., Adamik, R., Miedel, M. C., Pan, Y.-C. E., Kung, H.-F., Moss, J.. and Vaughan, M. (1986). Identification of the probable site of choleragen-catalyzed ADP-ribosylation in a G$_o\alpha$-like protein based on cDNA sequence. *Proc. Natl. Acad. Sci. U.S.A.* **83**, 5813–5816.

Baldassare, J. J., and Fisher, G. J. (1986). Regulation of membrane-associated and cytosolic phospholipase C activities in human platelets by guanosine triphosphate. *J. Biol. Chem.* **261**, 11942–11944.

Banno, Y., Nakashima, S., Tohmatsu, T., Nozawa, Y., and Lapetina, E. G. (1986). GTP and GDP will stimulate cytosolic phospholipase C independently of Ca^{2+} *Biochem. Biophys. Res. Commun.* **140**, 728–734.

Bar-Sagi, D., and Feramisco, J. R. (1985). Microinjection of the *ras* oncogene protein into PC12 cells induces morphological differentiation. *Cell* **42**, 841–848.

Beckner, S. K., Hattori, S., and Shih, T. Y. (1985). p21 does not function as a regulatory component of adenylate cyclase. *Nature (London)* **317**, 71–72.

Bell, J. D., and Brunton, L. L. (1986). Enhancement of adenylate cyclase activity in S49 lymphoma cells by phorbol esters. *J. Biol. Chem.* **261**, 12036–12041.

Bentley, J. K., Garbers, D. L., Domino, S. E., Noland, T. D., and Van Dop, C. (1986). Spermatozoa contain a guanine nucleotide-binding protein ADP-ribosylated by pertussus toxin. *Biochem. Biophys. Res. Commun.* **138**, 728–734.

Berridge, M. J., and Irvine, R. F. (1984). Inositol trisphosphate, a novel second messenger in signal transduction. *Nature (London)* **312**, 315–321.

Bigay, J., Deterre, P., Pfister, C., and Chabre, M. (1985). Fluoroaluminates activate transducin-GDP by mimicking the γ-phosphate of GTP in its binding site. *FEBS Lett.* **191**, 181–185.

Birnbaumer, L., Pohl, S. L., Rodbell, M., and Sunby, F. (1972). The glucagon-sensitive adenylate cyclase system in plasma membranes of rat liver. *J. Biol. Chem.* **247**, 2038–2043.

Bourne, H. R., Beiderman, B., Steinberg, F., and Brothers, V. M. (1982). Three adenylate cyclase phenotypes in S49 lymphoma cells produced by mutations of one gene. *Mol. Pharmacol.* **22**, 204–210.

Boyer, J. L., Garcia, A., Posadas, C., and Garcia-Sainz, A. (1984). Differential effect of pertussis toxin on the affinity state for agonists of renal α_1- and α_2-adrenoceptors *J. Biol. Chem.* **259**, 8076–8079.

Bray, P., Carter, A., Simons, C., Guo, V., Puckett, C., Kamholtz, J.. Spiegel, A., and Nirenberg, M. (1986). Human cDNA clones for four species of G-α_s signal transduction protein *Proc. Natl. Acad. Sci. U.S.A.* **83**, 8893–8897.

Bray, P., Carter, A., Guo, V., Puckett, C., Kamholz, J., Spiegel, A., and Nirenberg, M. (1987). Human cDNA clones for an alpha subunit of G_i signal transduction protein. *Proc. Natl. Acad. Sci. U. S. A.* **84**, 5115–5119.

Breitwieser, G. E., and Szabo, G. (1985). Upcoupling of cardiac muscarinic and β-adrenergic receptors from ion channels by a guanine nucleotide analogue. *Nature (London)* **317**, 538–540.

Broek, D., Samiy, N., Fasano, O., Fujiyama, A., Tamanoi, F., Northup, J., and Wigler, M. (1985). Differential activation of yeast adenylate cyclase by wild-type and mutant *ras* proteins. *Cell* **41**, 763–769.

Carter, A., Bardin, C., Collins, R., Simons, C., Bray, P., and Spiegel, A. (1987). Reduced expression of multiple forms of G_s-alpha in pseudohypoparathyroidism type Ia. *Proc. Natl. Acad. Sci. U. S. A.* **84**, 7266–7269.

Cassel, D., and Pfeuffer, T. (1978). Mechanism of cholera toxin action: Covalent modification of the guanyl nucleotide-binding protein of the adenylate cyclase system. *Proc. Natl. Acad. Sci. U.S.A.* **75**, 2669–2673.

Cassel, D., and Selinger, Z. (1977). Mechanism of adenylate cyclase activation by cholera toxin: inhibition of GTP hydrolysis at the regulatory site. *Proc. Natl. Acad. Sci. U.S.A.* **74**, 3307–3311.

Cerione, R. A., Sibley, D. R., Codina, J., Benovic, J. L., Winslow. J., Neer, E. J., Birnbaumer, L., Caron, M. G., and Lefkowitz, R. J. (1984). Reconstitution of a hormone-sensitive adenylate cyclase system. The pure β-adrenergic receptor and guanine nucleotide regulatory protein confer hormone responsiveness on the resolved catalytic unit. *J. Biol. Chem.* **259**, 9979–9982.

Cerione, R. A., Staniszewski, C., Benovic, J. L., Lefkowitz, R. J., Caron, M. F., Gierschik, P., Somers, R., Spiegel, A. M., Codina, J., and Birnbaumer, L. (1985). Specificity of the functional interactions of the β-adrenergic receptor and rhodopsin with guanine nucleotide regulatory proteins reconstituted in phospholipid vesicles. *J. Biol. Chem.* **260**, 1493–1500.

Cerione, R. A., Staniszewski, C., Gierschik, P., Codina, J., Somers, R. L., Birnbaumer, L., Spiegel, A. M., Caron, M. G., and Lefkowitz, R. J. (1986a). Mechanism of guanine nucleotide regulatory protein-mediated inhibition of adenylate cyclase. *J. Biol. Chem.* **261**, 9514–9520.

Cerione, R. A., Regan, J. W., Nakata, H., Codina, J., Benovic, J. L., Gierschik, P., Somers. R. L., Spiegel, A. M., Birnbaumer, L., Lefkowitz, R. J., and Caron, M. G. (1986b). Funcional reconstitution of the α_2-adrenergic receptor with guanine nucleotide regulatory proteins in phospholipid vesicles. *J. Biol. Chem.* **261**, 3901–3909.

Cerione, R. A., Gierschik, P., Stanizsewski, C., Benovic, J. L., Codina, J., Somers, R., Birnbaumer, L., Spiegel, A. M., Lefkowitz, R. J., and Caron, M. G. (1987). Functional differences in the β/γ complexes of transducin and the inhibitory guanine nucleotide regulatory protein. *Biochemistry* **26**, 1485–1491.

Chueh, S.-H., and Gill, D. L. (1986). Inositol 1,4,5-trisphosphate and guanine nucleotides activate calcium release from endoplasmic reticulum via distinct mechanisms. *J. Biol. Chem.* **261**, 13883–13886.

Cockcroft, S., and Gomperts, B. D. (1985). Role of guanine nucleotide binding protein in the activation of polyphosphoinositide phosphodiesterase. *Nature (London)* **314**, 534–536.

Codina, J., Hildebrandt, J., Iyengar, R., Birnbaumer, L., Sekura, R. D., and Manclark, C. R. (1983). Pertussis toxin substrate, the putative N_i component of adenylyl cyclases, is an α β heterodimer regulated by guanine nucleotide and magnesium. *Proc. Natl. Acad. Sci. U.S.A.* **80**, 4276–4280.

Codina, J., Stengel, D., Woo, S., and Birnbaumer, L. (1986). β-subunits of the human liver G_s/G_i signal-transducing proteins and those of bovine retinal rod cell transducin are identical. *FEBS Lett.* **207**, 187–193.

Cronin, M. J., Summers, S. T., Sortino, M. A., and Hewlett, E. L. (1986). Protein kinase C enhances growth hormone releasing factor(1–40)-stimulated cyclic AMP levels in anterior pituitary. *J. Biol. Chem.* **261**, 13932–13935.

Darfler, F. J., Mahan, L. C., Koachman, A. M., and Insel, P. A. (1982). Stimulation by forskolin of intact S49 lymphoma cells involves the nucleotide regulatory protein of adenylate cyclase. *J. Biol. Chem.* **256**, 11901–11907.

Deckmyn, H., Tu, S.-M., and Majerus, P. W. (1986). Guanine nucleotides stimulate soluble phosphoinositide-specific phospholipase C in the absence of membranes. *J. Biol. Chem.* **261**, 16553–16558.

DeFeo-Jones, D., Scolnick, E., Killer, R., and Dhar, R. (1983). Ras-related gene sequences identified and isolated from *Saccharomyces cerevisiae*. *Nature (London)* **306**, 707–709.

Deterre, P., Bigay, J., Pfister, C., and Chabre, M. (1984). Guanine nucleotides and magnesium dependence of the association states of the subunits of transducin. *FEBS Lett.* **178**. 228–232.

Dixon, R. A. F., Kobilka, B. K., Strader, D. J., Benovic, J. L., Dohlman, H. G., Frielle, T., Bolanowski, M. A., Bennett, C. D., Rands, E.. Diehl, R. E., Mumford, R. A., Slater, E. E., Sigal, I. S., Caron. M. G., Lefkowitz, R. J., and Strader, C. D. (1986). Cloning of the gene and cDNA for mammalian β-adrenergic receptor and homology with rhodopsin. *Nature (London)* **321**, 75–79.

Enjalbert, A., Sladeczek, F., Guillon, G., Bertrand, P., Shu, C.. Epelbaum, J., Garcia-Sainz, A., Jard, S.. Lombard, C., Kordon, C., and Bockaert, J. (1986). Angiotensin II and dopamine modulate both cAMP and inositol phosphate productions in anterior pituitary cells. *J. Biol. Chem.* **261**, 4071–4075.

Evans, T., Brown, M. L., Fraser, E. D., and Northup, J. K. (1986). Purification of the major GTP-binding proteins from human placental membranes. *J. Biol. Chem.* **261**, 7052–7059.

Falloon, J., Malech, H., Milligan, G., Unson, C., Kahn, R., Goldsmith, P., and Spiegel, A. (1986). Detection of the major pertussis toxin substrate of human leukocytes with antisera raised against synthetic peptides. *FEBS Lett.* **209**, 352–356.

Fein, A. (1986). Excitation and adaptation of *Limulus* photoreceptors by light and inositol 1,4,5-trisphosphate. *Trends NeuroSci.* **9**, 110–114.

Ferguson, K. M., Higashijima, T., Smigel, M. D., and Gilman, A. G. (1986). The influence of bound GDP on the kinetics of guanine nucleotide binding to G proteins. *J. Biol. Chem.* **261**, 7393–7399.

Fitzpatrick, L. A., Brandi, M. L., and Aurbach, G. D. (1986). Control of PTH secretion is mediated through calcium channels and is blocked by pertussis toxin treatment of parathyroid cells *Biochem. Biophys. Res. Commun.* **138**, 960–965.

Fleischman, L. F., Chahwala, S. B., and Cantley, L. (1986). *ras*-Transformed cells: Altered levels of phosphatidylinositol 4,5-bisphosphate and catabolites. *Science* **231**, 407–410.

Florio, V. A., and Sternweis, P. C. (1985). Reconstitution of resolved muscarinic cholinergic receptors with purified GTP-binding proteins. *J. Biol. Chem.* **260**, 3477–3483.

Fong, H. K. W., Hurley, J. B., Hopkins, R. S., Miake-Lye, R., Johnson, M. S., Doolittle, R. F., and Simon, M. I. (1986). Repetitive segmental structure of the transducin β subunit: Homology with the CDC4 gene and identification of related mRNAs. *Proc. Natl. Acad. Sci. U.S.A.* **83**, 2162–2166.

Fukui, Y., Kozasa, T., Kaziro, Y., Takeda, T., and Yamamoto, M. (1986). Role of a *ras* homolog in the life cycle of *Schizosaccharomyces pombe. Cell* **44**, 329–336.

Fung, B.-K. (1983). Characterization of transducin from bovine retinal rod outer segments. I. Separation and reconstitution of the subunits. *J. Biol. Chem.* **258**, 10495–10502.

Gibbs, J. B., Sigal, I. S., Poe, M., and Scolnick, E. M. (1984). Intrinsic GTPase activity distinguishes normal and oncogenic *ras* p21 molecules. *Proc. Natl. Acad. Sci. U.S.A.* **81**, 5704–5708.

Gierschik, P., and Spiegel, A. M. (1985). Chymotrypsin selectively decreases forskolin stimulation of adenylate cyclase. *Arch. Biochem. Biophys.* **242**, 457–463.

Gierschik, P., Codina, J., Simons, C., Birnbaumer, L., and Spiegel, A. (1985). Antisera against a guanine nucleotide binding protein from retina cross-react with the β subunit of the adenylyl cyclase associated guanine nucleotide binding proteins, N_s and N_i. *Proc. Natl. Acad. Sci. U.S.A.* **82**, 727–731.

Gierschik, P., Falloon, J., Milligan, G., Pines, M., Gallin, J. I., and Spiegel, A. (1986a). Immunochemical evidence for a novel pertussis toxin substrate in human neutrophils. *J. Biol. Chem.* **261**, 8058–8062.

Gierschik, P., Milligan, G., Pines, M., Goldsmith, P.. Codina, J., Klee, W., and Spiegel, A. (1986b). Use of specific antibodies to quantitate the guanine nucleotide-binding protein G_o in brain. *Proc. Natl. Acad. Sci. U.S.A.* **83**, 2258–2262.

Gierschik, P., Morrow, B., Milligan, G., Rubin, C., and Spiegel, A. (1986c). Changes in the guanine nucleotide-binding proteins, G_i and G_o, during differentiation of 3T3-L1 cells. *FEBS Lett.* **199**, 103–106.

Gill, D. M., and Meren, H. (1978). ADP-ribosylation of membrane proteins catalyzed by cholera toxin: Basis of the activation of adenylate cyclase. *Proc. Natl. Acad. Sci. U.S.A.* **75**, 3050–3054.

Gilman, A. G. (1984). G proteins and dual control of adenylate cyclase. *Cell* **36**, 577–579.

Glossman, H., Baukal, A., and Catt, K. J. (1974). Angiotensin II receptors in bovine adrenal cortex. *J. Biol. Chem.* **249**, 664–666.

Gomperts, B. D. (1983). Involvement of guanine nucleotide-binding protein in the gating of Ca^{2+} by receptors. *Nature (London)* **306**, 64–66.

Gomperts, B. D. (1986). Calcium shares the limelight in stimulus–secretion coupling. *Trends Biochem Sci.* **11**, 290–292.

Grunwald, G. B., Gierschik, P., Nirenberg, M., and Spiegel, A. (1986). Detection of α-transducin in retinal rods but not cones. *Science* **231**, 856–859.

Haga, T., Ross, E. M., Anderson, H. J., and Gilman, A. G. (1977). Adenylate cyclase permanently uncoupled from hormone receptors in a novel variant of S49 mouse lymphoma cells. *Proc. Natl. Acad. Sci. U.S.A.* **74**, 2016–2020.

Halliday, K. (1984). Regional homology in GTP-binding protooncogene products and elongation factors. *J. Cyclic Nucleotide Res.* **9**, 435–448.

Halvorsen, S. W., and Nathanson, N. M. (1984). Ontogenesis of physiological responsiveness and guanine nucleotide sensitivity of cardiac muscarinic receptors during chick embryonic development. *Biochemistry* **23**, 5813–5821.

Harris, B. A., Robishaw, J. D., Mumby, S. M., and Gilman, A. G. (1985). Molecular cloning of complementary DNA of the α subunit of the G protein that stimulates adenylate cyclase. *Science* **229**, 1274–1277.

Henne, V., and Soling, H.-D. (1986). Guanosine 5'-triphosphate releases calcium from rat liver and guinea pig parotid gland endoplasmic reticulum independently of inositol 1,4,5-trisphosphate. *FEBS Lett.* **202**, 267–272.

Hildebrandt, J. D., Hanoune, J., and Birnbaumer, L. (1982). Guanine nucleotide inhibition of cyc⁻ S49 mouse lymphoma cell membrane adenylyl cyclase. *J. Biol. Chem.* **257**, 14723–14725.

Hildebrandt, J. D., Codina, J., Rosenthal, W., Birnbaumer, L., Neer, E. J., Yamazaki, A., and Bitensky, M. W. (1985). Characterization by two-dimensional peptide mapping of the γ subunits of N_s and N_i, the regulatory proteins of adenylyl cyclase, and of transducin, the guanine nucleotide-binding protein of rod outer segments of the eye. *J. Biol. Chem.* **260**, 14867–14872.

Hinkle, P. M., and Phillips, W. J. (1984). Thyrotropin-releasing hormone stimulates GTP hydrolysis by membranes from GH_4C_1 rat pituitary tumor cells. *Proc. Natl. Acad. Sci. U.S.A.* **81**, 6183–6187.

Ho, Y.-K., and Fung, K.-K. (1984). Characterization of transducin from bovine retinal rod outer segments. *J. Biol. Chem.* **259**, 6694–6699.

Holz, G. G., IV, Rane, S. G., and Dunlap. K. (1986). GTP-binding proteins mediate transmitter inhibition of voltage-dependent calcium channels. *Nature (London)* **319**, 670–672.

Hsia, J. A., Moss, J., Hewlett, E. L., and Vaughan, M. (1984). ADP-ribosylation of adenylate cyclase by pertussis toxin. *J. Biol. Chem.* **259**, 1086–1090.

Huang, K.-S., Wallner, B. P., Mattaliano, R. J., Tizard, R., Burne, C., Frey, A., Hession, C., McGray, P., Sinclair, L. K., Chow, E. P., Browning, J. L., Ramachandran, K. L., Tang, J., Smart, J. E., and Pepinsky, R. B. (1986). Two human 35 kd inhibitors of phospholipase A_2 are related to substrates of pp60^{v-src} and of the epidermal growth factor receptor/kinase. *Cell* **46**, 191–199.

Hudson, T. H., Roeer, J. F., and Johnson, G. L. (1981). Conformational changes of adenylate cyclase regulatory proteins mediated by guanine nucleotides. *J. Biol. Chem.* **256**, 1459–1464.

Huff, R. M., Axton, J. M., and Neer, E. J. (1985). Physical and immunological characterization of a guanine nucleotide-binding protein purified from bovine cerebral cortex. *J. Biol. Chem.* **260**, 10864–10871.

Hughes, S. M. (1983). Are guanine nucleotide binding proteins a distinct class of regulatory proteins? *FEBS Lett.* **164**, 1–8.

Huque, T., and Bruch, R. C. (1986). Odorant- and guanine nucleotide-stimulated phosphoinositide turnover in olfactory cilia. *Biochem. Biophys. Res. Commun.* **137**, 36–42.

Hurley, J. B., Fong, H. K. W., Teplow, D. B., Dreyer, W. J., and Simon, M. I. (1984a). Isolation and characterization of a cDNA clone for the γ subunit of bovine retinal transducin. *Proc. Natl Acad. Sci. U.S.A.* **81**, 6948–6952.

Hurley, J. B., Simon, M. I., Teplow, D. B., Robishaw, J. D., and Gilman, A. G. (1984b).

Homologies between signal transducing G proteins and *ras* gene products. *Science* **226,** 860–862.

Hurwitz, R. L., Bunt-Milam, A. H., Chang, M. L., and Beavo, J. A. (1985). cGMP phosphodiesterase in rod and cone outer segments of the retina. *J. Biol. Chem.* **260,** 568–573.

Imboden, J. B., Shoback, D. M., Pattison, G., and Stobo, J. D. (1986). Cholera toxin inhibits the T-cell antigen receptor-mediated increases in inositol trisphosphate and cytoplasmic free calcium. *Proc. Natl. Acad. Sci. U.S.A.* **83,** 5673–5677.

Itoh, H., Kozasa, T., Nagata, S., Nakamura, S., Katada, T., Ui, M., Iwai, S., Ohtsuka, E., Kawasaki, H., Suzuki, K., and Kaziro, Y. (1986). (1986). Molecular cloning and sequence determination of cDNAs for α subunits of the guanine nucleotide-binding proteins G_s, G_i, and G_o from rat brain. *Proc. Natl. Acad. Sci. U.S.A.* **83,** 3776–3780.

Iyengar, R., and Birnbaumer, L. (1982). Hormone receptor modulates the regulatory component of adenylyl cyclase by reducing its requirement for Mg^{2+} and enhancing its extent of activation by guanine nucleotides. *Proc. Natl. Acad. Sci. U.S.A.* **79,** 5179–5183.

Jacquemin, C., Thibout, H., Lambert, B., and Correze, C. (1986). Endogenous ADP-ribosylation of G_s subunit and autonomous regulation of adenylate cyclase. *Nature (London)* **323,** 182–184.

Jakobs, K. H., Aktories, K., and Schultz, G. (1983). Mechanism of pertussis toxin action on the adenylate cyclase system: Inhibition of the turnon reaction of the inhibitory regulatory site. *Eur. J. Biochem.* **140,** 177–181.

Jakway, J. P., and DeFranco, A. L. (1986). Pertussis toxin inhibition of B cell and macrophage responses to bacterial lipopolysaccharide. *Science* **234.** 743–746.

Johnson, E. C., Robinson, P. R., and Lisman, J. E. (1986). Cyclic GMP is involved in the excitation of invertebrate photoreceptors. *Nature (London)* **324,** 468–470.

Johnson, G. L., Kaslow, H. R., and Bourne, H. R. (1978). Genetic evidence that cholera toxin substrates are regulatory components of adenylate cyclase. *J. Biol. Chem.* **253,** 7120–7123.

Johnson, J. D., and Davies, P. J. A. (1986). Pertussis toxin inhibits retinoic acid-induced expression of tissue transglutaminase in macrophages. *J. Biol. Chem.* **261,** 14982–19486.

Jurnak, F. (1985). Structure of the GDP domain of EF-Tu and location of the amino acids homologous to *ras* oncogene proteins. *Science* **230,** 32–36.

Kahn, R. A., and Gilman, A. G. (1986). The protein cofactor necessary for ADP-ribosylation of G_s by cholera toxin is itself a GTP binding protein. *J. Biol. Chem.* **261,** 7906–7911.

Kaibuchi, L., Miyajima, A., Arai, K.-I., and Matsumoto, K. (1986). Possible involvement of *RAS*-encoded proteins in glucose-induced inositol phospholipid turnover in *Saccharomyces cerevisiae*. *Proc. Natl. Acad. Sci. U.S.A.* **83,** 8172–8176.

Kamata, T., and Feramisco, J. R. (1984). Epidermal growth factor stimulates guanine nucleotide binding activity and phosphorylation of *ras* oncogene proteins. *Nature (London)* **310,** 147–150.

Kanaide, H., Matsumoto, T., and Nakamura, M. (1986). Inhibition of calcium transients in cultured vascular smooth muscle cells by pertussis toxin. *Biochem. Biophys. Res. Commun.* **140,** 195–203.

Katada, T., Bokoch, G. M., Northup, J. K., Ui, M., and Gilman, A. G. (1984a). The inhibitory guanine nucleotide-binding regulatory component of adenylate cyclase. Properties and function of the purified protein. *J. Biol. Chem.* **259,** 3568–3577.

Katada, T., Northup, J. K., Bokoch, G. M., Ui, M., and Gilman, A. G. (1984b). The inhibitory guanine nucleotide-binding and regulatory component of adenylate cyclase. Subunit dissociation and guanine nucleotide-dependent hormonal inhibition. *J. Biol. Chem.* **259**, 3578–3585.

Katada, T., Gilman, A. G., Watanabe, Y., Bauer, S., and Jakobs, K. H. (1985). Protein kinase C phosphorylates the inhibitory guanine nucleotide-binding regulatory component and apparently suppresses its function in hormonal inhibition of adenylate cyclase. *Eur. J. Biochem.* **151**, 431–437.

Katada, T., Oinuma, M., and Ui, M. (1986). Mechanisms for inhibition of the catalytic activity and adenylate cyclase by the guanine nucleotide-binding proteins serving as the substrate of islet-activating protein, pertussis toxin. *J. Biol. Chem.* **261**, 5215–5221.

Kataoka, T., Powers, S., Cameron, S., Fasano, O., Goldfarb, M., Broach, M., and Wigler, M. (1985). Functional homology of mammalian and yeast *RAS* genes. *Cell* **40**, 19–26.

Kikuchi, A., Kozawa, D., Kaibuchi, K., Katada, T., Ui, M., and Takai, Y. (1986). Direct evidence for involvement of a guanine nucleotide-binding protein in chemotactic peptide-stimulated formation of inositol bisphosphate and trisphosphate in differentiated human leukemic (HL-60) cells. *J. Biol. Chem.* **261**, 11558–11562.

Knight, D. E., and Baker, P. F. (1985). Guanine nucleotides and Ca-dependent exocytosis studies on two adrenal cell preparations. *FEBS Lett.* **189**, 345–349.

Koch, B. D., Dorflinger, L. J., and Schonbrunn, A. (1985). Pertussis toxin blocks both cyclic AMP-mediated and cyclic AMP-independent actions of somatostatin, evidence for coupling of N_i to decreases in intracellular free calcium. *J. Biol. Chem.* **260**, 13138–13145.

Kohno, K., Uchida, T., Ohkubo, H., Nakanishi, S., Nakanishi, T., Fukui, T., Ohtsuka, E., Ikehara, M., and Okada, Y. (1986). Amino acid sequence of mammalian elongation factor 2 deduced from the cDNA sequence: Homology with GTP-binding proteins. *Proc. Natl. Acad. Sci. U.S.A.* **83**, 4978–4982.

Kojima, I., Shibata, H.. and Ogata, E. (1986). Pertussis toxin blocks angiotensin II-induced calcium influx but not inositol trisphosphate production in adrenal glomerulosa cells. *FEBS Lett.* **204**, 347–351.

Kubo, T., Fukuda, K., Mikami, A., Maeda, A., Takahashi, H., Mishina, M., Haga, T., Haga, K., Ichiyama, A., Kangawa, K., Kojima, M., Matsuo, Y., Hirose, T., and Numa, S. (1986). Cloning, sequencing and expression of complementary DNA encoding the muscarinic acetylcholine receptor. *Nature (London)* **323**, 411–416.

Kuhn, H. (1980). Light- and GTP-regulated interaction of GTPase and other proteins with bovine photoreceptor membranes. *Nature (London)* **283**, 587–589.

Lai, E., Rosen, O. M., and Rubin, C. S. (1981). Differentiation-dependent expression of catecholamine-stimulated adenylate cyclase. *J. Biol. Chem.* **256**, 12866–12874.

Lerea, C. L., Somers, D. E., Hurley, J. B., Klock, I. B., and Bunt-Milan, A. H. (1986). Identification of specific transducin α subunits in retinal rod and cone photoreceptors. *Science* **234**, 77–80.

Letterio, J. J., Coughlin, S. R., and Williams, L. T. (1986). Pertussis toxin-sensitive pathway in the stimulation of *c-myc* expression and DNA synthesis by bombesin. *Science* **234**, 1117–1119.

Lewis, D., Weight, F. F., and Luini, A. (1986). A guanine nucleotide-binding protein mediates the inhibition of voltage-dependent calcium current by somatostatin in a pituitary cell line. *Proc. Natl. Acad. Sci. U.S.A.* **83**, 9035–9039.

Liang, B. T., Hellmich, M. R., Neer, E. J., and Galper, J. B. (1986). Development of muscarinic cholinergic inhibition of adenylate cyclase in embryonic chick heart. *J. Biol. Chem.* **261**, 9011–9021.

Litosch, I., Wallis, C., and Fain, J. N. (1985). 5-Hydroxytryptamine stimulates inositol phosphate production in a cell-free system from blowfly salivary glands. Evidence for a role of GTP in coupling receptor activation to phosphoinositide breakdown. *J. Biol. Chem.* **260,** 5464–5471.

Lochrie, M. A., Hurley, J. B., and Simon, M. I. (1985). Sequence of the α subunit of photoreceptor G protein: homologies between transducin, ras, and elongation factors. *Science* **228,** 96–99.

Logothetis, D. E., Kurachi, Y., Galper, J.. Neer, E. J., and Clapham, D. E. (1987). The β/γ subunits of GTP-binding proteins activate the muscarinic K+ channel in heart. *Nature (London)* **325,** 321–326.

Lowy, D. R., and Willumsen, B. M. (1986). The *ras* gene family. *Cancer Surv.* **5,** 274–289.

McCormick, F., Clark, B. F. C., LaCour, T. F. M., Kjeldgaard, M.. Norskov-Lauristen, L., and Nyborg, J. (1985). A model for the tertiary structure of p21, the product of the *ras* oncogene. *Science* **230,** 78–82.

McGrath, J. P., Capon, D. J., Goeddel, D. V., and Levinson, A. D. (1984). Comparative biochemical properties of normal and activated human *ras* p21 protein. *Nature (London)* **310,** 644–649.

Madaule, P., and Axel, R. (1985). A novel *ras*-related gene family. *Cell* **41,** 31–40.

Manning, D. R., and Gilman, A. G. (1983). The regulatory components of adenylate cyclase and transducin. A family of structurally homologous guanine nucleotide binding proteins. *J. Biol. Chem.* **258,** 7059–7063.

Masters, S. B., Martin, M. W., Harden, T. K., and Brown, J. H. (1985). Pertussis toxin does not inhibit muscarinic receptor-mediated phosphoinositide hydrolysis or calcium mobilization. *Biochem. J.* **227,** 933–937.

Mattera, R., Codina, J., Crozat, A., Kidd, V., Woo, S. L. C., and Birnbaumer, L. (1986). Identification by molecular cloning of two forms of the α-subunit of the human liver stimulatory (G$_s$) regulatory component of adenylyl cyclase. *FEBS Lett.* **206,** 36–41.

May, D. C., Ross, E. M., Gilman, A. G., and Smigel, M. D. (1985). Reconstitution of catecholamine-stimulated adenylate cyclase activity using three purified proteins. *J. Biol. Chem.* **260,** 15829–15833.

Medynski, D. C., Sullivan, K., Smith, D., Van Dop, C., Chang, F. H., Fung. B. K. K., Seeburg, P. H., and Bourne, H. R. (1985). Amino acid sequence of the α subunit of transducin deduced from the cDNA sequence. *Proc. Natl. Acad. Sci. U.S.A.* **82,** 4311–4315.

Michel, T., Winslow, J. W., Smith, J. A., Seidman, J. G., and Neer, E. J. (1986). Molecular cloning and characterization of cDNA encoding the GTP-binding protein α$_i$ and identification of a related protein α$_h$. *Proc. Natl. Acad. Sci. U.S.A.* **83,** 7663–7667.

Milligan, G., Streaty, R. A., Gierschik, P., Spiegel, A. M., and Klee, W. A. (1987). Development of opiate receptors and GTP-binding regulatory proteins in neonatal rat brain. *J. Biol. Chem.* **262,** 8626–8630.

Mumby, S. M., Kahn, R. A., Manning, D. R., and Gilman, A. G. (1986). Antisera of designed specificity for subunits of guanine nucleotide-binding regulatory proteins. *Proc. Natl. Acad. Sci. U.S.A.* **83,** 265–269.

Naghshineh, S., Noguchi, M., Huang, K.-P., and Londos, C. (1986). Activation of adipocyte adenylate cyclase by protein kinase C. *J. Biol. Chem.* **261,** 14534–14538.

Nakamura, T., and Ui, M. (1985). Simultaneous inhibitions of inositol phospholipid breakdown, arachidonic acid release, and histamine secretion in mast cells by islet-activating protein, pertussis toxin. *J. Biol. Chem.* **260,** 3584–3593.

Nathans, J., Thomas, D., and Hogness, D. S. (1986). Molecular genetics of human color vision: The genes encoding blue, green, and red pigments. *Science* **232,** 193–202.

Neer, E. J., Lok, J. M., and Wolf, L. G. (1984). Purification and properties of the inhibitory guanine nucleotide regulatory unit of brain adenylate cyclase. *J. Biol. Chem.* **259**, 14222–14229.

Nielsen, T. B., Downs, R. W., Jr., and Spiegel, A. M. (1980). Restoration of guanine nucleotide- and fluoride-stimulated activity to an adenylate cyclase-deficient cell line with affinity-purified guanine nucleotide regulatory protein. *Biochem. J.* **190**, 439–443.

Nukada, T., Tanabe, T., Takahashi, H., Noda, M., Hirose, T., Inayama, S., and Numa, S. (1986a). Primary structure of the α-subunit of bovine adenylate cyclase-stimulating G-protein deduced from the cDNA sequence. *FEBS Lett.* **195**, 220–224.

Nukada, T., Tanabe, T., Takahashi, H., Noda, M., Haga, K., Haga, T., Ichiyama, A., Kangawa, K., Hiranaga, M., Matsuo, H., and Numa, S. (1986b). Primary structure of the α-subunit of bovine adenylate cyclase-inhibiting G-protein deduced from the cDNA sequence. *FEBS Lett.* **197**, 305–310.

Oetting, M., LeBoff, M., Swiston, L., Preston, J., and Brown, E. (1986). Guanine nucleotides are potent secretagogues in permeabilized parathyroid cells. *FEBS Lett.* **208**, 99–98.

Oinuma, M., Katada, T., Yokosawa, H., and Ui, M. (1986). Guanine nucleotide-binding protein in sea urchin eggs serving as the specific substrate of islet-activating protein, pertussis toxin. *FEBS Lett.* **207**, 28–34.

Okajima, F., and Ui, M. (1984). ADP-ribosylation of the specific membrane protein by islet-activating protein, pertussis toxin, associated with inhibition of a chemotactic peptide-induced arachidonate release in neutrophils. *J. Biol. Chem.* **259**, 13863–13871.

Orly, J., and Schramm, M. (1976). Coupling of catecholamine receptor from one cell with adenylate cyclase from another cell by cell fusion. *Proc. Natl. Acad. Sci. U.S.A.* **73**, 4410–4411.

Ovchinnikow, Y. A., Lipkin, V. M., Shuvaeva, T. M., Bogachuk, A. P., and Shemyakin, V. V. (1985). Complete amino acid sequence of γ-subunit of the GTP-binding protein from cattle retina. *FEBS Lett.* **179**, 107–110.

Owens, J. R., Frame, L. T., Ui, M., and Cooper, D. M. F. (1985). Cholera toxin ADP-ribosylates the islet-activating protein substrate in adipocyte membranes and alters its function. *J. Biol. Chem.* **260**, 15946–15952.

Pace, U., and Lancet, D. (1986). Olfactory GTP-binding protein: Signal-transducing polypeptide of vertebrate chemosensory neurons. *Proc. Natl. Acad. Sci. U.S.A.* **83**, 4947–4951.

Pace, U., Hanski, E., Salomon, Y., and Lancet, D. (1985). Odorant-sensitive adenylate cyclase may mediate olfactory reception. *Nature (London)* **316**, 255–258.

Pedersen, S. E., and Ross, E. M. (1982). Functional reconstitution of β-adrenergic receptors and the stimulatory GTP-binding protein of adenylate cyclase. *Proc. Natl. Acad. Sci. U.S.A.* **79**, 7228–7232.

Pellman, D., Garber, E. A., Cross, F. R., and Hanafusa, H. (1985). An N-terminal peptide from p60[src] can direct myristylation and plasma membrane localization when fused to heterologous proteins. *Nature (London)* **314**, 374–377.

Pfaffinger, P. J., Martin, J. M., Hunter, D. D., Nathanson, N. M.. and Hille, B. (1985). GTP-binding proteins couple cardiac muscarinic receptors to a K channel. *Nature (London)* **317**, 536–538.

Pfeuffer, T. (1977). GTP-binding proteins in membranes and the control of adenylate cyclase activity. *J. Biol. Chem.* **252**, 7224–7234.

Pfeuffer, E., Dreher, R.-M., Metzger, H., and Pfeuffer, T. (1985). Catalytic unit of adenylate cyclase: Purification and identification by affinity cross-linking. *Proc. Natl Acad. Sci. U.S.A.* **82**, 3086–3090.

Pines, M., Gierschik, P., and Spiegel, A. (1985). The tryptic and chymotryptic fragments of the β-subunit of guanine nucleotide binding proteins in brain are identical to those of retinal transducin. *FEBS Lett.* **182**, 355–359.

Pines, M., Santora, A., and Spiegel, A. (1986). Effects of phorbol esters and pertussis toxin on agonist-stimulated cyclic AMP production in rat osteosarcoma cells. *Biochem. Pharmacol.* **35**, 3639–3641.

Poe, M., Scolnick, E. M., and Stein, R. B. (1985). Viral harvey *ras* p21 expressed in *Escherichia coli* purifies as a binary one-to-one complex with GDP. *J. Biol. Chem.* **260**, 3906–3909.

Preiss, J., Loomis, C. R., Bishop, W. R., Stein, R., Niedel, J. E., and Bell, R. M. (1986). Quantitative measurement of *sn*-1,2-diacylglycerols present in platelets hepatocytes, and *ras*- and *sis*-transformed normal rat kidney cells. *J. Biol. Chem.* **261**, 8597–8600.

Robishaw, J. D., Russell, D. W., Harris, B. A., Smigel, M. D., and Gilman, A. G. (1986a). Deduced primary structure of the α subunit of the GTP-binding stimulatory protein of adenylate cyclase. *Proc. Natl. Acad. Sci. U.S.A.* **83**, 1251–1255.

Robishaw, J. D., Smigel, M. D., and Gilman, A. G. (1986b). Molecular basis for two forms of the G protein that stimulates adenylate cyclase. *J. Biol. Chem.* **261**, 9587–9590.

Rodbell, M. (1980). The role of hormone receptors and GTP-regulatory proteins in membrane transduction. *Nature (London)* **284**, 17–21.

Rodbell, M. (1985). Programmable messengers: A new theory of hormone action. *Trends Biochem. Sci.* **119**, 461–464.

Roof, D. J., Applebury, M. L., and Sternweis, P. C. (1985). Relationships within the family of GTP-binding proteins isolated from bovine central nervous system. *J. Biol. Chem.* **260**, 16242–16249.

Ross, E. M., Howlett, A. C., Ferguson, K. M., and Gilman, A. G. (1978). Reconstitution of hormone-sensitive adenylate cyclase activity with resolved components of the enzyme. *J. Biol. Chem.* **253**, 6401–6412.

Salomon, M. R., and Bourne, H. R. (1981). Novel S49 lymphoma variants with aberrant cyclic AMP metabolism. *Mol. Pharmacol.* **19**, 109–116.

Schlegel, W., Wuarin, F., Zbaren, C., Wollheim, C. B., and Zahnd, G. R. (1985). Pertussis toxin selectively abolishes hormone induced lowering of cytosolic calcium in GH₃ cells. *FEBS Lett.* **189**, 27–32.

Schleifer, L. S., Garrison, J. C., Sternweis, P. C., Northup, J. K., and Gilman, A. G. (1981). The regulatory component of adenylate cyclase from uncoupled S49 lymphoma cells differs in charge from the wild-type protein. *J. Biol. Chem.* **255**, 2641–2644.

Seamon, K. B., Vaillancourt, R., Edwards, M., and Daly, J. W. (1984). Binding of [³H]forskolin to rat brain membranes. *Proc. Natl. Acad. Sci. U.S.A.* **81**, 5081–5085.

Sibley, D. R., Nambi, P., Peters, J. R., and Lefkowitz, R. J. (1984). Phorbol diesters promote β-adrenergic receptor phosphorylation and adenylate cyclase densensitization in duck erythrocytes. *Biochem. Biophys. Res. Commun.* **121**, 973–979.

Schmitt, H. D., Wagner, P., Pfaff, E., and Gallwitz, D. (1986). The *ras*-related YPT1 gene product in yeast: A GTP-binding protein that might be involved in microtubule organization. *Cell* **47**, 401–412.

Shinozawa, T., Uchida, S., Martin, E., Cafiso, D., Hubbell, W., and Bitensky, M. (1980). Additional component required for activity and reconstitution of light-activated vertebrate photoreceptor GTPase. *Proc. Natl. Acad. Sci. U.S.A.* **77**, 1408–1411.

Sklar, P. B., Anholt, R. R. H., and Snyder, S. H. (1986). The odorant-sensitive adenylate cyclase of olfactory receptor cells differential stimulation by distinct classes of odorants. *J. Biol. Chem.* **261**, 15538–15543.

Smith, C. D., Lane, B. C., Kusaka, I., Verghese, M. W., and Snyderman, R. (1985). Chemoattractant receptor-induced hydrolysis of phosphatidyl 4,5-bisphosphate in human polymorphonuclear leukocyte membranes. Requirement for a guanine nucleotide regulatory protein. *J. Biol. Chem.* **260**, 5875–5878.

Spiegel, A. M., Downs. R. W., Jr., and Aurbach, G. D. (1979). Separation of a guanine nucleotide regulatory unit from the adenylate cyclase complex with GTP affinity chromatography. *J. Cyclic Nucleotide Res.* **5**, 3–17.

Spiegel, A. M., Gierschik, P., Levine, M. A., and Downs, R. W., Jr. (1985). Clinical implications of guanine nucleotide-binding proteins as receptor–effector couplers. *New Engl. J. Med.* **312**, 26–33.

Steinberg, S. F., Drugge, E. D., Bilezikian, J. P., and Robinson, R. B. (1985). Acquisition by innervated cardiac myocytes of a pertussis toxin-specific regulatory protein linked to the α_1-receptor. *Science* **230**, 186–188.

Sternweis, P. C. (1986). The purified α subunits of G_o and G_i from bovine brain require β/γ for association with phospholipid vesicles. *J. Biol. Chem.* **261**, 631–637.

Sternweis, P. C., and Gilman, A. G. (1979). Reconstitution of catecholamine-sensitive adenylate cyclase. *J. Biol. Chem.* **254**, 3333–3340.

Sternweis, P. C., and Gilman, A. G. (1982). Aluminum: A requirement for activation of the regulatory component of adenylate cyclase by fluoride. *Proc. Natl. Acad. Sci. U.S.A.* **79**, 4888–4891.

Sternweis, P. C., and Robishaw, J. D. (1984). Isolation of two proteins with high affinity for guanine nucleotides from membranes of bovine brain. *J. Biol. Chem.* **259**, 13806–13813.

Sternweis, P. C., Northup, J. K., Smigel, M. D., and Gilman, A. G. (1981). The regulatory component of adenylate cyclase. *J. Biol. Chem.* **256**, 11517–11526.

Stryer, L. (1986). Cyclic GMP cascade of vision. *Annu. Rev. Neurosci.* **9**, 87–119.

Sugimoto, K., Nukada, T., Tanabe, T., Takahashi, H., Noda, M.. Minamino, N., Kangawa, K., Matsuo, H., Hirose, T., Inayama, S., and Numa, S. (1985). Primary structure of the β-subunit of bovine transducin deduced from the cDNA sequence. *FEBS Lett.* **191**, 235–240.

Sullivan, K. A., Liao, Y.-C., Alborzi, A., Beiderman. B., Chang, F.-H., Masters, S. B., Levinson, A. D., and Bourne, H. R. (1986). Inhibitory and stimulatory G proteins of adenylate cyclase: cDNA and amino acid sequences of the α chains. *Proc. Natl. Acad. Sci. U.S.A.* **83**, 6687–6691.

Swanson, M. E., Elste, A. M., Greenberg, S. M., Schwartz, J. H., Aldrich, T. H., and Furth, M. E. (1986). Abundant expression of *ras* proteins in *Aplysia* neurons. *J. Cell Biol.* **103**, 485–492.

Sweet, R. W., Yokoyama, S., Kamata, T., Feramisco, J. R., Rosenberg, M., and Gross, M. (1984). The product of *ras* is a GTPase and the T24 oncogenic mutant is deficient in this activity. *Nature (London)* **311**, 273–275.

Tanabe, T., Nukada, T., Nishikawa, Y., Sugimoto, K., Suzuki, H., Takahashi, H., Noda, M., Haga, T., Ichiyama, A.. Kangawa, K., Minamino, N., Matsuo, H., and Numa, S. (1985). Primary structure of the α subunit of transducin and its relationship to *ras* proteins. *Nature (London)* **315**, 242–245.

Taparowsky, E., Shimizu, K., Goldbarb. M., and Wigler, M. (1983). Structure and activation of the human *N-ras* gene. *Cell* **34**, 581–586.

Tsai, S.-C., Adamik, R., Kanaho, Y., Hewlett, E. L., and Moss, J. (1984). Effects of guanyl nucleotides and rhodopsin on ADP-ribosylation of the inhibitory GTP-binding component of adenylate cyclase by pertussis toxin. *J. Biol. Chem.* **259**, 15320–15323.

Tsuda, M., Tsuda, T., Terayama, Y., Fukada, Y., Akino, T., Yamanaka, G., Stryer, L.,

Katada, T., Ui, M., and Ebrey, T. (1986). Kinship of cephalopod photoreceptor G-protein with vertebrate transducin. *FEBS Lett.* **198**, 5–10.

Turner, P. R., Jaffe, L. A., and Fein, A. (1986). Regulation of cortical vesicle exocytosis in sea urchin egs by inositol 1,4,5-trisphosphate and GTP-binding protein. *J. Cell Biol.* **102**, 70–76.

Ui, M. (1984). Islet-activating protein, pertussis toxin: A probe for functions of the inhibitory guanine nucleotide regulatory component of adenylate cyclase. *Trends Pharmacol. Sci.* **5**, 277–279.

Urumow, T., and Wieland, O. H. (1986). Stimulation of phosphatidylinositol 4-phosphate phosphorylation in human placenta membranes by GTPγS. *FEBS Lett.* **207**, 253–254.

Valentine-Braun, K. A., Northup, J. K., and Hollenberg, M. D. (1986). Epidermal growth factor (urogastrone)-mediated phosphorylation of a 35-kDa substrate in human placental membranes: Relationship to the β subunit of the guanine nucleotide regulatory complex. *Proc. Natl. Acad. Sci. U.S.A.* **83**, 236–240.

Van Dop, C., Medynski, D., Sullivan, K., Wu, A. M., Fung, B.-K., and Bourne, H. R. (1984a). Partial cDNA sequence of the γ subunit of transducin. *Biochem. Biophys. Res. Commun.* **124**, 250–255.

Van Dop, C., Yamanaka, G., Steinberg, F., Sekura, R. D., Manclark, C. R., Stryer, L., and Bourne, H. R. (1984b). ADP-ribosylation of transducin by pertussis toxin blocks the light-stimulated hydrolysis of GTP and cGMP in retinal photoreceptors. *J. Biol. Chem.* **259**, 23–26.

Van Veen, T., Ostholm, T., Gierschik, P., Spiegel, A., Somers, R., Korf, H.W., and Klein, D. C. (1986). Alpha-transducin immunoreactivity in retinae and sensory pineal organs of adult vertebrates. *Proc. Natl. Acad. Sci. U.S.A.* **83**, 912–916.

Verghese, M., Uhing, R. J., and Snyderman, R. (1986). A pertussis/cholera toxin-sensitive N protein may mediate chemoattractant receptor signal tansduction. *Biochem. Biophys. Res. Commun.* **138**, 887–894.

Wakelam, M. J. O., Davies. S. A., Houslay, M. D., McKay, I., Marshall, C. J., and Hall, A. (1986). Normal p21$^{N\text{-}ras}$ couples bombesin and other growth factor receptors to inositol phosphate production. *Nature (London)* **323**, 173–176.

Weinstock, R. S., Wright, H. N., Spiegel, A. M., Levine, M. A., and Moses, A. M. (1986). Olfactory dysfunction in humans with deficient guanine nucleotide-binding protein. *Nature (London)* **322**, 635–636.

West, R. E., Jr., Moss, J., Vaughan, M.. Liu, T., and Liu, T.-Y. (1985). Pertussis toxin-catalyzed ADP-ribosylation of transducin. Cysteine 347 is the ADP–ribose acceptor site. *J. Biol. Chem.* **260**, 14428–14430.

Williamson, J. R. (1986). Role of inositol lipid breakdown in the generation of intracellular signals. *Hypertension* **8**, II140–II156.

Willumsen, B. M., Norris, K., Papageorge, A. G., Hubbert, N. L., and Lowy, D. R. (1984). Harvey murine sarcoma virus p21 *ras* protein: biological and biochemical significance of the cysteine nearest the carboxy terminus. *EMBO J.* **3**, 2581–2585.

Winslow, J. W., Van Amsterdam, J. R.. and Neer, E. J. (1986). Conformations of the α_{39}, α_{41}, and β/γ components of brain guanine nucleotide-binding proteins. *J. Biol. Chem.* **261**, 7571–7579.

Wistow, G. J., Katial, A., Craft, C., and Shinohara, T. (1986). Sequence analysis of bovine retinal S-antigen: Relationships with α-transducin and G-proteins. *FEBS Lett.* **196**, 23–28.

Worley, P. F., Baraban, J. M., Van Dop, C., Neer, E. J., and Snyder, S. H. (1986). G_o, a guanine nucleotide-binding protein: Immunohistochemical localization in rat brain resembles distribution of second messenger systems. *Proc. Natl. Acad. Sci. U.S.A.* **83**, 4561–4565.

Yamazaki, A., Stein, P. J., Chernoff, N., and Bitensky, M. W. (1983). Activation mechanism of rod outer segment cyclic GMP phosphodiesterase. Release of inhibitor by the GTP-binding protein. *J. Biol. Chem.* **258**, 8188–8194.

Yarden, Y., Rodriguez, H., Wong, S. K.-F., Brandt, D. R., May, D. C., Burnier, J., Harkins, R. N., Chen, E. Y., Ramachandran, J., Ullrich, A., and Ross, E. M. (1986). The avian β-adrenergic receptor: Primary structure and membrane topology. *Proc. Natl. Acad. Sci. U.S.A.* **83**, 6795–6799.

Yatani, A., Codina, J., Brown, A. M., and Birnaumer, L. (1987). Direct activation of mammalian atrial muscarinic potassium channels by GTP regulatory protein G_k. *Science* **235**, 207–211.

Yatsunami, K., and Khorana, G. (1985). GTPase of bovine rod outer segments: the amino acid sequence of the α subunit as derived from the cDNA sequence. *Proc. Natl. Acad. Sci. U.S.A.* **82**, 4316–4320.

Yatsunami, K., Pandya, B. V., Oprian, D. D., and Khorana, H. G. (1985). cDNA-derived amino acid sequence of the γ subunit of GTPase from bovine rod outer segments. *Proc. Natl. Acad. Sci. U.S.A.* **82**, 1936–1940.

Zick, Y., Eisenberg, R. S., Pines, M., Gierschik, P., and Spiegel, A. M. (1986). Multi-site phosphorylation of the α subunit of transducin by the insulin receptor kinase and protein kinase C. *Proc. Natl. Acad. Sci. U.S.A.* **83**, 9294–9297.

Insulin-Sensitive Glucose Transport

TETSURO KONO

Department of Molecular Physiology and Biophysics
School of Medicine
Vanderbilt University
Nashville, Tennessee 37232

I. Introduction

In spite of decades of investigation, the molecular mechanisms of insulin action remain obscure. The hormone regulates a number of metabolic activities, but in this article only one facet of insulin action, namely, the stimulation of glucose transport across the plasma membrane, is discussed. As is well known, insulin was discovered by Banting and Best (1922) as a hypoglycemic factor. and its major site of action in glucose metabolism was determined by Levine and Goldstein (1955) to be the membrane transport of the hexose. Since that time, a great number of studies have been done, and many excellent review articles have been published. For example, the early studies were summarized by Levine and Goldstein (1955) and by Randle and Morgan (1962); more recent work was covered by Pilkis and Park (1974) as well as by Czech (1977); the most recent developments were discussed by Levine (1982) and also by Simpson and Cushman (1986); and recent observations on the early events in insulin actions in general were concisely summarized by Denton (1986). In addition, various aspects of insulin actions, including its action on glucose transport, are discussed in depth in two recently published books, entitled "Molecular Basis of Insulin Action" (edited by Czech, 1985) and "Mechanisms of Insulin Action" (edited by Belfrage *et al.*, 1986).

It would appear, therefore, that there is no point in adding another review article at this time. I feel, however, that because such a huge quantity of information has been accumulated over such a long period of time no single review published in recent years adequately covers the entire subject. Therefore, in this article, I have attempted to place the whole subject in perspective by limiting citations to critical "strategic points" in the immense field of insulin studies. I hope that this review article will be useful to investigators who are new in the field as well as to those outsiders who are interested in the subject but too busy to read many articles that describe in depth certain limited aspects of the insulin-dependent regulation of glucose transport.

II. CLASSIFICATION OF INSULIN EFFECTS

As mentioned in the introduction, the effects of insulin on cellular metabolism are diverse; some effects are chronic, others acute and complete within 5 to 20 minutes. The chronic effects of insulin include many complex processes, such as the stimulation of protein synthesis, cell growth and mitosis. The acute effects are also complex but may be classified into subgroups, as listed in Table I. The first four systems in Table I, designated as Type A, are known to be either stimulated or inhibited by phosphorylation or dephosphorylation of the enzyme proteins (Greengard, 1978; Krebs and Beavo, 1979). The effects of insulin on these enzymes are consistent with the interpretation that the hormone promotes dephosphorylation of the enzymes (Pilkis and Park, 1974; Czech, 1977). This view is further supported by the fact that the effects of insulin on Type A enzymes are reversed by phosphorylation mediated by either cAMP-dependent protein kinase or protein kinase C.

In contrast, the insulin-dependent stimulation of cAMP phosphodiesterase (Type B) is observable only in the presence of ATP (Kono *et al.*, 1977), and the effect of the hormone on this enzyme is reversed in the absence of ATP (Vega *et al.*, 1980). Furthermore, the effect of insulin on this enzyme is mimicked, rather than reversed, by

TABLE I
CLASSIFICATION OF ACUTE TYPES OF INSULIN ACTIONS

Enzyme	Insulin effect	Type	Ref.[a]
Glycogen synthase	Stimulation	A	a
Hormone-sensitive lipase	Inhibition	A	b
Pyruvate dehydrogenase	Stimulation	A	c
Pyruvate kinase	Inhibition	A	d
cAMP phosphodiesterase	Stimulation	B	e
Glucose transporter	Stimulation	C	f
Insulin-like growth factor II receptor	Stimulation	C	g
Transferrin receptor	Stimulation	C	h
Phosphoenolpyruvate carboxykinase	Inhibition	D	i

[a] Key to references: a, Villar-Palasi and Larner (1961); b, Jungas and Ball (1963); c, Coore et al. (1971), Jungas (1971); Claus et al. (1979); e, Loten and Sneyd (1970), Manganiello and Vaughan (1973); f, Cushman and Wardzala (1980), Suzuki and Kono (1980); g, Oppenheimer et al. (1983), Wardzala et al. (1984); h, Davis et al. (1986); i, Sasaki et al. (1984).

the action of agents that increase the cellular concentration of cAMP (Zinman and Hollenberg, 1974; Makino and Kono, 1980). It would appear, therefore, that insulin might stimulate cAMP phosphodiesterase by promoting its phosphorylation. However, no solid experimental evidence is available to substantiate this view. Incidentally, it was recently reported from two laboratories that both glycogen synthase (Type A) and cAMP phosphodiesterase (Type B) are activated in a cell-free system by a putative insulin mediator, which may be either a peptide (Jarett et al., 1985) or a carbohydrate-containing substance (Saltiel, 1987). Therefore, insulin might regulate both Type A and Type B enzymes by a common underlying mechanism which is yet to be delineated.

Insulin appears to regulate the activities of the glucose transport system (Cushman and Wardzala, 1980; Suzuki and Kono, 1980), the insulin-like growth factor II receptor (Oppenheimer et al., 1983; Wardzala et al., 1984), and the transferrin receptor (Davis et al., 1986) (Type C systems) primarily by relocating either the transport system or the receptors from an intracellular site to the plasma membrane, as described later in detail (see Section VI). Apparently, ATP is involved in both the insulin-dependent translocation (i.e., externalization) of the glucose transport system (Korbl *et al.*, 1977; Chandramouli *et al.*, 1977; Kano *et al.*, 1977) and the reversal of the hormonal effect on the system (i.e., relocation of the system back into the intracellular site by endocytosis), at least in adipocytes (Vega *et al.*, 1980; Ciaraldi and Olefsky, 1981; Laursen *et al.*, 1981). However, the situation mav be somewhat different in muscle (Gould, 1984), as explained in Section V,G. In the Type D effect, insulin reduces the cellular activity of phosphoenolpyruvate carboxykinase by inhibiting the *de novo* synthesis of the enzyme protein at the level of transcription, that is, at the step of mRNA synthesis (Sasaki *et al.*, 1984). At present, it is entirely unknown how insulin exerts these four types of acute biochemical effects, which are apparently distinct from one another, in addition to the chronic biological effects mentioned earlier.

III. Classification of Glucose Transport Systems

The glucose transport systems that are found in nature can be classified as shown in Table II. The first group, namely, nonspecific, physical diffusion, is almost negligible in the plasma membrane under physiologic conditions. Since glucose is a highly hydrophilic compound, its free diffusion into living cells is effectively blocked by the lipid bilayers of the plasma membrane. As a result, the uptake of glucose by living cells is almost entirely dependent on some sort of carrier-mediated mechanism. Some of these mechanisms are "active" in the sense that they transport glucose against its concentration gradient. The energy that is needed for an active transport is supplied in the form of either a Na^+ concentration gradient (Crane *et al.*. 1965) or phosphoenolpyruvate (Kundig and Roseman, 1971). Most animal cell types,

TABLE II

Classification of Glucose Transport Systems

A. Nonspecific, physical diffusion
B. Carrier-mediated diffusion or transport
   1. Active transport
      a. Dependent on Na^+ concentration gradient (e.g., those in small intestine and kidney)
      b. Dependent on phosphoenolpyruvate (e.g., in *Escherichia coli*)
   2. Passive transport
      a. Insulin insensitive (e.g., those in liver and erythrocytes)
      b. Insulin sensitive (e.g., those in muscle and fat cells)

---

however, do not require active glucose transport; these cells are equipped with "passive" transport systems. The function of passive transport systems is to facilitate translocation of selected substrates across the plasma membrane according to its concentration gradient.

The passive transport systems can be further divided into insulin-sensitive and -insensitive systems. In animals, muscle (Levine and Goldstein. 1955) and adipose tissue cells (Winegrad and Renold, 1958) are the major types equipped with the insulin-sensitive system, although fibroblasts (Cynober et al., 1986) and some other cell types fall within this group. Other cells are equipped with the insulin-insensitive glucose transport system. It is of interest that liver cells, although highly insulin sensitive in many other respects, bear a perpetually active insulin-insensitive transport system for glucose. Hence liver cells can discharge glucose into the bloodstream under starved conditions (when the insulin concentration is low) in order to maintain glucose homeostasis. It is also important physiologically that the glucose uptake by muscle and fat cells is minimized under starved conditions because of the lack of insulin. In fact, it would be diastrous if these cell types rapidly took up glucose under starved conditions and converted it to fat and glycogen.

In general, the carrier-mediated transport systems show the following common features: (1) saturable transport kinetics, (2) stereospecificity, (3) competitive inhibition, and (4) counter-transport (Morgan et al., 1964). The kinetic properties of a carrier-mediated transport process are mathematically identical to those of an enzyme-mediated chemical reaction. The stereospecificity of the glucose transport system is such that it mediates the translocation of certain hexoses, such as D-glucose, D-galactose, 2-deoxy-D-glucose, and 3-O-methyl-D-glucose, as well as selected pentoses, such as D-xylose and L-arabinose (see Randle and Morgan, 1962). The system does not support translocation of the optical antipodes of the aforementioned sugar isomers, such as L-glucose or D-arabinose, sugar alcohols, such as sorbitol or mannitol, nor disaccharides, such as sucrose. The transport of fructose, a ketohexose, appears to be mediated by both insulin-sensitive and -insensitive mechanisms (Battaglia and Randle, 1960; Froesch and Ginsberg, 1962; Halperin and Cheema-Dhadli, 1982). On the other hand, D-galactose is rapidly taken up by adipocytes, as well as by muscle, via an insulin-dependent process (Vega and Kono, 1978), contrary to some earlier observations. Those sugar isomers that share the same transport carrier competitively inhibit the transport of other members. In a counter-transport reaction, a trace quantity of a labeled sugar, e.g., 3-O-[^{3}H]methyl-D-glucose, is translocated across the plasma membrane against the concentration gradient of the same, but unlabeled, sugar isomer. This paradoxical reaction can be readily explained once it is realized that the interaction of the tracer with the transport system is competitively inhibited by the unlabeled compound to different degrees at the outer and inner surfaces of the plasma membrane (Morgan *et al.*, 1964).

Historically, the insulin-sensitive and -insensitive glucose transport systems were studied by separate groups of investigators. The insulin-sensitive system was studied by investigators who were mainly interested in the action of insulin, while the hormone-insensitive system was studied by those researchers who were fascinated by the transport process itself. The glucose transport system ideally suited for the latter study is found in human erythrocytes. Human erythrocytes are readily available and readily pipetted quantitatively. Plasma membranes (the so-called ghosts) are easy to prepare, and as much as 4–5% of the ghost protein is said to be the glucose transporter itself. Thus, not surprisingly, the glucose transporter in erythrocytes is the best characterized transport system available.

Although characteristics of the insulin-sensitive and -insensitive glucose transport systems differ, such differences are becoming less and less obvious. Most important was the finding by Wheeler *et al.* (1982) that the antibody developed against human erythrocyte glucose transporter cross-reacts with the insulin-sensitive transporter from rat adipocytes. It would appear, therefore, (1) that peptide sequences are conserved among transport systems of different species and (2) that significant chemical similarities exist between the insulin-sensitive and -insensitive glucose transport systems. Since the basic properties of the two types of glucose transport systems are similar, if not identical, we shall briefly review in the next section the biochemical properties of the glucose transport system in human erythrocytes.

IV. GLUCOSE TRANSPORT SYSTEM IN ERYTHROCYTES

The general characteristics of the glucose transport system in erythrocytes are described in chapters of several books, such as "Membrane Transport in Red Cells," edited by Ellory and Lew (1977); recent progress in the field was reviewed by Wheeler and Hinkle (1985). The glucose transport system (or transporter) in human erythrocytes has been purified to apparent homogeneity by washing ghosts (plasma membranes) with EDTA at alkaline pH, solubilizing with Triton X-100, and chromatographing on DEAE–cellulose (Kasahara and

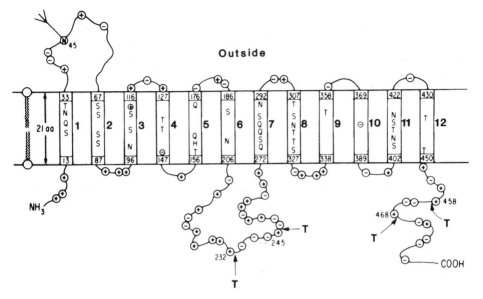

FIG. 1. Proposed model for orientation of the glucose transport in the human hepatoma cell membrane. The 12 putative membrane-spanning domains are numbered and shown as rectangles. The relative positions of acidic (Glu, Asp) and basic (Lys, Arg) amino acid residues are indicated by circled plus and minus signs, respectively. Uncharged polar residues within the membrane-spanning domains are indicated by their single-letter abbreviations: S, serine; T, threonine; H, histidine; N, asparagine; Q, glutamine. The predicted position of the N-linked oligosaccharide at Asn-45 is shown. The arrows point to positions of known tryptic cleavage sites in the active, membrane-bound enzyme. (From Mueckler *et al.*, 1985, with permission.)

Hinkle, 1977). Further purification of the transporter was achieved by Allard and Lienhard (1985) with the use of a monoclonal antibody; the molecular weight of the purified transporter estimated by these investigators was 55,000. The complete amino acid sequence of the transporter has been determined by Mueckler *et al.* (1985) from the cDNA sequence. The latter study indicates that the transporter is a long single-chain polypeptide containing 12 distinct hydrophobic regions. Thus the protein may contain 12 membrane-spanning segments, as shown in Fig. 1. The transporter peptide is adorned with a single chain of polysaccharide, which is localized on the outer surface of the cell. At approximately the middle of the transporter molecule, there trypsin-sensitive peptide linkages. These linkages must be exposed to the cytosolic side of the plasma membrane since the glucose transporter in erythrocytes is known to be attacked by trypsin exclusively from the cytosolic side.

The glucose transporter purified from human erythrocytes was successfully reconstituted into phospholipid liposomes by Kasahara and Hinkle (1977). They solubilized the transporter with Triton X-100, removed the latter with Bio-Beads SM-2, and incorporated the transporter into liposomes by sonication after a cycle of freezing and thawing. The function of freezing and thawing in the reconstitution procedure is not clear, but it is essential for success. Both native and reconstituted glucose transport activity is inhibited by $HgCl_2$, phloretin. and cytochalasin B but not by antitransporter antibodies tested so far.

The binding of cytochalasin B is not specific to the glucose transporter. The binding is high affinity (K_m = 0.5 μM; Bloch, 1973), however, and is competitively inhibited by high concentrations of D-glucose (e.g., 500 mM) in a cell-free system (Cushman and Wardzala, 1980). Therefore, the D-glucose-inhibitable cytochalasin B-binding activity is a useful index to determine the number of glucose transporters. Unlike the case in the cell-free system, however, the binding of cytochalasin B to glucose transporter in intact cells is competitively inhibited only when D-glucose is added to the cytosol (Basketter and Widdas, 1978; Deve's and Krupka 1978). Thus, the efflux of glucose is competitively inhibited by cytochalasin B, while the influx of the sugar is noncompetitively blocked. This asymmetry is interpreted as indicating that cytochalasin B binds to the glucose transport system not at the active center for transport, but at an unidentified location in the vicinity but definitely on the cytosolic side of the active center (Krupka and Devés, 1986). This site is designated as X_i in Fig. 2B. By the same token, phloretin, another potent inhibitor of glucose transport, appears to bind in the vicinity, but on the outside, of the active center (Krupka, 1985; Krupka and Devés, 1986). This site is referred to as X_o in Fig. 2B.

Years ago when the molecular structure of glucose transporter was still unknown, the kinetics of glucose transport were conveniently explained by the mobile-carrier model (e.g., Morgan et al.. 1964), as schematically illustrated in Fig. 2A. In this model, a carrier molecule shuttles back and forth between the outer and inner surfaces of the plasma membrane. This model is now obsolete as it has been established that glucose transporter is a large protein that must be anchored in the lipid bilayer of the plasma membrane (Mueckler et al., 1985). Currently, it is generally assumed that the transporter molecule is folded in such a way that it forms a hydrophilic channel in the plasma membrane. The transport channel must be equipped with a stereospecific active center (the carrier or the glucose-binding site) and

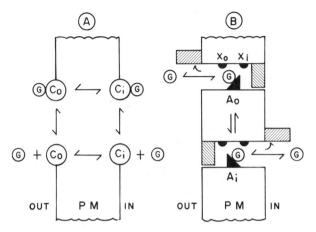

FIG. 2. Two models of the glucose transport system. (A) In the mobile carrier model, which is now obsolete, glucose is transported across the plasma membrane (PM) being bound to a mobile carrier (C). The carrier at the outer surface (C_o) and that at the inner surface (C_i) of the plasma membrane may have different properties, for example, affinity for glucose. (B) In the stationary carrier model, glucose is transported through a channel equipped with two gates (hatched area) and an active center facing either outside (A_o) or inside (A_i). The channel is also equipped with specific sites for the binding of transport inhibitors both outside (X_o) and inside (X_i) of the active center. Based on information published by Morgan *et al.* (1964), Devés and Krupka (1978), Gorga and Lienhard (1981), and Krupka and Devés (1986).

two gates. These gates, it is believed, alternately open and close, thereby making the active center accessible to a glucose molecule from either the extracellular or intracellular surfaces of the plasma membrane but not from both surfaces simultaneously (Fig. 2B). This stationary carrier model, first proposed by Vidaver (1966) and discussed by a number of investigators, including Gorga and Lienhard (1981) and Krupka and Devés (1986), appears to explain all the experimental data satisfactorily, although the actual molecular structure of the transport channel is yet to be ascertained.

The kinetics of glucose transport in the stationary carrier model are difficult to depict on paper and hence are usually explained by the mobile-carrier model (Fig. 2A) with the tacit agreement that $C_o \leftrightarrow C_i$ indicates not the shuttling of the transport carrier. but the conformational change in the transporter protein. It should be noted in this model that the transport carrier (or the active center) can assume different affinities for glucose when located at the inside versus the outside of the cell. The K_m estimated by Bloch (1974) for human erythrocytes is 0.4–0.8 mM for the influx and 15 mM for the efflux, and

1.0–1.5 mM for the influx with exchange and 20–30 mM for the efflux with exchange. In other words, the apparent K_m for efflux is approximately 20-fold greater than that for influx. If so, the rate of efflux must also be greater than that of influx since, at the equilibrium point, the glucose concentrations at the two sides of the erythrocyte plasma membrane are equal. In mathematical terms, this means that the K_m/V_{max} for the influx must be equal to the K_m/V_{max} value of the efflux (Naftalin and Holman, 1977).

In the past, it was generally thought that the insulin-sensitive glucose transport system in muscle and adipocytes is symmetric (e.g.. May and Mikulecky, 1982). However, it was recently reported by Vinten (1984) that the transport system in rat adipocytes is asymmetrical. If so, another apparent distinction between the insulin-sensitive and -insensitive glucose transport systems has been eliminated.

V. INSULIN-SENSITIVE GLUCOSE TRANSPORT SYSTEMS

A. EXPERIMENTAL MODELS

The dog represented the model for the classic studies of Banting and Best (1922), who discovered insulin, and those of Levine and Goldstein (1955), who found that insulin stimulates glucose transport in muscle. Dogs are still used in some insulin studies, but simpler models have evolved with time. Thus, in the 1950s and early 1960s, the most popular model system was the rat diaphragm, consisting of thin layers of muscle fibers, or cells. In the first studies, the diaphragm membrane was removed from the rib cage prior to incubation with the substrate sugar; such preparations gave only weak responses to insulin, presumably because some muscle fibers were cut. The apparent response of the diaphragm to insulin was considerably increased with the introduction of the "intact diaphragm" by Kipnis and Cori (1957). In this preparation, the diaphragm was taken out of the animal together with a part of the rib cage and detached from the latter after the incubation with sugar. The precision of the diaphragm experiments was significantly improved by the use of a pair of "intact hemidiaphragms" for an experiment and its control (Kono and Colowick, 1961). The intact hemidiaphragms were prepared by cutting an intact diaphragm at the center.

With the whole or hemidiaphragm preparations, many fundamental observations were made: stereospecificity of the transport system (see Randle and Morgan, 1962), insulin-like effects of anoxia (Randle and

Smith, 1958), effects of cold (Brown *et al.* 1952) and of hypertonicity (Kuzuya *et al.*, 1965), preliminary studies on binding of insulin (Stadie *et al.*, 1952), inhibition of insulin action with dinitrophenol (Kono and Colowick, 1961), and insulin-dependent stimulation of glycogen synthesis (Villar-Palasi and Larner, 1961). In the mid-1960s, Morgan *et al.* (1964) discovered the counter-transport phenomenon with the use of perfused rat hearts.

Toward the end of the 1950s, Winegrad and Renold (1958) demonstrated that rat epididymal adipose tissue is highly suitable for studies of insulin action. Then, Rodbell (1964) reported that free adipocytes prepared by collagenase treatment of rat epididymal adipose tissue are very sensitive to diverse hormones. In general, isolated cell preparations are highly suitable to quantitative studies of cellular metabolism since the preparations can be divided into identical aliquots for studies on effects of oxygen, insulin, glucose, etc. Not surprisingly isolated adipocytes have been widely used in insulin studies.

Major discoveries made with adipose tissue or cell preparations of the physiological actions of insulin include the existence of the cellular insulin receptor (Kono, 1969b,c; Freychet *et al.*, 1971), the significance of spare receptors (Kono and Barham, 1971b), negative cooperativity in the interaction of insulin with its receptor (De Meyts *et al.*, 1973), internalization (Terris and Steiner, 1976; Gorden *et al.*, 1980) and intracellular processing of insulin (Marshall and Olefsky, 1979; Suzuki and Kono, 1979), recycling of the internalized insulin receptor (Marshall *et al.*, 1981; Smith and Jarett, 1983), requirements for ATP (Chandramouli *et al.*, 1977; Kono *et al.*, 1977) and Mg^{2+} (Ueda *et al.*, 1984) in the actions of insulin on glucose transport and phosphodiesterase, involvement of cAMP in the action of lipolytic hormones (Butcher *et al.*, 1965), antilipolytic action of insulin (Jungas and Ball, 1963), involvement of cAMP phosphodiesterase in the antilipolytic action of insulin (Loten and Sneyd, 1970; Manganiello and Vaughan, 1973; Zinman and Hollenberg, 1974), insulin-dependent stimulation of pyruvate dehydrogenase (Coore *et al.*, 1971; Jungas, 1971), effects of insulin on the kinetic parameters of glucose transport (Vinten *et al.*, 1976; Whitesell and Gliemann, 1979), and the translocation hypothesis of insulin action on glucose transport (Cushman and Wardzala, 1980; Suzuki and Kono, 1980).

During the period when many investigators were using adipocytes, Gould and associates continued their studies with rat soleus muscle. They found, among other things, that the action of insulin on glucose transport in muscle, as in adipocytes, requires ATP (Korbl *et al.*, 1977) and Mg^{2+} (Hall *et al.*, 1982). In addition, they discovered that the properties of glucose transporter in muscle are somewhat different from those of the transporter in adipocytes, especially in response to ATP (Kaldawi et al., 1983; Gould, 1984; see discussion Section V,G). Isolated cardiac myocytes of adult rats were first prepared by treatment of the tissue with trypsin and then collagenase (Kono, 1969a). The earlier preparations were insulin insensitive and easily damaged by Ca^{2+} at physiologic concentrations. Insulin-sensitive and Ca^{2+}-tolerant preparations of cardiac myocytes were recently introduced and used for insulin studies by Haworth et al. (1980), Lindgren et al. (1982), Eckel et al. (1983), and Bihler et al. (1984). Other muscle preparations used in insulin studies include frog sartorius muscle (e.g., Wohltmann and Narahara, 1967; Narahara and Green, 1983) and rat epitrochlearis muscle (e.g., Wallberg-Henriksson and Holloszy, 1985).

More recently, several groups have found cultured cell lines useful for investigating actions of insulin and other hormones. The cell lines often used in insulin studies include fibroblasts from human skin and chick embryos (Cynober et al., 1986), 3T3-L1 adipocytes (Frost and Lane, 1985; Gibbs et al., 1986), Swiss 3T3 preadipocytes (Kitagawa et al., 1986), cardiac myocytes (Eckel et al., 1985), L-6 skeletal muscle cells (Klip and Ramlal, 1987), and BC3H-1 myocytes (Farese et al., 1985; Cooper et al., 1987). The glucose transport activity of cultured cells can be assessed easily with cells grown on sections of glass plate which are then dipped in a solution of 2-deoxy-D-[^{14}C]glucose for a given period. Using cultured cells, Farese and associates (Farese et al., 1985; Cooper et al., 1987) found that protein kinase C may be involved in the action of insulin on glucose transport in BC3H-1 myocytes. On the other hand, Kitagawa et al. (1986) reported that two different mechanisms may be involved in the stimulation of glucose transport in Swiss 3T3 preadipocytes by insulin and by PMA (phorbol 12-myristyl-13-acetate), an activator of protein kinase C. This problem is considered in Section V,H.

In the following sections, I describe the actions of insulin in rat epididymal adipocytes and discuss observations made in other cell types.

B. INSULIN RECEPTOR

The first step of insulin action on glucose transport and other metabolic processes is the binding of the hormone to the cellular receptor, which is a specific peptide localized on the cell surface. This fundamental concept was empirically substantiated by the observation that cellular capacities to bind insulin and to respond to the hormone are concomitantly abolished on treatment of cells with trypsin (Kono, 1969b,c). Subsequently, the cellular receptor for insulin was purified by Jacobs *et al.* (1977) from the liver plasma membrane by affinity chromatography. A purer preparation that could bind one molecule of insulin per molecule of the receptor was later obtained by Fujita-Yamaguchi *et al.* (1983) from human placenta, using sequential affinity chromatography on wheat germ agglutinin–Sepharose and on insulin–Sepharose.

The chemical structure of the insulin receptor was determined by the efforts of many investigators, as reviewed by Czech and Massague (1982) and Pessin *et al.* (1985). The results of these studies indicate that the insulin receptor is a tetramer consisting of two α subunits (M_r 125,000) and two β subunits (M_r 90,000). The four subunits are bound together with S–S linkages in the order β–α–α–β; the α subunits are localized outside of the cell surface, being held by the β subunits that are transfixed across the plasma membrane. The entire amino acid sequence of the insulin receptor (from human placenta) has been elucidated from the nucleic acid sequence of its cDNA (Ullrich *et al.*, 1985; Ebina *et al.*, 1985). Portions of the amino acid sequence in the receptor, including the tyrosine kinase region (see below), bear striking similarities to those of the epidermal growth factor receptor (EGF receptor) and certain members of the *src* family of oncogene products. Kasuga *et al.* (1982a,b) found that the insulin receptor is an insulin-sensitive tyrosine kinase and that the tyrosine within the receptor molecule is one of the substrates. Later, this receptor kinase was localized in the intracellular portion of the β subunit of the insulin receptor (Ullrich *et al.*, 1985; Ebina *et al.*, 1985).

The physiological function of the receptor kinase is currently controversial. Ellis *et al.* (1986) and Ebina *et al.* (1987) concluded that the kinase must be involved in the action of insulin on glucose transport. Their conclusion was based on the observation that a modified insulin receptor lacking kinase activity was inert on glucose transport. Similarly, Morgan and Roth (1987) found that there was no effect of insulin on glucose transport in CHO cells microinjected with monoclonal antibodies specific for insulin receptor kinase. In contrast, Simpson and Hedo (1984) and Forsayeth *et al.* (1987) reported that the receptor kinase may not be involved in the action of insulin on glucose transport since certain antireceptor antibodies (both monoclonal and polyclonal) that are specific to the extracellular regions of the insulin receptor clearly stimulated the glucose transport activity in rat adipocytes without stimulating the receptor kinase activity.

The interaction of insulin with its receptor has been studied with the

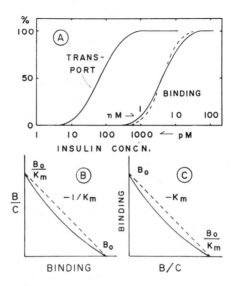

FIG. 3. Relationship between binding of insulin to adipocytes and insulin-dependent stimulation of glucose transport. The binding of insulin to adipocytes is half-maximal at 3–7 nM (solid line on the right-hand side in A). Binding is negatively cooperative; hence, data yield curvilinear plots with Scatchard (B) or Hofstee analyses (C). Noncooperative binding would yield steeper plots as shown by the dashed line in A, with rectilinear plots as indicated by dashed lines in B and C. Although most investigators analyze their binding data by the Scatchard method (B), the Hofstee plot is preferable in some cases because the binding data appear in the ordinate and the K_m can be read directly from the slope of the line. The insulin-dependent stimulation of glucose transport is half-maximal at hormone concentrations of 60–70 pM. Thus, glucose transport is stimulated maximally when less than 5% of the cellular receptors is occupied by hormone. See text for the physiological significance of the unoccupied ("spare") receptors. Based on information provided by Kono (1969a,b), Kono and Barham (1971a,b), De Meyts *et al.* (1973), and Gammeltoft and Gliemann (1973); the plots do not represent actual data.

use of [125]monoiodoinsulin as a tracer. Insulin maintains biological activity on iodination at 1 mol per mole of peptide (Freychet *et al.,* 1971). As may be expected from the nature of hormone actions, binding of [125]monoiodoinsulin to its cellular receptor is reversible and competitively inhibited by unlabeled insulin (Freychet *et al.,* 1971; Kono and Barham, 1971b). Nevertheless, the insulin–receptor complex does not have any fixed dissociation constant. Binding data for insulin analyzed by the method of Scatchard or Hofstee give curvilinear plots (solid lines in Figs. 3B and 3C) rather than rectilinear as expected for interaction with a single class of binding site. De Meyts *et al.* (1973) interpreted the curvilinear plot as indicating that the binding of insulin to its receptor is negatively cooperative. Some investigators, however, interpret this result as reflecting multiple insulin receptors with different dissociation constants.

Although the insulin–receptor complex displays no constant K_d (see above), the actual binding of insulin to its adipocyte receptor is half-maximal at hormone concentrations of approximately 3–7 nM (Kono and Barham, 1971b; Gammeltoft and Gliemann, 1973) (see Fig. 3A). It is important to note that this value (i.e., the apparent K_d) is higher than the physiological concentration of insulin, which is roughly between 10 pM and 1 nM in peripheral blood (1 nM = 150 μU/ml = 6 ng/ml). Consequently, (1) the cellular insulin receptors would never be occupied in full by the hormone under physiologic conditions, whereas (2) the glucose transport activity in adipocytes is half-maximally activated at hormone concentrations of approximately 60–70 pM and maximally activated at 250 pM (Kono 1969b; Kono and Barham, 1971b). In other words, glucose transport in adipocytes is maximally stimulated with only 5% of the cellular insulin receptors occupied, as depicted in Fig. 3A (Kono and Barham, 1971b). Hence, 95% of the cellular insulin receptors remain unoccupied with glucose transport activity maximally stimulated. This does not mean, however, that these unoccupied receptors are simply in excess; on the contrary, these so-called spare receptors are essential to make the cellular glucose transport system highly sensitive to insulin. Thus, according to the law of mass action, the concentration (or number per milliliter) of insulin–receptor complexes, which generate the (hypothetical) hormonal signal is proportional to the concentration (or number per milliliter) of spare receptors at a given insulin concentration [Eqs. (1)–(3)]. That is, according to the law of mass action,

$$[I][R] = [IR] \times K \tag{1}$$

Therefore,

$$[\text{Unbound insulin}] \times [\text{unoccupied receptor}] = [\text{insulin–receptor complex}] \times K \tag{2}$$

Therefore,

$$[\text{Insulin in solution}] \times [\text{spare receptor}] = [\text{hormonal signal}] \times K \tag{3}$$

This relationship was first verified empirically modulating the number of insulin receptors in adipocytes by treating the latter with trypsin (Kono and Barham, 1971b). As predicted by the above equations, the insulin sensitivity of adipocytes, but not their maximum response to the hormone, was reduced when the number of cellular insulin receptors was reduced.

The optimum pH for the binding of insulin to its receptor is not 7.4, but approximately 7.8 (e.g., Gavin *et al.*, 1973; Ginsberg *et al.*, 1976). As a result, the binding of the hormone to the cellular receptor is rather sensitive to small changes in pH value around 7.4. In the fat cell system, no significant binding is detectable at a pH of 6.0 or less (M. Ueda and T. Kono, unpublished data).

C. CELLULAR PROCESSING OF INSULIN

The insulin–receptor complex formed on the cell surface is rapidly internalized (Terris and Steiner, 1976) by endocytosis (e.g., Gorden *et al.*, 1080; Smith and Jarett, 1983). Most of the hormone internalized by adipocytes is associated with slow-sedimenting vesicles that are separable from the plasma membrane by sucrose density gradient centrifugation (Kono *et al.*, 1975, 1977; Suzuki and Kono, 1979). Insulin labeled with ^{125}I bound to the plasma membrane and internalized is associated with slow-sedimenting vesicles and is separable into two peaks, as depicted in Fig. 4. The formation of peak 2 is ATP dependent, temperature sensitive (Kono *et al.*, 1977), and completed in approximately 10 min at 37°C (Ezaki and Kono, 1984). Peak 2 is not an artifact of cell homogenization; instead, it is formed during the incubation of the hormone with adipocytes in a time-dependent manner, by

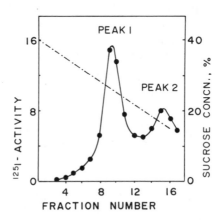

FIG. 4. Distribution of [^{125}I]iodoinsulin in subcellular fractions of adipocytes. When adipocytes incubated with labeled insulin for 10 minutes were homogenized and fractionated, the label was found not only in the plasma membrane fraction (peak 1) but also in a slow-sedimenting microsomal fraction (peak 2). In this experiment, fractionation of the subcellular components was carried out by sucrose density gradient centrifugation. (From Hashimoto *et al.*, 1987, with permission from the publisher.)

relocation of the hormone that was initially associated with the plasma membrane (Suzuki and Kono, 1979). At a steady state, the ratio of peaks 1 and 2 is approximately 2 to 1 (Kono *et al.*, 1977; Suzuki and Kono, 1979). This is almost identical to the ratio of surface-bound and intracellular insulin molecules estimated by washing off the surface-bound insulin with acidic buffer (Marshall, 1985).

Of the internal insulin–receptor complexes, approximately one-third becomes externalized, presumably by route A in Fig. 5, without any apparent modification (Suzuki and Kono, 1979; Marshall, 1985). The physiologic significance of this seemingly wasteful, energy-dependent recycling of insulin is still unknown. The balance of the internalized hormone is thought to be dissociated from the receptor as the endocytic vesicles are acidified (Ueda *et al.*, 1985). Vesicles at the stage of acidification have not been identified in fat cells, but they were detected in liver cells and designated by Geuze *et al.* (1983) as CURLs (compartments of uncoupling of receptor and ligand). The hormone released from its receptor is transported into lysosomes and degraded there by a process sensitive to chloroquine (Marshall and Olefsky, 1979; Suzuki and Kono, 1979), dibucaine, or tetracaine (Suzuki and Kono, 1979). The degradation products are eliminated from the cells via route B (Fig. 5). On the other hand, internalized receptor freed from insulin is recycled back onto the cell surface by route C without significant modification (Marshall *et al.*, 1981; Smith and Jarett, 1983).

The acidification of CURLs mentioned above is blocked by monensin (Ueda *et al.*, 1985), an ionophore for monovalent cations. The insulin–receptor complexes accumulated in cells by the effect of monensin show weak, but significant, physiological activity on both glucose transport and phosphodiesterase (Ueda *et al.*, 1985). In contrast, the hormone accumulated in cells (presumably in a specific type of lysosomes; Suzuki and Kono, 1979) by the effect of chloroquine does not show any physiologic activity *in situ* (i.e., in lysosomes; T. Kono, unpublished data), although it is still immunoreactive (Suzuki and Kono, 1979). It may be concluded, therefore, that the degradative pathway (i.e., the pathway that includes CURLs and lysosomes, Fig. 5) may not be involved in the physiologic actions of insulin, such as the stimulation of glucose transport.

The above consideration leads us to an important question of whether internalized insulin–receptor complexes are involved in the physiological actions of the hormones. Although it is generally assumed that the (hypothetical) signal of insulin is generated and transmitted from the hormone–receptor complex in the plasma membrane,

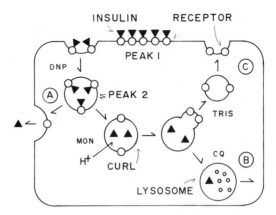

INSULIN   RECEPTOR

Fig. 5. Processing of cell-bound insulin. Insulin binds to its receptor on the surface of adipocytes, forming a hormone–receptor complex that corresponds to peak 1 shown in Fig. 4. The insulin complex is then internalized by endocytosis, which is ATP dependent and, therefore, inhibitable with 2,4-dinitrophenol (DNP). The internalized insulin–receptor complex is associated with certain microsomal vesicles that form peak 2 as shown in Fig. 4. Approximately one-third of the hormone in peak 2 is externalized via route A. The rest of the hormone is dissociated from its receptor when the inside of the vesicles (designated as CURLs) is acidified. The acidification of CURLs and, therefore, the dissociation of insulin from its receptor are blocked by monensin (MON). Insulin dissociated from the receptor is decomposed in lysosomes by a chloroquine (CQ)-sensitive process. The degradation products are eliminated from cells via route B. On the other hand, the freed insulin receptor is recycled back to the cell surface via route C. Recycling of receptor is blocked if incubation is carried out in Tris buffer. Based on information provided by Suzuki and Kono (1979), Marshall and Olefsky (1979), Marshall et al. (1981), Smith and Jarett (1983), Geuze et al. (1983), Marshall (1985), and Ueda et al. (1985).

the complex associated with the intracellular, slow-sedimenting vesicles (peak 2 in Figs. 4 and 5) is also a legitimate candidate for the signal generator. In fact, both internalization of insulin and its action on glucose transport are (1) initiated rapidly (Ezaki and Kono, 1984; Kono et al., 1982), (2) completed in approximately 10 minutes at 37°C (Ezaki and Kono, 1984; Kono et al., 1981). (3) ATP dependent (Kono et al., 1977, 1981), and (4) temperature sensitive (Ezaki and Kono, 1982; Kono et al., 1977). In addition, if the internalized hormone is not involved in the action of insulin, what could be the physiological significance of the energy-dependent internalization? Naturally. internalization of the hormone–receptor complex induces a down-regulation of the receptor, and this may be the important mechanism for the development of insulin resistance under chronic conditions. However, the acute and large down-regulation reported earlier by some investigators was later found to be an artifact of Tris buffer (Marshall and Olefsky, 1981; Rennie and Gliemann, 1981), and no such large down-regulation is detectable in the experiments carried out in bicarbonate or HEPES buffer (K. Suzuki and T. Kono, unpublished data). Also, the degradation of insulin in lysosomes may have some physiological significance; however, the amount of insulin degraded in lysosomes is negligible compared to that decomposed by "insulinase" on the cell surface (Suzuki and Kono, 1979). Moreover, as mentioned earlier, approximately 30% of the hormone internalized by an energy-dependent process is rapidly recycled back into the extracellular buffer without making any apparent contribution to the cellular metabolism (via route A in Fig. 5).

In agreement with the view that internalization of insulin might be involved in its physiologic actions, it was recently reported by Jochen and Berhanu (1986, 1987a,b) that both internalization of insulin and its action on glucose transport are blocked by certain oligopeptides. In addition, we previously found that the two reactions were concomitantly inhibited by treatment of adipocytes with 1 mM bromophenacyl bromide, 3.3 mM phenylglyoxal, or 1 mM iodoacetamide (O. Ezaki and T. Kono, unpublished). It should be noted, however, that these data are still highly preliminary since the agents used in the studies may inhibit the hormonal action at a step or steps other than the internalization process.

D. Determination of Glucose Transport Activity

Although isolated adiopocytes are highly advantageous for quantitative studies of hormone actions in general, the determination of glucose transport in this cell type requires some considerations. First, glucose itself cannot be used as the substrate since it is rapidly metabolized in adipocytes, as well as in other cell types. Therefore, the transport of glucose must be estimated from that of a nonmetabolized analogs, such as 3-O-methyl-D-glucose, which is taken up by cells via the glucose transport system at approximately the same rate as glucose (Cheung et al., 1978; Whitesell and Gliemann, 1979). Second, there are technical problems in the assay of 3-O-methyl-D-glucose transport in adipocytes since (1) the intracellular water space of this cell type is only 1–2% of the total cell volume (Whitesell and Gliemann, 1979; Toyoda et al., 1987) and (2) this space in insulin-treated cells is rapidly equilibrated with 3-O-methyl-D-glucose ($t_{1/2}$ 2.7 seconds; Whitesell and Gliemann, 1979). Therefore, most of the earlier "transport studies" were carried out by measuring the rate of appearance of glucose carbon in CO_2 and lipid fractions (e.g., Winegrad and Renold, 1958; Rodbell, 1964). The rationale of this practice was the observation made by Crofford and Renold (1965) that membrane transport is the rate-limiting step in the overall metabolism of glucose in adipocytes, under physiologic conditions. Some investigators like to compromise by using 2-deoxy-D-glucose, which is taken up by adipocytes via the glucose transport system, converted to its 6-phosphate, and accumulated in cells without any further metabolism. With labeled 2-deoxy-D-glucose at very low concentrations (i.e., without added unlabeled carrier hexose) intracellular accumulation is proportional to time, at least for the first several minutes of incubation (Foley et al. 1980). It should be noted, however, that the intracellular accumulation of this hexose is dependent on hexokinase and ATP as well as the transport activity.

The first reliable method for the assay of 3-O-methyl-D-glucose transport in adipocytes was introduced by Whitesell and Gliemann (1979). These investigators incubated cells with 3-O-[^{14}C]methyl-D-glucose and timed the incubation period (1 to several seconds) with a metronome set at 2 beats/second. They stopped the reaction by diluting the incubation mixture with more than 50 volumes of 0.3 mM phloretin and collected cells by a two-step oil-flotation technique, developed earlier by Gliemann et al. (1972) for the separation of adipocytes from the bulk of the incubation mixture. In this technique, a cell suspension is centrifuged together with a selected oil which is heavier than adipocytes but lighter than water. The oil used in their original study (Gliemann et al., 1972) was dinonylphthalate (d 0.981), but silicone oil with a similar specific gravity (e.g., d 0.960, from Thomas, Cat. No. 6428-R15) can also be used.

The above method of Whitesell and Gliemann (1979) has been widely used, either in its original form or with some modifications. Significant modifications include (1) estimation of the total and apparent extracellular water spaces in the same cell preparation by incubating cells with a mixture of 3-O-[^{3}H]methyl-D-glucose and [^{14}C]sucrose and by diluting the reaction mixture with an approximately equal volume of phloretin (Toyoda et al., 1986), (2) use of a small amount (30 μl) of a concentrated cell suspension (40% by the cytocrit assay; Whitesell and Gliemann, 1979) with subsequent dilution with approximatelv 10 volumes of phloretin (Toyoda et al., 1987), (3) increase in the final phloretin concentration to 0.9 mM (Toyoda et al., 1987), (4) use of an infant incubator (37°C) for the incubation of adipocytes with the substrate sugar (Toyoda et al., 1987), and (5) mechanical swirling of the cell suspension with an adjustable orbit shaker (600 rpm; $r = 2$ mm) (Toyoda et al., 1987).

The purpose of the modifications described above in (1) and (2) is to minimize the volume of the reaction mixture after dilution with phloretin. With these modifications, the cells can be recovered by a single centrifugation in a 400-μl microfuge tube. As for the modification described in (3), Toyoda et al. (1987) reported that 0.9 mM phloretin effectively inhibited glucose transport in 0.06 second even in the presence of 1.4 mg/ml albumin (1 mM phloretin remains in solution for a few hours if its 100 mM solution in ethanol is diluted with 154 mM NaCl and kept at 37°C). The use of an infant incubator (4, above), or a similar device in which all the reagents and pipet tips needed for the assay can be kept at 37°C, is essential for serious kinetic studies. The selection of the swirling conditions (5, above) is important for three reasons: the membrane transport of glucose is a rapid reaction that occurs in a heterogeneous system; on a per mole basis, the glucose transporter in basal cells must be as active as its counterpart in insulin-treated adipocytes since it appears that changes in cellular transport activity are mainly caused by changes in the number of transport systems in the plasma membrane (see Section VI); and the basal glucose transport activity is stimulated by a certain type of mechanical agitation of adipocytes (Vega and Kono, 1979; Toyoda et al., 1987), as described later in detail (Section V,H). The incubation time estimated by the sound of a metronome (Whitesell and Gliemann, 1979) is amazingly consistent. According to the data published by Toyoda et al. (1987), the 1-second transport assay could be done with a standard coefficient (SD/average) of 6.0% ($n = 26$). Note that this figure includes not only the timing error but also other errors involved in the entire transport assay.

Conventionally, transport of labeled sugar, such as 3-O-methyl-D-glucose, is determined under four different conditions. Thus, in equilibrium–exchange experiments, either the influx or the efflux of a tracer quantity of a labeled sugar is determined while the concentrations of the unlabeled carrier sugar are kept equal on both sides of the membrane. In contrast, in zero-transport experiments, either the net influx or the net efflux of the substrate sugar is determined by placing both the labeled and unlabeled sugar molecules on the same side of the plasma membrane. It is important to note that time courses for movement of labeled sugar are different in the equilibrium–exchange and zero-transport experiments. The integrated rate equation derived by May and Mikulecky (1982) for equilibrium–exchange reactions is shown in Eq. (4), while that formulated by Taylor and Holman (1981) for zero-trans experiments is presented in Eq. (5),

$$-\ln(1 - C/C_{eq}) = V_o \times t/S \qquad (4)$$

$$(A + BS)[\ln(1 - C/S) + C/S]/C - A/S = -t/C \qquad (5)$$

where C is the intracellular hexose concentration at time t, C_{eq} the intracellular hexose concentration at equilibrium, V_0 the initial velocity, S the hexose concentration in buffer, and A and B constants.

In theory, then, one can calculate the initial rate of transport from the data obtained at time t even with a curvilinear time course. It should be noted, however, that these equations are applicable only if (1) the intracellular water space for distribution of the labeled sugar is in one compartment and (2) (in the equilibrium–exchange experiments) the system has been thoroughly equilibrated. Unfortunately, the actual situation is rather complex. Toyoda et al. (1987) found that the intracellular water space available for the distribution of 3-O-methyl-D-glucose is not a single compartment and that a major compartment in insulin-stimulated adipocytes is saturated with the hexose in 20 seconds. The equilibration of adipocytes with the substrate sugar is also tricky since (1) the basal transport activity is elevated transiently in cells with very low basal transport activity exposed to 20–60 mM 3-O-methyl-D-glucose and (2) the stimulated transport activity gradually returns to its initial level during a course of approximately 2 hours (N. Toyoda and T. Kono, unpublished). This phenomenon is found even when the osmolarity of the solution is adjusted by reducing the NaCl concentration. As a result, the Hanes' plot of the transport data obtained in equilibrium–exchange experiments is often curvilinear (Vinten et al., 1976; Toyoda et al., 1987). The estimation of an exact initial velocity from a curvilinear time course of zero-trans experiments is also difficult when the number of available data is limited, as discussed elsewhere (Toyoda et al., 1987).

E. INSULIN EFFECTS ON THE KINETICS OF GLUCOSE TRANSPORT

As shown earlier in Fig. 3, glucose transport in adipocytes is half-maximally stimulated at insulin concentrations of 60–70 pM and almost maximal at 250 pM (e.g., Kono and Barham, 1971b). Unlike some other insulin-sensitive systems (e.g., cAMP phosphodiesterase; Kono et al., 1975), the effect of insulin on glucose transport is not suppressed by supramaximal concentrations of the hormone (e.g., Kono and Barham, 1971b). With insulin at 1 nM, glucose transport activity is stimulated maximally in 5–10 minutes at 37°C (e.g., Vega and Kono, 1979). This reaction is temperature dependent (Häring et al., 1981); it is very slow at temperatures below 20°C, although significant stimulation can still be detected at 10°C (Ezaki and Kono, 1982).

Some investigators contend that there is a 30 to 45-second absolute lag period before the appearance of an insulin effect on glucose transport (Häring et al., 1979, 1981). According to Häring et al. (1979), this lag period is increased to approximately 5 min with millimolar concentrations of colchicine or vinblastine; the latter at micromolar concentrations inhibit functions of cytoskeletal and microfilamentous proteins. In contrast, the data obtained in our laboratory suggest that the insulin-dependent stimulation of glucose transport is very slow at the beginning and gradually accelerates with time, rather than starting abruptly after a certain length of an absolute lag period (T. Kono, unpublished).

The effects of insulin on the kinetic parameters of glucose transport were first seriously studied by Vinten et al. (1976). They concluded that insulin stimulates glucose transport in fat cells by increasing V_{max} for transport without significantly changing the K_m value, 4–8 mM. Their observations were supported by several subsequent studies, as reviewed elsewhere (see Toyoda et al., 1987). It was then reported by Whitesell and Abumrad (1985) that the predominant effect of insulin on glucose transport in adipocytes is suppression of K_m, rather than elevation of V_{max}, as shown in Table III. Their report prompted several researchers to reinvestigate the problem. Martz et al. (1986) reconfirmed the old notion that insulin does not change the K_m. In contrast, Toyoda et al. (1987), Okuno and Gliemann (1987), and Suzuki (1987)

TABLE III

TRANSPORT PARAMTERS OF 3-O-METHYL-D-GLUCOSE AND GLUCOSE IN ISOLATED ADIPOCYTES

Reference	K_m or K_i (mM)[a]		$V_i/V_b{}^b$	Exp.[c]
	Basal	+Insulin		
Whitesell and Abumrad (1985)				
3OMG (K_m)	35 ± 5	3 ± 0	5	EE
Glucose (K_m)	75 ± 10	8 ± 3	2	EE
Glucose (K_i)	105 ± 15	10 ± 2	2	EE
Martz et al. (1986)	6.4 ± 0.3	6.3 ± 0.5	21	EE
Toyoda et al. (1987)	11.7 ± 1.3	5.4 ± 0.6	16	EE
Toyoda et al. (1987)	9.7 ± 0.5	4.8 ± 0.4	18	ZT
Okuno and Gliemann (1987)[d]				
3OMG (K_m)	8.1 ± 1.6	3.3 ± 0.8	18	ZT
Glucose (K_m)	7.0 ± 2.8	4.2 ± 1.7	19	ZT
Suzuki (1987)	12.8 ± 1.1	7.3 ± 0.6	?	EE

[a] Unless otherwise specified, the data show the K_m values of 3-O-methyl-D-glucose (3OMG) ± SE.

[b] Ratio of V_{max} values for insulin-stimulated and basal transport activities.

[c] Experimental conditions: either equilibrium–exchange (EE) or zero-transport (ZT).

[d] Data before correction for a minor leakage.

reported that insulin does lower the K_m (Table III). The decrease in the K_m value observed, however, was only approximately one-half of basal, and the predominant effect of the hormone was on V_{max} rather than K_m.

Although it has been generally thought that the glucose transport system in erythrocytes is not insulin-sensitive, it was recently reported by Dustin et al. (1984) that insulin decreased the K_m for glucose transport in erythrocytes from 1.8 to 1.1 mM in infinite-cis influx experiments, and from 25 to 13 mM in zero-trans efflux experiments, in both cases without changing V_{max}. These data suggest that insulin might reduce the K_m for glucose transport to approximately one-half of basal not only in adipocytes (as shown in Table III), but also in other cell types currently thought to be insulin insensitive.

F. ATP AND DIVALENT CATIONS IN INSULIN ACTIONS

The action of insulin on glucose transport in adipocytes appears to be ATP dependent since the hormonal action is blocked on reduction of ATP concentrations by treatment of cells with 1 mM 2,4-dinitrophenol, 1 mM dicumarol, 1–2 mM KCN, or 10 mM sodium azide (Chandramouli et al., 1977; Kono et al., 1977). Note that dinitrophenol and dicumarol are uncouplers of oxidative phosphorylation, whereas KCN and sodium azide are inhibitors of cellular respiration. and that the common feature of these two types of agents is to lower the cellular level of ATP. Similarly, the effects of insulin on glucose transport in rat diaphragm and soleus muscle are also blocked in tissue preparations treated with 1 mM dinitrophenol (Kono and Colowick, 1961; Korbl et al., 1977) or deprived of oxygen for a prolonged period (Korbl et al., 1977). Interestingly, however, basal glucose transport activity in muscle preparations, including that in perfused rat hearts (Morgan et al., 1961), is considerably elevated on addition of low concentrations of dinitrophenol (e.g., 0.1 mM; Kono and Colowick, 1961) or 1 mM dinitrophenol or induction of anoxic conditions for a short time (Randle and Smith, 1958; Korbl et al., 1977). No such stimulation, which may be induced by a slight loss of ATP, has been observed in the adipocyte system.

The inhibitory effects of the above agents are reversible, at least in adipocytes. For example, in cells exposed to dinitrophenol for 5 minutes, washed, and kept in fresh buffer with glucose (but without dinitrophenol) for 10 minutes, the ATP concentration is restored almost to normal, and the cells regain responsiveness to insulin (Kono et al., 1977). The reversal of the insulin effect on glucose transport is also ATP dependent in adipocytes (Vega et al., 1980; Ciaraldi and Olefsky,

1981; Laursen et al., 1981). Thus, when insulin-treated cells are deprived of ATP by incubation with dinitrophenol or KCN for 5 minutes, washed, and suspended in fresh buffer containing the same inhibitor without insulin, the glucose transport activity remains stimulated for at least 1 hour (Vega et al., 1980). Again, the situation appears to be different in muscle, since it was reported by Kaldawi et al. (1983) that the insulin-stimulated glucose transport activity in soleus muscle is reduced rapidly and considerably by the addition of dinitrophenol. Apparently, ATP is involved in more than one step in the cascade of insulin actions (Gould, 1984); however, details are yet to be obtained. Witters et al. (1985) discovered that protein kinase C catalyzes phosphorylation of the glucose transporter. However, there appears to be no correlation between the level of phosphorylation and that of transport (Gibbs et al., 1986; Joost et al., 1987).

As expected with reactions dependent on ATP, either Mg^{2+} or Mn^{2+} is required for the action of insulin on glucose transport. Thus, Hall, et al. (1982) and Eckel et al. (1983) found that the action of insulin on glucose transport in muscle is inhibited by the joint actions of A 23187 (an ionophore for divalent cations) plus EDTA (a chelator specific to divalent cations in general) but not by those of A 23187 plus EGTA (a chelator specific for Ca^{2+}). Parallel results were also obtained in experiments with adipocytes (Ueda et al., 1984) and cultured Swiss 3T3 fibroblasts (Kitagawa et al., 1986). In addition, Ueda et al. (1984) found that the inhibitory effect of A 23187 plus EDTA in adipocytes is reversed by the addition of 0.3 mM Mn^{2+} or 1 mM Mg^{2+} but not by Ca^{2+}. These studies indicate that either Mn^{2+} may be involved in the action of insulin, but Ca^{2+} may not be required in the action of the hormone on glucose transport. In agreement with this view, Klip et al. (1983) observed that stimulation of glucose transport in muscle by serum was not blocked by Quin2 ester (the latter is taken up by cells and hydrolyzed to Quin2, which is a potent Ca^{2+}-specific chelator). In contrast, Pershadsingh et al. (1987) concluded that Ca^{2+} is essential for the action of insulin on glucose transport in adipocytes as the hormonal effect was blocked by 90–150 μM of Quin2 ester (see also McDonald and Pershadsingh, 1985). In addition, Clausen and associates (see Clausen, 1975, 1980) have found several lines of indirect evidence that strongly imply Ca^{2+} involvement in the action of insulin.

G. TERMINATION OF INSULIN EFFECT

In insulin-treated cells washed with insulin-free buffer and maintained at 37°C, insulin dissociates rather rapidly (Ciaraldi and Olefsky,

1980), but the stimulated glucose transport declines only gradually for 45–60 minutes (Vega and Kono, 1979; Karnieli *et al.*, 1981). The dissociation of insulin from the cell surface receptor is not accelerated by the addition of trypsin (K. Suzuki and T. Kono, unpublished), although some investigators assume that the trypsin resistance of cell-bound insulin is the sign of its internalization. Apparently, both insulin and the cellular receptor are rendered trypsin resistant as a result of mutual binding (K. Suzuki and T. Kono, unpublished). Likewise, dissociation of insulin from frog muscle is not facilitated by the addition of anti-insulin antibody (Wohltmann and Narahara, 1967).

As described earlier, reversal of the insulin effect on glucose transport is apparently ATP dependent in adipocytes (Vega *et al.*, 1980; Ciaraldi and Olefsky, 1981; Laursen *et al.*, 1981). In adipocytes, the decline of glucose transport activity that has been stimulated by mechanical agitation of cells (see below) also requires metabolic energy (Vega and Kono, 1979). In contrast, insulin-stimulated glucose transport in soleus muscle is partially deactivated by the addition of 2,4-dinitrophenol (Kaldawi *et al.*, 1983), as mentioned earlier.

H. INSULINOMIMETIC SUBSTANCES AND FACTORS

Insulin-sensitive glucose transport activity is stimulated, if not maximally, by a number of factors as described below.

1. *Low Temperature*

The stimulatory effect of low temperature was first observed in the 1950s in muscle experiments (Brown *et al.*, 1952). Nevertheless, the same effect in adipocytes was first erroneously interpreted as indicating that the basal and insulin-stimulated transport activities have different temperature coefficients (Czech, 1976a; Vega and Kono, 1979). Later, Ezaki and Kono (1982) found that the basal glucose transport activity in adipocytes is stimulated at low temperatures by an ATP-dependent reaction and that the temperature coefficients of the basal and insulin-stimulated transport activities are identical if they are determined in the presence of dinitrophenol.

2. *Oxidants*

The glucose transport system in adipocytes is stimulated by a variety of oxidants, including hydrogen peroxide (Czech *et al.*, 1974a,b). As might be expected, hydrogen peroxide can stimulate glucose transport in cells whose insulin receptor (or insulin-binding capacity) has been modified by trypsin treatment (Kono *et al.*, 1982). Interestingly, it was recently observed by Kadota *et al.* (1987) that, in media containing vanadate, hydrogen peroxide stimulates both insulin-receptor kinase and the translocation of the insulin-like growth factor II receptor.

3. *Vanadate*

Although vanadate is an established inhibitor of Na,K-ATPase, it stimulates the insulin-sensitive glucose transport system by an unknown mechanism (Dubyak and Kleinzeller, 1980). Kadota *et al.* (1987) found that vanadate and hydrogen peroxide synergistically stimulate insulin-receptor kinase and the translocation of the receptor for insulin-like growth factor II (see above). Their data suggest that the receptor kinase activity *may* be important in physiological actions of insulin.

4. *Proteolytic Enzymes*

A number of proteolytic enzymes stimulate glucose transport activity in both muscle and adipocytes at low enzyme concentrations (e.g., 1–10 µg/ml; Kuo *et al.,* 1966). Glucose transport activity in adipocytes is also stimulated in cells exposed to 1 mg/ml trypsin for 15 seconds (Kono and Barham, 1971a); such a short trypsin treatment is feasible with addition of soybean trypsin inhibitor. Apparently, the action of trypsin on the transport system is indirect because activity is elevated gradually, reaching the maximum 20–25 minutes after a brief (15-second) exposure of cells to the enzyme (Kono and Barham, 1971a).

5. *Phospholipase*

Blecher (1965), Rodbell (1966), and Rosenthal and Fain (1971) observed that phospholipase C mimics the physiologic actions of insulin. In addition, Koepfer-Hobelsberger and Wieland (1984) found that insulin stimulates phospholipase C activity in the plasma membrane of adipocytes. These observations are of interest as it was recently reported by Saltiel (1987) that a putative insulin-mediator substance is generated by treatment of liver plasma membranes with a phospholipase C specific for lipid containing phosphatidylinositol.

6. *Divalent Cations*

Either Mn^{2+} or Mg^{2+} is essential for the action of insulin on glucose transport (Hall *et al.*, 1982; Eckel *et al.*, 1983; Ueda *et al.*, 1984). In cells treated with A 23187 and exposed to high concentrations of cations (i.e., 1 m*M* Mn^{2+} or 10 m*M* Mg^{2+}), cellular glucose transport and cAMP phosphodiesterase are both stimulated without insulin (Ueda *et al.*, 1984). It would appear, therefore, that the cells have an intrinsic capacity to increase both glucose transport and phosphodiesterase activities in response to either Mn^{2+} or Mg^{2+} and that the function of insulin is to make the cellular system more sensitive to these cations. Incidentally, increasing Mn^{2+} concentrations still further (e.g., to 10 mM), stimulates glucose transport even without A 23187 (Saggerson *et al.*. 1976; Ueda *et al.*, 1984).

7. *SH Blockers*

The SH blockers (or sulfhydryl reagents) have several different effects on insulin-sensitive glucose transport activity (Kozka and Gould, 1982). Thus, iodoacetamide partially stimulates basal glucose transport activity in rat diaphragm and, at the same time, blocks the action of insulin (Kono and Colowick, 1961). In rat adipocytes, *p*-chloromercuribenzene sulfate stimulates basal transport activity as strongly as insulin does (Minemura and Crofford, 1969). In contrast. *N*-ethylmaleimide and phenylarsine oxide inhibit, the action of insulin on glucose transport, as described in Section V,I.

8. *Mechanical Agitation*

Glucose transport activity in adipocytes is considerably stimulated by centrifuging, e.g., for 1 to 10 minutes at 127 *g*, or strenuously shaking cells for 6 minutes (Vega and Kono, 1969). This stimulation is apparently ATP dependent as the reaction is prevented by preliminary treatment of the cells with 2,4-dinitrophenol or KCN. Significantly, however, ATP-dependent stimulation is not observed with rapid motion (600 cycles/min) on a mechanical device that makes a small circular motion (*r* 2 mm) (Toyoda *et al.*, 1987). Since the centrifugal force developed by this swirling motion is 0.2 *g*, it is suggested that glucose transport in adipocytes is stimulated by an elevated *g* value, rather than by a rapid movement of cells or buffer. Could this stimulation be secondary to the stretching of adipocytes or their plasma membranes? Since fat cells contain a fat droplet (which is light) and a nucleus (which is heavy), the cells should be stretched when exposed to increased centrifugal or gravitational force. Could the suggested "stretching effect" contribute to some extent to the stimulation of glucose transport in exercised muscle described below?

9. *Muscle Exercise*

Glucose transport activity in muscle is stimulated by exercise independent of insulin (e.g., Garthwaite and Holloszy, 1982; Wallberg-Henriksson and Holloszy, 1985). Narahara and Green (1983) found that certain peptides are lost from the muscle plasma membrane during exercise. Garthwaite and Holloszy (1982) reported that protein synthesis is required for recovery of the transport system from the exercise-induced stimulation.

10. *Antireceptor Antibody*

Some anti-insulin receptor antibodies stimulate glucose transport (Kahn *et al.*, 1977). As mentioned earlier, Simpson and Hedo (1984) and Forsayeth *et al.* (1987) reported that certain antireceptor antibodies activate glucose transport in adipocytes without stimulating receptor kinase activity.

11. *Phorbol Ester*

Kirsch *et al.* (1985) and Martz *et al.* (1986) reported that PMA, a phorbol ester which stimulates protein kinase C (Nishizuka, 1984), weakly stimulates glucose transport in adipocytes. The maximum effect of PMA is only approximately one tenth that of insulin (Martz *et al.*, 1986), and the agent significantly inhibits the action of insulin (Kirsch *et al.*, 1985). Klip and Ramlal (1987) found that the effect of PMA is negligible on glucose transport in L-6 skeletal muscle cells. Kitagawa *et al.* (1986) observed that the glucose transport activity in cultured Swiss 3T3 fibroblasts is considerably stimulated by both insulin and PMA, but apparently via two different mechanisms. They found that the PMA-dependent stimulation is mediated by protein kinase C and Ca^{2+} but the insulin-dependent reaction is not. In contrast, in cultured BC3H-1 myocytes Farese and associates found that not only does PMA stimulate cellular glucose transport (Farese *et al.*, 1985), but also that insulin activates intracellular protein kinase C (Cooper *et al.*, 1987).

Other factors known to stimulate glucose transport include hypertonicity (Kuzuya *et al.*, 1965) and high pH (Sonne *et al.*. 1981).

I. INHIBITORS OF INSULIN ACTION

1. *SH Blockers*

As mentioned in the previous section, SH blockers produce complex effects on glucose transport. While some SH blocking agents mimic the actions of insulin (see above), *N*-ethylmaleimide blocks the hormonal action on glucose transport (Mirsky and Perisutti, 1962) and, at the same time, inhibits reversal of the hormonal effect on transport (Czech, 1976b). Phenylarsine oxide, which forms a pentagonal ring with vicinal SH residues, also inhibits insulin action on glucose transport (Frost and Lane, 1985). Recently, Bernier *et al.* (1987) reported that phenylarsine oxide plus insulin produce a phosphorylated compound (M_r 15,000) in cultured 3T3-L1 adipocytes. They suggested that the compound might be involved in the intracellular signaling of insulin.

2. *Catecholamines*

Under "normal" conditions, catecholamines, such as isoproterenol, slightly stimulate basal glucose transport in adipocytes (U. Smith *et al.*, 1984; Joost *et al.*, 1985). However, isoproterenol strongly inhibits both basal and insulin-stimulated glucose transport activities when endogenous adenosine (which is secreted from adipocytes) is eliminated by the addition of adenosine deaminase (Green, 1983; U. Smith *et al.*, 1984). Joost *et al.* (1986, 1987) found that this inhibition is caused by deactivation of the intrinsic glucose transport activity, rather than by relocation of the transport system, as discussed in Section V,I.

3. *Peptides*

As mentioned earlier, Jochen and Berhanu (1986, 1987a,b) found that certain peptides inhibit both internalization of insulin and its action on glucose transport. The peptides found to be inhibitory happened to be substrates of chymotrypsin. PKCL, a specific inhibitor of chymotrypsin, however, did not affect insulin action. On the other hand, Kikuchi *et al.* (1981) noted that the actions of insulin on both glucose transport and glycogen synthase were blocked by TLCK, a specific inhibitor of trypsin. Based on this and other observations, Kikuchi *et al.* (1981) suggest that a proteolytic enzyme might be involved in the production of a putative insulin-mediator substance.

4. *Extracellular ATP*

The action of insulin on glucose transport in adipocytes is strongly inhibited by extracellular ATP at 1 m*M*, as first reported by Chang and Cuatrecasas (1974). ATP added to extracellular buffer partially inhibits the binding of insulin to its receptor (Trischitta *et al.*, 1984) but does not significantly affect internalization of the hormone–receptor complex (Hashimoto *et al.*, 1987). Nevertheless, ATP almost completely abolishes the chloroquine-dependent as well as the monensin-dependent accumulation of insulin in adipocytes (Hashimoto *et al.*, 1987). Hashimoto *et al.* (1987) suggest that this ATP effect may be secondary to its effect on blocking the degradative pathway for intra-cellular processing of insulin (see Fig. 5).

J. OTHER FACTORS AFFECTING GLUCOSE TRANSPORT ACTIVITY

The basal and insulin-stimulated glucose transport activities in fat cells reported from different laboratories are often quite different. Some of the factors known to cause such variations are described below.

1. *Collagenase*

Cells in adult rat adipose tissue are dispersed by the joint action of (1) two types of collagenolytic enzymes (Types A and B), which are capable of solubilizing native collagen by synergistic actions (Kono, 1968), and (2) another proteolytic enzyme that hydrolyzes an uniden-tified cell-binding protein (Kono, 1969a). This proteolytic enzyme can be trypsin, chymotrypsin, papain, or ficin if the aim of the operation is to obtain a viable cell preparation (Kono, 1969a,b). However, none of these enzymes can be used for insulin studies as they modify the cel-lular insulin receptor (Kono, 1969b). To date, only an acidic proteinase associated with crude bacterial collagenase (Kono, 1968) allows sol-ubilization of the cell-binding protein without modification of the in-sulin receptor (T. Kono, unpublished data). A problem with crude bac-terial collagenase is that it often contains another trypsinlike enzyme which, depending on its concentration, either mimics or blocks the actions of insulin (Kono, 1969b; Kono and Barham, 1971a).

2. *Bovine Serum Albumin*

Isolated adipocytes are prepared and suspended in a buffer contain-ing 2–4% crude bovine serum albumin (e.g., Rodbell, 1964) that corre-sponds to Fraction V of Cohn *et al.* (1946). This albumin preparation effectively (1) prevents the adsorption of insulin to the container wall (Ferrebee *et al.*, 1951), (2) takes up free fatty acid from the incubation mixture (Morrisett *et al.*, 1975), (3) prevents degradation of iodinated insulin (Yalow and Berson, 1960), and (4) protects isolated cells from lysis (Rinaldini, 1959). Although the mechanism of this lysis is not clear, up to 50% of cells are destroyed in 20-minute incubations in Krebs–Henseleit bicarbonate buffer free of albumin (T. Kono, un-published observation). A problem with Fraction V albumin is that it sometimes contains either an "insulin-like" activity or an "anti-in-sulin" factor. The insulin-like activity, which may be insulin itself,

can usually be eliminated by trypsin treatment of the albumin preparation followed by the addition of either soybean or egg trypsin inhibitor (Jordan and Kono, 1980). On the other hand, no effective method
has been found for elimination of the anti-insulin factor. Some investigators recommend an overnight dialysis, but this is rarely effective.

3. Rats

To demonstrate a large insulin effect on overall glucose utilization
in adipocytes, one must use young rats less than 150 g. However, the
effect of the hormone on glucose transport per se is not significantly
affected by the age of animals until body weight approaches 250 g (T.
Kono, unpublished observation).

4. Handling of Isolated Adipocytes

Before use in the transport assay, freshly prepared aipocytes should
be incubated at 37°C for 30 minutes or more with gentle shaking (30
strokes/minute) in 2–5 mM pyruvate. As reported elsewhere, basal
glucose transport activity is stabilized at the minimal level during this
incubation (Vega and Kono, 1979). The concentration of pyruvate can
be anywhere between 2 and 5 mM; 2 mM glucose may be substituted
for pyruvate, but lactate or acetate are ineffective for lowering the
basal transport activity (T. Kono, unpublished data). Although adjust-
ment of the adenosine concentration is important in stabilizing the
cAMP-dependent protein kinase activity (Honnor et al., 1985), it has
little effect in stabilizing the insulin effect on glucose transport (T.
Kono, unpublished).

VI. TRANSLOCATION HYPOTHESIS OF INSULIN ACTION

The translocation hypothesis, which was proposed in 1980 by Cushman and Wardzala (1980) and Suzuki and Kono (1980) on the basis of
two independent experimental observations, has been extensively reviewed during the last several years (e.g., Kahn and Cushman, 1985;
Simpson and Cushman, 1986; Kono, 1983, 1985). According to the
hypothesis, insulin increases cellular glucose transport activity by fa-
cilitating relocation of the transport system from an intracellular site
to the plasma membrane. This concept is schematically illustrated in
Fig. 6. Under basal conditions, most of the glucose transport systems
are associated with intracellular vesicles, the so-called slow-sedimenting vesicles. On stimulation with insulin. the glucose transport systems
are translocated to the plasma membrane.

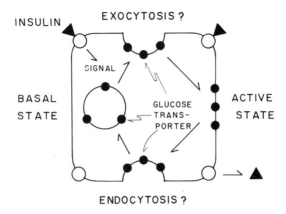

FIG. 6. Translocation hypothesis of insulin action on glucose transport. When adipocytes are stimulated by insulin (triangle). the glucose transporter (filled circle) is translocated from an intracellular site (specific vesicles?) to the plasma membrane, presumably by exocytosis. Subsequently, when insulin is dissociated from its receptor (open circle), the glucose transporter is relocated from the plasma membrane back into the intracellular site, possibly by endocytosis. Based on information published by Cushman and Wardzala (1980), Suzuki and Kono (1980), Karnieli *et al.,* (1981), and Kono *et al.* (1981).

Empirically, the plasma membrane and the slow-sedimenting vesicles are readily separable by differential and sucrose density gradient centrifugations, as described later. The amounts of glucose transport systems associated with the two membrane fractions have been determined by measuring (1) the D-glucose-inhibitable cytochalasin B-binding activity (Cushman and Wardzala, 1980; Wardzala and Jeanrenaud, 1981), (2) the glucose transport activity after reconstitution of the transport systems into egg lecithin liposomes (Suzuki and Kono, 1980; Robinson *et al.,* 1982), (3) the amount of photoaffinity-labeled [^{3}H]cytochalasin B (Horuk *et al.,* 1983; Oka and Czech, 1984), and (4) the level of immunoreactivity toward the anti-glucose transporter antibody prepared for the transporter from human erythrocytes (Wheeler *et al.,* 1982; Joost *et al.,* 1987). An example of such an experiment is shown in Fig. 7; the plasma membrane and slow-sedimenting fractions are separated by sucrose density gradient centrifugation (Kono *et al.,* 1982). In this experiment, the quantity of glucose transport systems was estimated by measuring the glucose transport activity after the transport systems had been reconstituted into egg lecithin liposomes (Robinson *et al.,* 1982). As may be seen in Fig. 7, (1) the glucose transport activities associated with the plasma membrane and the slow-sedimenting vesicles were clearly separated, and (2) insulin increased the

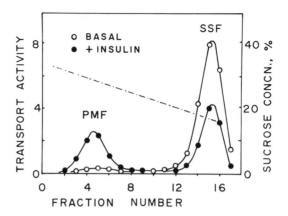

FIG. 7. Insulin-dependent changes in the intracellular distribution of glucose transport activity. Under basal conditions, most of the glucose transport activity is found in the slow-sedimenting fraction (SSF) whereas a small amount is detectable in the plasma membrane fraction (PMF). When cells are stimulated by insulin, the glucose transport activity in the slow-sedimenting fraction is decreased whereas the activity in the plasma membrane fraction is increased. In this experiment, the glucose transport activity was determined after reconstitution into egg lecithin liposomes. (From Kono et al., 1982, with permission from the publisher.)

glucose transport activity in the plasma membrane fraction (PMF) while decreasing the activity in the slow-sedimenting fraction (SSF). It should be noted in Fig. 7 that the insulin-dependent decrease in the glucose transport activity in the slow-sedimenting fraction was only about one-half of basal, even under optimum conditions. An explanation for this limited insulin effect is provided later in this section.

The above insulin effects are all reversible. Insulin-treated cells washed and incubated with fresh buffer show decreased glucose transport activity in the plasma membrane whereas activity in the slow-sedimenting fraction is increased (Karnieli et al., 1981; Kono et al., 1981). As for the insulin-dependent forward reaction, changes in the glucose transport activity in the two membrane fractions are complete in approximately 5–10 minutes at 37°C (Karnieli et al., 1981; Kono et al., 1981). All of these changes are temperature sensitive (Ezaki and Kono, 1982), ATP dependent, and protein synthesis independent (Kono et al., 1981). The effects of insulin on glucose transport activities in the two subcellular fractions are mimicked by a number of factors known to stimulate cellular glucose transport, such as low concentrations of trypsin, Mn^{2+} or Mg^{2+}, hydrogen peroxide, vanadate, SH blocking agents (Kono et al., 1982) low temperature (Ezaki and Kono, 1982), hyperosmolarity (Toyoda et al., 1986), and high pH (Toyoda et al.,

1986). An insulinomimetic agent that shows a large insulin-like effect in the plasma membrane fraction also exhibits a strong insulin-like effect in the slow-sedimenting fraction, and vice versa (Kono *et al.*, 1982).

The biochemical properties of the glucose transport activities in the plasma membrane and the slow-sedimenting fractions have been indistinguishable (M. Smith *et al.*, 1984). Nevertheless, the transport systems in the slow-sedimenting fraction are separated into two subfractions by isoelectric focusing. The sizes of the two subfractions are approximately equal, and their isoelectric points (pI) are 5.6 and 6.4 (Horuk *et al.*, 1986; Matthaei *et al.*, 1987). In contrast, the transport system in the plasma membrane fraction is apparently homogeneous, and its pI is 5.6. These data suggest that there are two types of glucose transport systems in adipocytes and that the more acidic component (pI 5.6) is recycled between the two membrane fractions whereas the more basic component is localized exclusively in the slow-sedimenting fraction. This suggestion is consistent with the earlier observation that the glucose transport activity in the slow-sedimenting fraction is suppressed only about one-half by the action of insulin even under optimum conditions (see Fig. 7).

The insulin-dependent apparent translocation of the glucose transport system was observed not only in rat adipocytes but also in rat diaphragm (Wardzala and Jeanrenaud, 1981) and cardiac muscle (Watanabe *et al.*, 1984). In addition, the apparent insulin-dependent translocation was detected not only in the glucose transport activity, but also in the activity of the insulin-like growth factor II receptor (Wardzala *et al.*, 1984; Kadota *et al.*, 1987) and that of the transferrin receptor (Oppenheimer *et al.*, 1983). Possible mechanisms involved in the translocation of these membrane components are exo- and endocytosis, as schematically illustrated in Fig. 6 above. The experimental basis for this suggestion is the observation that the characteristics of the insulin-dependent stimulation of the cellular glucose transport are similar to those of the endocytotic internalization of the insulin–receptor complex. Thus, both reactions are temperature sensitive, ATP dependent, and completed in approximately 10 minutes (see Kono, 1983). It should be noted, however, that these data can also be explained by the hypothesis that the action of insulin on glucose transport is secondary to the internalization of the hormone–receptor complex.

Although the translocation hypothesis is now generally accepted, it has yet to be established (1) where the slow-sedimenting vesicles are located in the cell, (2) whether the glucose transport system is actually recycled between the two subcellular fractions, and (3) what percentage of the insulin effect on glucose transport can be accounted for by the translocation mechanism. The first problem must be solved morphologically. During the initial phase of the translocation studies, the slow-sedimenting vesicles were consistently recovered in low-density microsomal fraction (Cushman and Wardzala, 1980; Karnieli et al., 1981), which was enriched with a Golgi marker enzyme (Suzuki and Kono, 1980; Kono et al., 1982). For this reason, the fraction was often referred to as the "low-density microsomal" fraction (e.g., Karnieli et al., 1981) or the "Golgi-rich" fraction (e.g., Kono et al., 1982). However, these earlier results were obtained with centrifugation of the membrane preparations under relatively mild conditions, e.g., 45 minutes at 35,000 rpm in a Beckman SW41 rotor (Kono et al., 1982). More recently, Shibata et al. (1987) reported that membrane preparations subjected to a long, isopycnic centrifugation (e.g., for 18 hours at 40.000 rpm in an SW41 rotor) yield plasma membrane and slow-sedimenting vesicles (as well as marker enzymes of the Golgi apparatus) concentrated into the same fraction (d 1.118–1.122). Shibata et al. (1987) also noted that if the centrifugation is discontinued at 3–4 hours, the glucose transport activity and the activity of a Golgi marker enzyme are partially separated. It would appear. therefore, that the slow-sedimenting vesicles which are associated with intracellular glucose transporter do not belong to the low-density microsomal fraction and are not entirely identical to the Golgi complex. In a separate study, Oka and Czech (1984) concluded that under basal conditions the slow-sedimenting transport system must be sequestered from the extracellular environment since the system is not accessible to ethylidene glucose (a nontransportable sugar isomer) added to the extracellular buffer. Their results are consistent with the translocation hypothesis but do not exclude the possibility (however unlikely) that the slow-sedimenting transport systems might te associated with the plasma membrane but are "masked" under basal conditions.

The second problem (2, above) should be solved biochemically. As mentioned earlier, it is now established that the levels of glucose transport activities in the two subcellular fractions are reciprocally changed by the action of insulin or other factors. Nevertheless, it has yet to be ascertained whether these changes are indeed induced by the shuttling of the transport systems. Although highly unlikely, transport systems in the two subcelluar fractions might change their numbers reciprocally by a seesaw mechanism, without moving back and forth between the two fractions. This problem might be solved in theory were it possible to label the glucose transport system in one fraction and follow the translocation of the label from one fraction to the other.

The third problem (3, above) is currently controversial. Our earlier data indicated that the effect of insulin in intact cell systems may be largely accounted for by the translocation hypothesis. According to the data, the insulin-dependent stimulation of 2-deoxy-D-glucose uptake observed in intact cell systems was 10.0-fold whereas that detected in the reconstituted system was 8.6-fold (Kono et al., 1982). In contrast, Joost et al. (1986) found that the insulin-dependent increase in the cellular transport activity for 3-O-methyl-D-glucose was 26-fold whereas that in the glucose transport activity in the resealed plasma membrane fraction was 8-fold. However, a precise comparison of insulin effects that expressed as "-fold increase" is not easy when the hormone-dependent stimulation is 10-fold or more, since the apparent insulin effect [namely, (plus insulin activity)/(basal activity)] is greatly affected by small changes in the observed basal activity.

Perhaps the strongest experimental evidence that translocation may not be the only mechanism of insulin action on glucose transport is the observation that the apparent K_m is modulated by insulin (Section V,E). Since the changes in K_m cannot be explained by the classic translocation hypothesis, the following two alternative models have been proposed by Toyoda et al. (1987). In one model, insulin recruits a large number of low K_m transport systems from an intracellular site to the plasma membrane, which is equipped with a small number of stationary, high K_m transporters. In another model, insulin increases the V_{max} of cellular glucose transport activity by the translocation mechanism and, at the same time, lowers the K_m of the intrinsic glucose transport activity by an unknown mechanism.

VII. MODULATION OF INTRINSIC GLUCOSE TRANSPORT ACTIVITY

As mentioned earlier in Section V,I, isoproterenol (a catecholamine) strongly inhibits both basal and insulin-stimulated glucose transport activities in adipocytes incubated with adenosine deaminase, that is, without adenosine (Green, 1983; Smith et al., 1984). The inhibitory effect of isoproterenol is blocked by phenylisopropyladenosine (PIA), which is a deaminase-resistant analog of adenosine (U. Smith et al., 1984). It would appear, therefore, that isoproterenol can inhibit glucose transport activity and that this action of isoproterenol is blocked by adenosine or its analogs. Joost et al. (1986, 1987) found that isoproterenol reduces the glucose transport activity in plasma membranes in situ, without changing the number of the transport systems in the membrane (as determined by the cytochalasin B-binding method). The effect of isoproterenol is specific to the transporter in the plasma membrane; neither the activity nor the number of the transport systems in the slow sedimenting fraction is affected. Kuroda *et al.* (1987) concluded that the isoproterenol effect is not mediated by cAMP. Taken together, these observations appear to indicate that the glucose transport system in plasma membranes is located in close proximity to receptors for isoproterenol and adenosine and that transport activity is affected by the two effectors through unknown mechanisms which may involved G-proteins (see Section VIII).

Kahn and Cushman (1987) discovered that diabetic rats given insulin for several days show glucose transport activity in adipocytes considerably greater than predicted from cytochalasin B-binding data. These observations are of interest but must be interpreted with caution since the site of the binding of cytochalasin B is apparently distinct from the active center for glucose transport (Gorga and Lienhard, 1981; Krupka and Devés, 1986).

Hyslop *et al.* (1985) reported that the insulin-dependent percent stimulation [(plus insulin/basal) × 100] of glucose transport in adipocytes was identical regardless of whether or not the transport activity was partially inhibited by fluorescein isothiocyanate. Baly and Horuk (1987) found that insulin stimulated glucose transport in cycloheximide-inhibited adipocytes without affecting distribution of glucose transport systems in subcellular fractions. These two sets of observations are difficult to reconcile with the translocation hypothesis of insulin action discussed earlier in Section VI.

VIII. POSSIBLE MECHANISMS OF INSULIN ACTION ON GLUCOSE TRANSPORT

As mentioned earlier, ATP is apparently involved in the actions of insulin on glucose transport in both muscle and adipocytes as well as in actions on phosphodiesterase in adipocytes (see Section II). Therefore, it can be postulated that the actions of insulin on these metabolic activities are mediated by a series of reactions which involve phosphorylation (see Kono, 1983). In agreement with this view, Kasuga *et al.* (1982a,b) discovered that the insulin receptor itself is an insulin-sensitive protein kinase. Nevertheless, as was also considered earlier, the role of the insulin-receptor kinase on the hormone-dependent stimulation of glucose transport is currently controversial (see Section V,B).

A current major problem of the phosphorylation theory of insulin action is a lack of information on the physiological substrate for the receptor kinase, other than the insulin receptor itself (Denton, 1986). Although Witters *et al.* (1985) found that glucose transporter can be phosphorylated by the action of protein kinase C, there appears to be no correlation between the level of phosphorylation and that of the transport activity (Gibbs *et al.*, 1985; Joost *et al.*, 1987). Naturally, these latter observations do not necessarily rule out the possibility that phosphorylation at a selected site in the transporter molecule is important for its activation. Also, as mentioned elsewhere, Bernier *et al.* (1987) reported that a specific phosphopeptide accumulated in cultured 3T3-L1 adipocytes which had been incubated with insulin in the presence of phenylarsine oxide, a potent inhibitor of the insulin action on glucose transport (Frost and Lane, 1985). Their observation is suggestive though still preliminary. Although Cooper *et al.* (1987) and Farese *et al.* (1985) found that the action of insulin on glucose transport in cultured BC3H-1 myocytes may be mediated by protein kinase C, the mechanism appears to be applicable only to a limited number of cell types or cell lines (see Section V,H).

A number of investigators have reported that several kinds of putative insulin-mediator substances are generated from either cells or plasma membranes which have been treated with insulin (e.g., see Jarett and Kiechle, 1984). Jarett *et al.* (1985) found that their mediator substance, when administered to intact adipocytes, stimulated both glycogen synthase and cAMP phosphodiesterase but not glucose transport. No other information is available on the effects of other mediator substances on cellular glucose transport activity. This lack of information is not surprising since no cell-free system has been developed for the evaluation of the effectiveness of a potential insulin-mediator substance on glucose transport.

If the major effect of insulin on glucose transport is indeed to facilitate the exocytotic translocation of glucose transport systems, how can we study the mechanism of hormonal action on glucose transport? The potential problems involved in answering this question are formidable since, by definition, one cannot demonstrate an exocytotic reaction once the cells are homogenized. Because of the lack of any other good idea. we previously asked a naive question: Can the internalized insulin–receptor complex "communicate" with the intracellular slow-sedimenting vesicles? Although the answer to this question has yet to be obtained, we found that the internalized insulin and the intracellular glucose transport systems are apparently associated with different vesicles (Ezaki and Kono, 1984). We also examined whether cytoskeletal and/or microfilamentous proteins might be involved in the intracellular movement of the slow-sedimenting vesicles. The results of this experiment simply indicated that cytochalasin B, vinblastine, and colchicine (at millimolar levels) extended the apparent lag period (T. Kono, unpublished), as previously reported by Häring et al. (1979) (see Section V,E).

Perhaps the best characterized models of exocytosis are (1) the secretion of neurotransmitters at the synaptic junction and (2) the secretion of insulin from pancreatic islet cells. In both cases, the exocytotic secretion is said to be triggered by increases in the intracellular level of Ca^{2+}. As discussed earlier, Ca^{2+} has also been implicated in the actions of insulin, but the problem is still controversial (see Section V,F).

Recently, we were encouraged by three lines of information that appeared in literature. First, Baxter et al. (1983) and Mundy and Strittmatter (1985) reported that a metalloendopeptidase is involved in the exocytotic secretion of neurotransmitters. Second, Burgoyne (1987) and Burgoyne and Cheek (1987) suggested that cytoskeletons and microfilaments may exist as intracellular obstacles which would hinder, rather than promote, exocytosis and that the elimination of the obstacles may be facilitated by a reaction involving GTP. Third, Vallar et al. (1987) found that there is a Ca^{2+}-independent mechanism for the secretion of insulin from cultured RINm5F cells and that this reaction is promoted by the action of guanine nucleotides. The first piece of information is suggestive since, as considered earlier (see Section V,I), the action of insulin on glucose transport is strongly inhibited by several substrates of endopeptidase (Jochen and Berhanu, 1986, 1987a,b) and TLCK (Kikuchi et al., 1981). The second and third findings are intriguing since it is now known that the actions of a large number of hormones are mediated by GTP and G-proteins (Dohlman et al., 1987; Levitzki, 1987). In addition, it was recently shown that glucose transport in adipocytes is inhibited by isoproterenol through a cAMP-dependent reaction (Kuroda et al., 1987) and that this inhibition is blocked by adenosine (U. Smith et al., 1984), which is known to exert its physiological effects by modulating an inhibitory G-protein. Although the action of insulin on glucose transport (Moreno et al., 1983) and phosphodiesterase activities (Weber et al., 1987) in adipocytes are not inhibited by pertussis toxin. there may be G-proteins that are insensitive to the toxin. The possible existence of an insulin-sensitive G-protein has been suggested by Houslay et al. (1984) and Espinal (1987). It is quite possible that the function of ATP, mentioned at the beginning of this section, may not be phosphorylation of protein, but maintenance of the GTP level in the cell.

All the above arguments are only speculative since the molecular mechanism of insulin actions is still elusive. In addition to the few possibilities considered above, a great number of theories and hypotheses have been proposed by many investigators. Although none of these theories is entirely convincing at the present stage of investigation, many of them are still being considered, as discussed in the books edited by Czech (1985) and by Belfrage *et al.* (1986), and also reviewed by, e.g.. Pilkis and Park (1974) and Czech (1977).

ACKNOWLEDGMENTS

I thank the editors of *Vitamins and Hormones* for giving me the opportunity to write this review article, which was not easy but was enjoyable. I also thank Dr. James May for critical reading of the manuscript. Our original studies on the actions of insulin cited in this article were conducted in collaboration with many investigators and technicians and were financed mainly by grants from the National Institutes of Health (DK 06725 and 19925). I am also grateful to Mrs. Frances W. Robinson, Miss Jo Ellen Flanagan, Mrs. Maylene Long, and Mrs. Patsy Raymer for their help in preparation of the manuscript.

REFERENCES

Allard, W. J., and Lienhard, G. E. (1985). Monoclonal antibodies to the glucose transporter from human erythrocytes. *J. Biol. Chem.* **260**, 8668–8675.

Baly, D. L., and Horuk, R. (1987). Dissociation of insulin-stimulated glucose transport from the translocation of glucose carriers in rat adipose cells. *J. Biol. Chem.* **262**, 21–24.

Banting, F. G., and Best, C. H. (1922). The internal secretion of the pancreas. *J. Lab. Clin. Med.* **7**, 251–266, 464–472.

Basketter, D. A., and Widdas, W. F. (1978). Asymmetry of the hexose transfer system in human erythrocytes. *J. Physiol. (London)* **278**, 389–401.

Battaglia, F. C., and Randle, P. J. (1960). Regulation of glucose uptake by muscle: The specificity of transport systems. *Biochem. J.* **75**, 408–416.

Baxter, D. A., Johnston, D., and Strittmatter, W. J. (1983). Protease inhibitors implicate metalloendoprotease in synaptic transmission at the mammalian neuromuscular junction. *Proc. Natl. Acad. Sci. U.S.A.* **80**, 4174–4178.

Belfrage, P., Donnér, J., and Stralförs, P., eds. 1986). "Mechanisms of Insulin Action." Elsevier, Amsterdam.

Bernier, M., Laird, D. M., and Lane, M. D. (1987). Insulin-activated tyrosine phosphorylation of a 15-kilodalton protein in intact 3T3-L1 adipocytes. *Proc. Natl. Acad. Sci. U.S.A.* **84**, 1844–1848.

Bihler, I., Ho, T. K., and Sawh, P. C. (1984). Isolation of Ca^{2+}-tolerant myocytes from adult rat heart. *Can. J. Physiol. Pharmacol.* **62**, 581–588.

Blecher, M. (1965). Phospholipase C and mechanisms of action of insulin and cortisol on glucose entry into free adipose cells. *Biochem. Biophys. Res. Commun.* **21**. 202–209.

Bloch, R. (1973). Inhibition of glucose transport in human erythrocytes by cytochalasin B. *Biochemistry* **12**, 4799–4801.

Bloch, R. (1974). Human erythrocyte sugar transport. *J. Biol. Chem.* **249**, 3543–3550.

Brown, D. H., Park, C. R., Daughaday, W. H., and Cornblath, M. (1952). The influence of preliminary soaking on glucose utilization by diaphragm. *J. Biol. Chem.* **197**, 167–174.

Burgoyne, R. D. (1987). Control of exocytosis. *Nature (London)* **328,** 112–113.

Burgoyne, R. D., and Cheek, T. R. (1987). Role of fodrin in secretion. *Nature (London)* **326,** 448.

Butcher, R. W., Ho, R. J., Meng, H. C., and Sutherland, E. W. (1965). cAMP in biological materials. II. The measurement of cAMP and its role in lipolysis. *J. Biol. Chem.* **240,** 4515–4523.

Chandramouli, V., Milligan, M., and Carter, J. R., Jr. (1977). Insulin stimulation of glucose transport in adipose cells: An energy-dependent process. *Biochemistry* **16,** 1151–1158.

Chang, K.-J., and Cuatrecasas, P. (1974). ATP-dependent inhibition of insulin-stimulated glucose transport in fat cells. *J. Biol. Chem.* **249,** 3170–3180.

Cheung, J. Y., Conover, C., Regen, D. M., Whitfield, C. F., and Morgan, H. E. (1978). Effect of insulin on kinetics of sugar transport in heart muscle. *Am. J. Physiol.* **234,** E70–E78.

Ciaraldi, T. P., and Olefsky, J. M. (1980). Relationship between deactivation of insulin-stimulated glucose transport and insulin dissociation in isolated rat adipocytes. *J. Biol. Chem.* **255,** 327–330.

Ciaraldi, T. P., and Olefsky, J. M. (1981). Metabolic requirements for deactivation of insulin-stimulated glucose transport in isolated rat adipocytes. *Arch. Biochem. Biophys.* **208,** 502–507.

Claus, T. H., El-Maghrabi, M. R., and Pilkis, S. J. (1979). Modulation of the phosphorylation state of rat liver pyruvate kinase by allosteric effectors and insulin. *J. Biol. Chem.* **254,** 7855–7864.

Clausen, T. (1975). The effect of insulin on glucose transport in muscle cells. *Curr. Top. Membr. Transp.* **6,** 169–226.

Clausen, T. (1980). The role of calcium in the activation of the glucose transport system. *Cell Calcium* **1,** 311–325.

Cohn, E. J., Strong, L. E., Hughes, W. L., Jr., Mulford, D. J., Ashworth, J. N., Melin, M., and Taylor, H. L. (1946). Preparation and properties of serum and plasma proteins. *J. Am. Chem. Soc.* **68,** 459–475.

Cooper, D. R., Konda, T. S., Standaert, M. L., Davis, J. S., Pollet, R. J., and Farese, R. V. (1987). Insulin increases membrane and cytosolic protein kinase C activity in BC3H-1 myocytes. *J. Biol. Chem.* **262,** 3633–3639.

Coore, H. G., Denton, R. M., Martin, B. R., and Randle, P. J. (1971). Regulation of adipose tissue pyruvate dehydrogenase by insulin and other hormones. *Biochem. J.* **125,** 115–127.

Crane, R. K., Forstner, G., and Eicholz, A. (1965). Studies on the mechanism of the intestinal absorption of sugars: An effect of Na^+ concentration on the apparent Michaelis constants. *Biochim. Biophys. Acta* **109,** 467–477.

Crofford, O. B., and Renold, A. E. (1965). Glucose uptake by incubated rat epididymal adipose tissue. *J. Biol. Chem.* **240,** 14–21.

Cushman, S. W., and Wardzala, L. J. (1980). Potential mechanism of insulin action on glucose transport in the isolated rat adipose cell. *J. Biol. Chem.* **255,** 4758–4762.

Cynober, L., Capeau, J., and Ekindjian, O. G. (1986). Cultured fibroblasts as a suitable model for studying insulin action on glucose uptake. *Diab. Metabol. (Paris)* **12,** 308–314.

Czech, M. P. (1976a). Regulation of the D-glucose transport system in isolated fat cells. *Mol. Cell. Biochem.* **11,** 51–63.

Czech, M. P. (1976b). Differential effects of sulfhydryl reagents on activation and deactivation of the fat cell hexose transport system. *J. Biol. Chem.* **251,** 1164–1170.

Czech, M. P. (1977). Molecular basis of insulin action. *Annu. Rev. Biochem.* **46,** 359–384.

Czech, M. P., ed. (1985). "Molecular Basis of Insulin Action." Plenum, New York.

Czech, M. P., and Massague, J. (1982). Subunit structure and dynamics of the insulin receptor. Fed. Proc., Fed. Am. Soc. Exp. Biol. 41, 2719–2723.

Czech, M. P., Lawrence J. C., Jr., and Lynn, W. S. (1974a). Evidence for electron transfer reactions involved in the Cu^{2+}-dependent thiol activation of fat cell glucose utilization. J. Biol. Chem. 249, 1001–1006.

Czech, M. P., Lawrence, J. C., Jr., and Lynn, W. S. (1974b). Hexose transport in isolated brown fat cells. J. Biol. Chem. 249, 5421–5427.

Davis, R. J., Corvera, S., and Czech, M. P. (1986). Insulin stimulates cellular iron uptake and causes the redistribution of intracellular transferrin receptors to the plasma membrane. J. Biol. Chem. 261, 8708–8711.

De Meyts, P., Roth, J., Neville, D. M., Jr., Gavin, J. R., III, and Lesniak, M. A. (1973). Insulin interactions with its receptors: Experimental evidence for negative cooperativity. Biochem. Biophys. Res. Commun. 55, 154–161.

Denton, R. M. (1986). Early events in insulin actions. Adv. Cyclic Nucleotide Protein Phosphorylat. Res. 20, 293–341.

Devés, R., and Krupka, R. M. (1978). Cytochalasin B and the kinetics of inhibition of biological transport: A case of asymmetric binding to the glucose carrier. Biochim. Biophys. Acta 510, 339–348.

Dohlman, H. G., Caron, M. G., and Lefkowitz, R. J. (1987). A family of receptors coupled to guanine nucleotide regulatory proteins. Biochemistry 26, 2657–2664.

Dubyak, G. R., and Kleinzeller, A. (1980). The insulin-mimetic effects of vanadate in isolated rat adipocytes. J. Biol. Chem. 255, 5306–5312.

Dustin, M. L., Jacobson, G. R., and Peterson, S. W. (1984). Effects of insulin receptor down-regulation on hexose transport in human erythrocytes. J. Biol. Chem. 259, 13660–13663.

Ebina, Y., Ellis, L., Jarnagin, K., Edery, M., Graf, L., Clauser, E., Ou, J.-H., Masiarz, F., Kan, Y. W., Goldfine, I. D., Roth, R. A., and Rutter, W. J. (1985). The human insulin receptor cDNA: The structural basis for hormone-activated transmembrane signalling. Cell 40, 747–758.

Ebina, Y., Araki, E., Taira, M., Shimada, F., Mori, M., Craik, C. S.. Siddle, K., Pierce, S. B., Roth, R. A., and Rutter, W. J. (1987). Replacement of lysine residue 1030 in the putative ATP-binding region of the insulin receptor abolishes insulin- and antibody-stimulated glucose uptake and receptor kinase activity. Proc. Natl. Acad. Sci. U.S.A. 84, 704–708.

Eckel, J., Pandalis, G., and Reinauer, H. (1983). Insulin action on the glucose transport system in isolated cardiocytes from adult rat. Biochem. J. 212, 385–392.

Eckel, J., Van Echten, G., and Reinauer, H. (1985). Adult cardiac myocytes in primary culture. Am. J. Physiol. 249, H212–H221.

Ellis, L., Clauser, E., Morgan, D. O., Edery, M., Roth, R. A., and Rutter, W. J. (1986). Replacement of insulin receptor tyrosine residues 1162 and 1163 compromises insulin-stimulated kinase activity and uptake of 2-deoxyglucose. Cell 45, 721–732.

Ellory, J. C., and Lew, V. L., eds. (1977). "Membrane Transport in Red Cells." Academic Press, New York.

Espinal, J. (1987). Mechanism of insulin action. Nature (London) 328, 574–575.

Ezaki, O., and Kono, T. (1982). Effects of temperature on basal and insulin-stimulated glucose transport activities in fat cells. J. Biol. Chem. 257, 14306–14310.

Ezaki, O., and Kono, T. (1984). Sedimentation characteristics of subcellular vesicles associated with internalized insulin and those bound with intracellular glucose transport activity. Arch. Biochem. Biophys. 231, 280–286.

Farese, R. V., Standaert, M. L., Barnes, D. E., Davis, J. S., and Pollet, R. J. (1985).

Phorbol ester provokes insulin-like effects on glucose transport, amino acid uptake, and pyruvate dehydrogenase activity in BC3H-1 cultured myocytes. *Endocrinology* **116**, 2650–2655.

Ferrebee, J. W., Johnson, B. B., Mithoefer, J. C., and Gardella, J. W. (1951). Insulin and adrenocorticotropin labeled with radioiodine. *Endocrinology* **48**, 277–283.

Foley, J. E., Foley, R., and Gliemann, J. (1980). Rate-limiting steps of 2-deoxyglucose uptake in rat adipocytes. *Biochim. Biophys. Acta* **599**, 689–698.

Forsayeth, J. R., Caro, J. F., Sinha, M. K., Maddux, B. A., and Goldfine, I. D. (1987). Monoclonal antibodies to the human insulin receptor that activate glucose transport but not insulin receptor kinase activity. *Proc. Natl. Acad. Sci. U.S.A.* **84**, 3448–3451.

Freychet, P., Roth, J., and Neville, D. M., Jr. (1971). Monoiodoinsulin: Demonstration of its biological activity and binding to fat cells and liver membranes. *Biochem. Biophys. Res. Commun.* **43**, 400–408.

Froesch, E. R., and Ginsberg, J. L. (1962). Fructose metabolism of adipose tissue. *J. Biol. Chem.* **237**, 3317–3324.

Frost, S. C., and Lane, M. D. (1985). Evidence for the involvement of vicinal sulfhydryl groups in insulin-activated hexose transport by 3T3-L1 adipocytes. *J. Biol. Chem.* **260**, 2646–2652.

Fujita-Yamaguchi, Y., Choi, S., Sakamoto, Y., and Itakura, K. (1983). Purification of insulin receptor with full binding activity. *J. Biol. Chem.* **258**, 5045–5049.

Gammeltoft, S., and Gliemann, J. (1973). Binding and degradation of ^{125}I-labelled insulin by isolated rat fat cells. *Biochim. Biophys. Acta* **320**, 16–32.

Garthwaite, S. M., and Holloszy, J. O. (1982). Increased permeability to sugar following muscle contraction. *J. Biol. Chem.* **257**, 5008–5012.

Gavin, J. R., III, Gorden, P., Roth, J.. Archer, J. A., and Buell, D. N. (1973). Characteristics of the human lymphocyte insulin receptor. *J. Biol. Chem.* **248**, 2202–2207.

Geuze, H. J., Slot, J. W., Strous, G. J. A. M., Lodish, H. F., and Schwartz, A. L. (1983). Intracellular site of asialoglycoprotein receptor–ligand uncoupling. *Cell* **32**, 277–287.

Gibbs, E. M., Allard, W. J., and Lienhard, G. E. (1986). The glucose transporter in 3T3-L1 adipocytes is phosphorylated in response to phorbol ester but not in response to insulin. *J. Biol. Chem.* **261**, 16597–16603.

Ginsberg, B. H., Kahn, C. R., and Roth, J. (1976). The insulin receptor of the turkey erythrocyte. *Biochim. Biophys. Acta* **443**, 227–242.

Gliemann, J., Østerlind, K., Vinten, J., and Gammeltoft, S. (1972). A procedure for measurement of distribution spaces in isolated fat cells. *Biochim. Biophys. Acta* **286**, 1–9.

Gorden, P., Carpentier, J.-L., Freychet, P., and Orci, L. (1980). Internalization of polypeptide hormones. *Diabetologia* **18**, 263–274.

Gorga, F. R., and Lienhard, G. E. (1981). Equilibria and kinetics of ligand binding to the human erythrocyte glucose transporter: Evidence for an alternating conformation model for transport. *Biochemistry* **20**, 5108–5113.

Gould, M. K. (1984). Multiple roles of ATP in the regulation of sugar transport in muscle and adipose tissue. *Trends Biol. Sci.* **9**, 524–527.

Green, A. (1983). Catecholamines inhibit insulin-stimulated glucose transport in adipocytes, in the presence of adenosine deaminase. *FEBS Lett.* **152**, 261–264.

Greengard, P. (1978). Phosphorylated proteins as physiological effectors. *Science* **199**, 146–152.

Hall, S., Keo, L., Yu, K. T., and Gould, M. K. (1982). Effect of ionophore A23187 on basal and insulin-stimulated sugar transport by rat soleus muscle. *Diabetes* **31**, 846–850.

Halperin, M. L., and Cheema-Dhadli, S. (1982). Comparison of glucose and fructose transport into adipocytes of the rat. *Biochem. J.* **202,** 717–721.

Häring, H. U., Kemmler, W., and Hepp, K. D. (1979). Effect of colchicine and vinblastine on the coupling of insulin binding and insulin actions in fat cells. *FEBS Lett.* **105,** 329–332.

Häring, H. U., Biermann, E., and Kemmler, W. (1981). Coupling of insulin binding and insulin action on glucose transport in fat cells. *Am. J. Physiol.* **240,** E556–E565.

Hashimoto, N., Robinson, F. W., Shibata, Y., Flanagan, J. E., and Kono, T. (1987). Diversity in the effects of extracellular ATP and adenosine on the cellular processing and physiologic actions of insulin in rat adipocytes. *J. Biol. Chem.* **262,** 15026–15032.

Haworth, R. A., Hunter, D. R., and Berkoff, H. A. (1980). The isolation of Ca^{2+}-resistant myocytes from the adult rat. *J. Mol. Cell. Cardiol.* **12,** 715–723.

Honnor, R. C., Dhillon, G. S., and Londos, C. (1985). cAMP-dependent protein kinase and lipolysis in rat adipocytes. I & II. *J. Biol. Chem.* **260,** 15122–15129, 15130–15138.

Horuk, R., Rodbell, M., Cushman, S. W., and Simpson, I. A. (1983). Identification and characterization of the rat adipocyte glucose transporter by photoaffinity crosslinking. *FEBS Lett.* **164,** 261–266.

Horuk, R., Matthaei, S., Olefsky, J. M., Baly, D. L., Cushman, S. W., and Simpson, I. A. (1986). Biochemical and functional heterogeneity of rat adipocyte glucose transporters. *J. Biol. Chem.* **261,** 1823–1828.

Houslay, M. D., Wallace, A. V., Cooper. M. E., Payne, N. J., Wilson, S. R., and Heyworth, C. M. (1984). Does insulin exert certain of its actions through a distinct species of guanine nucleotide regulatory protein? *Biochem. Soc. Trans.* **12,** 766–768.

Hyslop, P. A., Kuhn, C. E., and Sauerheber, R. D. (1985). Insulin stimulation of glucose transport in isolated rat adipocytes: Functional evidence for insulin activation of intrinsic transporter activity within the plasma membrane. *Biochem. J.* **232,** 245–254.

Jacobs, S., Shechter, Y., Bissell, K., and Cuatrecasas, P. (1977). Purification and properties of insulin receptors from rat liver membranes. *Biochem. Biophys. Res. Commun.* **77,** 981–988.

Jarett, L., and Kiechle, F. L. (1984). Intracellular mediators of insulin action. *Vitam. Horm.* **41,** 51–78.

Jarett, L., Wong, E. H. A., Macaulay, S. L., and Smith, J. A. (1985). Insulin mediators from rat skeletal muscle have differential effects on insulin-sensitive pathways of intact adipocytes. *Science* **227,** 533–535.

Jochen, A. L., and Berhanu, P. (1986). Chymotrypsin substrate analogues inhibit endocytosis of insulin and insulin receptors in adipocytes. *J. Cell Biol.* **103,** 1807–1816.

Jochen, A. L., and Berhanu, P. (1987a). Insulin-stimulated glucose transport and insulin internalization share a common postbinding step in adipocytes. *Diabetes* **36,** 542–545.

Jochen, A. L., and Berhanu, P. (1987b). Effects of metalloendoprotease inhibitors on insulin binding, internalization and processing. *Biochem. Biophys. Res. Commun.* **142,** 205–212.

Joost, H.-G., Göke, R., and Steinfelder, H.-J. (1985). Dual effect of isoprenaline on glucose transport and response to insulin in isolated adipocytes. *Biochem. Pharmacol.* **34,** 649–653.

Joost, H. G., Weber, T. M., Cushman, S. W., and Simpson, I. A. (1986). Insulin-stimulated glucose transport in rat adipose cells: Modulation of transporter intrinsic activity by isoproterenol and adenosine. *J. Biol. Chem.* **261,** 10033–10036.

Joost, H. G., Weber, T. M., Cushman, S. W., and Simpson, I. A. (1987). Activity and phosphorylation state of glucose transporters in plasma membranes from insulin-, isoproterenol-, and phorbol ester-treated rat adipocytes. *J. Biol. Chem.* **262,** 11261–11267.

Jordan, J. E., and Kono, T. (1980). Elimination of insulin-like activity present in certain batches of crude bovine serum albumin by trypsin treatment. *Anal. Biochem.* **104,** 192–195.

Jungas, R. L. (1971). Hormonal regulation of pyruvate dehydrogenase. *Metabolism* **20,** 43–53.

Jungas, R. L., and Ball, E. G. (1963). Studies on the metabolism of adipose tissue. XII. The effects of insulin and epinephrine on free fatty acid and glycerol production. *Biochemistry* **2,** 383–388.

Kadota, S., Fantus, I. G., Deragon, G., Guyda, H. J., and Posner, B. I. (1987). Stimulation of insulin-like growth factor II receptor binding and insulin receptor kinase activity in rat adipocytes. *J. Biol. Chem.* **262,** 8252–8256.

Kahn, B. B., and Cushman, S. W. (1985). Subcellular translocation of glucose transporters: Role in insulin action and its perturbation in altered metabolic states. *Diabet. Metab. Rev.* **1,** 203–227.

Kahn, B. B., and Cushman, S. W. (1987). Mechanism for markedly hyperresponsive insulin-stimulated glucose transport activity in adipose cells from insulin-treated streptozotocin diabetic rats. *J. Biol. Chem.* **262,** 5118–5124.

Kahn, C. R., Baird, K., Flier, J. S., and Jarrett, D. B. (1977). Effects of autoantibodies to the insulin receptor on isolated adipocytes. *J. Clin. Invest.* **60,** 1094–1106.

Kaldawi, R. E., Yu, K. T., and Gould, M. K. (1983). ATP depletion promotes deactivation of insulin-stimulated sugar transport in rat soleus muscle. *Arch. Biochem. Biophys.* **226,** 612–617.

Karnieli, E., Zarnowski, M. J., Hissin, P. J., Simpson, I. A., Salans, L. B., and Cushman, S. W. (1981). Insulin-stimulated translocation of glucose transport systems in the isolated rat adipose cell. *J. Biol. Chem.* **256,** 4772–4777.

Kasahara, M., and Hinkle, P. C. (1977). Reconstitution and purification of the D-glucose transporter from human erythrocytes. *J. Biol. Chem.* **252,** 7384–7390.

Kasuga, M., Karlsson, F. A., and Kahn, C. R. (1982a). Insulin stimulates the phosphorylation of the 95,000-dalton subunit of its own receptor. *Science* **215,** 185–187.

Kasuga, M., Zick. Y., Blithe, D. L., Crettaz, M.. and Kahn. C. R. (1982b). Insulin stimulates tyrosine phosphorylation of the insulin receptor in a cell-free system. *Nature (London)* **298,** 667–669.

Kikuchi, K., Schwartz, C., Creacy, S., and Larner, J. (1981). Independent control of selected insulin-sensitive cell membrane and intracellular functions. III. The influence of trypsin. *Mol. Cell. Biochem.* **37,** 125–130.

Kipnis, D. M., and Cori, C. F. (1957). The effect of insulin on pentose uptake by the diaphragm. *J. Biol. Chem.* **224,** 681–693.

Kirsch, D., Obermaier, B., and Häring, H. U. (1985). Phorbol esters enhance basal D-glucose transport but inhibit insulin stimulation of D-glucose transport and insulin binding in isolated rat adipocytes. *Biochem. Biophys. Res. Commun.* **128,** 824–832.

Kitagawa, K., Nishino, H., and Iwashima, A. (1986). Effect of protein kinease C activation and Ca^{2+} mobilization on hexose transport in Swiss 3T3 cells. *Biochim. Biophys. Acta* **887,** 100–104.

Klip, A., and Ramlal, T. (1987). Protein kinase C is not required for insulin stimulation of hexose uptake in muscle cells in culture. *Biochem. J.* **242,** 131–136.

Klip, A., Li, G., and Logan, W. J. (1983). Role of Ca in serum–stimulation of hexose transport in muscle cells. *FEBS Lett.* **162,** 329–333.

Koepfer-Hobelsberger, B., and Wieland, O. H. (1984). Insulin activates phospholipase C in fat cells. *Mol. Cell. Endocrinol.* **36,** 123–129.

Kono, T. (1968). Purification and partial characterization of collagenolytic enzymes from *Cl. histolyticum. Biochemistry* **7**, 1106–1114.

Kono, T. (1969a). Roles of collagenases and other proteolytic enzymes in the dispersal of animal tissues. *Biochim. Biophys. Acta* **178**, 397–400.

Kono, T. (1969b). Destruction of insulin effector system of adipose tissue cells by proteolytic enzymes. *J. Biol. Chem.* **244**, 1772–1778.

Kono, T. (1969c). Destruction and restoration of the insulin effector system of isolated fat cells. *J. Biol. Chem.* **244**, 5777–5784.

Kono, T. (1983). Actions of insulin on glucose transport and cAMP phosphodiesterase in fat cells. *Recent Prog. Horm. Res.* **39**, 519–557.

Kono, T. (1985). Insulin-dependent apparent translocation of glucose transport activity. *In* "Molecular Basis of Insulin Action" (M. P. Czech, ed.), pp. 423–431. Plenum, New York.

Kono, T., and Barham, F. W. (1971a). Insulin-like effects of trypsin on fat cells. *J. Biol. Chem.* **246**, 6204–6209.

Kono, T., and Barham, F. W. (1971b). The relationship between the insulin-binding capacity of fat cells and the cellular response to insulin. *J. Biol. Chem.* **246**, 6210–6216.

Kono, T., and Colowick, S. P. (1961). Stereospecific sugar transport caused by uncouplers and SH-inhibitors. *Arch. Biochem. Biophys.* **93**, 514–519.

Kono, T., Robinson, F. W., and Sarver, J. A. (1975). Insulin-sensitive phosphodiesterase. *J. Biol. Chem.* **250**, 7826–7835.

Kono, T., Robinson, F. W., Sarver, J. A., Vega, F. V., and Pointer, R. H. (1977). Actions of insulin in fat cells. *J. Biol. Chem.* **252**, 2226–2233.

Kono, T., Suzuki, K., Dansey, L. E., Robinson, F. W., and Blevins, T. L. (1981). Energy-dependent and protein synthesis-independent recycling of the insulin-sensitive glucose transport mechanism in fat cells. *J. Biol. Chem.* **256**, 6400–6407.

Kono, T., Robinson, F. W., Blevins, T. L., and Ezaki, O. (1982). Evidence that translocation of the glucose transport activity is the major mechanism of insulin action on glucose transport in fat cells. *J. Biol. Chem.* **257**, 10942–10947.

Korbl, G. P., Sloan, I. G., and Gould, M. K. (1977). Effect of anoxia, 2,4-dinitrophenol and salicylate on xylose transport by isolated rat soleus muscle. *Biochim. Biophys. Acta* **465**, 93–109.

Kozka, I. J., and Gould, M. K. (1982). Multiple effects of sulfhydryl reagents on sugar transport by rat soleus muscle. *Biochim. Biophys. Acta* **689**, 210–218.

Krebs, E. G., and Beavo, J. A. (1979). Phosphorylation–dephosphorylation of enzymes. *Annu. Rev. Biochem.* **48**, 923–959.

Krupka, R. M. (1985). Asymmetrical binding of phloretin to glucose transport system of human erythrocytes. *J. Membr. Biol.* **83**, 71–80.

Krupka, R. M., and Devés, R. (1986). Looking for probes of glucose and choline transport in erythrocytes. *Biochem. Cell. Biol.* **64**, 1099–1107.

Kundig, W., and Roseman, S. (1971). Sugar transport. I & II. *J. Biol. Chem.* **246**, 1393–1406, 1407–1418.

Kuo, J. F., Holmlund, C. E., and Dill, I. K. (1966). The effect of proteolytic enzymes on isolated adipose cells. *Life Sci.* **5**, 2257–2262.

Kuroda, M., Honnor, R. C., Cushman, S. W., Londos, C., and Simpson, I. A. (1987). Regulation of insulin-stimulated glucose transport in the isolated rat adipocyte. *J. Biol. Chem.* **262**, 245–253.

Kuzuya, T., Samols, E., and Williams, R. H. (1965). Stimulation by hyperosmolarity of glucose metabolism in rat adipose tissue and diaphragm *in vitro. J. Biol. Chem.* **240**, 2277–2283.

Laursen, A. L., Foley, J. E., Foley, R., and Gliemann, J. (1981). Termination of insulin-induced hexose transport in adipocytes. *Biochim. Biophys. Acta* **673**, 132–136.

Levine, R. (1982). Insulin: The effects and mode of action of the hormone. *Vitam. Horm.* **39**, 145–173.

Levine, R., and Goldstein, M. S. (1955). On the mechanism of action of insulin. *Recent Prog. Horm. Res.* **11**, 343–380.

Levitzki, A. (1987). Regulation of adenylate cyclase by hormones and G-proteins. *FEBS Lett.* **211**, 113–118.

Lindgren, C. A., Paulson, D. J., and Shanahan, M. F. (1982). Isolated cardiac myocytes. *Biochim. Biophys. Acta* **721**, 385–393.

Loten, E. G., and Sneyd, J. G. T. (1970). An effect of insulin on adipose-tissue cAMP phosphodiesterase. *Biochem. J.* **120**, 187–193.

McDonald, J. M., and Pershadsingh, H. A. (1985). The role of calcium in the transduction of insulin action. *In* "Molecular Basis of Insulin Action" (M. P. Czech, ed.), pp. 103–118. Plenum, New York.

Makino, H., and Kono, T. (1980). Characterization of insulin-sensitive phosphodiesterase in fat cells. (2) Comparison of enzyme activities stimulated by insulin and by isoproterenol. *J. Biol. Chem.* **255**, 7850–7854.

Manganiello, V., and Vaughan, M. (1973). An effecf of insulin on cAMP phosphodiesterase in fat cells. *J. Biol. Chem.* **248**, 7164–7170.

Marshall, S. (1985). Dual pathways for the intracellular processing of insulin. *J. Biol. Chem.* **260**. 13524–13531.

Marshall, S., and Olefsky, J. M. (1979). Effects of lysosomotropic agents on insulin interactions with adipocytes. *J. Biol. Chem.* **254**, 10153–10160.

Marshall, S., and Olefsky, J. M. (1981). Tris(hydroxymethyl)aminomethane permits the expression of insulin-induced receptor loss in isolated adipocytes. *Biochem. Biophys. Res. Commun.* **102**, 646–653.

Marshall, S., Green, A., and Olefsky, J. M. (1981). Evidence for recycling of insulin receptors in isolated rat adipocytes. *J. Biol. Chem.* **256**, 11464–11470.

Martz, A., Mookerjee, B. K., and Jung, C. Y. (1986). Insulin and phorbol esters affect the maximum velocity rather than the half-saturation constant of 3-O-methylglucose transport in rat adipocytes. *J. Biol. Chem.* **261**, 13606–13609.

Matthaei, S., Garvey, W. T., Horuk, R., Hueckstaedt, T. P., and Olefsky, J. M. (1987). Human adipocyte glucose transport system. *J. Clin. Invest.* **79**, 703–709.

May, J. M., and Mikulecky, D. C. (1982). The simple model of adipocyte hexose transport. *J. Biol. Chem.* **257**, 11601–11608.

Minemura, T., and Crofford, O. B. (1969). Insulin-receptor interaction in isolated fat cells. I. The insulin-like properties of *p*-chloromercuribenzene sulfonic acid. *J. Biol. Chem.* **244**, 5181–5188.

Mirsky, I. A., and Perisutti, G. (1962). The inhibition of the action of insulin on rat epididymal adipose tissue by sulfhydryl blocking agents. *Biochim. Biophys. Acta* **62**, 490–496.

Moreno, F. J., Mills, I., Gracia-Sáinz, J. A., and Fain, J. N. (1983). Effects of pertussis toxin treatment on the metabolism of rat adipocytes. *J. Biol. Chem.* **258**, 10938–10943.

Morgan, D. O., and Roth, R. A. (1987). Acute insulin action requires insulin receptor kinase activity. *Proc. Natl. Acad. Sci. U.S.A.* **84**, 41–45.

Morgan, H. E., Henderson, M. J., Regen, D. M., and Park, C. R. (1961). Regulation of glucose uptake in muscle. *J. Biol. Chem.* **236**, 253–261.

Morgan, H. E., Regen, D. M., and Park, C. R. (1964). Identification of a mobile carrier-mediated sugar transport system in muscle. *J. Biol. Chem.* **239**, 369–374.

Morrisett, J. D., Pownall, H. J., and Gotto, A. M., Jr. (1975). Bovine serum albumin: Study of the fatty acid and steroid binding sites. *J. Biol. Chem.* **250**, 2487-2494.

Mueckler, M., Caruso, C., Baldwin, S. A., Panico, M., Blench, I.. Morris, H. R., Allard, W. J., Lienhard, G. E., and Lodish, H. F. (1985). Sequence and structure of human glucose transporter. *Science* **229**, 941-945.

Mundy, D. I., and Strittmatter, W. J. (1985). Requirement for metalloendoprotease in exocytosis: Evidence in mast cells and adrenal chromaffin cells. *Cell* **40**, 645-656.

Naftalin, R. J., and Holman, G. D. (1977). Transport of sugars in human red cells. *In* "Membrane Transport in Red Cells" (J. C. Ellory and V. L. Lew, eds.), pp. 257-300. Academic Press. New York.

Narahara, H. T., and Ozand, P. (1963). The effect of insulin on the penetration of 3-methylglucose in frog muscle. *J. Biol. Chem.* **238**, 40-49.

Narahara, H. T., and Green, J. D. (1983). Selective loss of a plasma membrane protein associated with contraction of skeletal muscle. *Biochim. Biophys. Acta* **730**, 71-75.

Nishizuka, Y. (1984). Role of protein kinase C in cell surface signal transduction and tumour promotion. *Nature (London)* **308**, 693-698.

Oka, Y., and Czech, M. P. (1984). Photoaffinity labeling of insulin-sensitive hexose transporters in intact rat adipocytes. *J. Biol. Chem.* **259**, 8125-8133.

Okuno, Y., and Gliemann, J. (1987). Enhancement of glucose transport by insulin at 37°C in rat adipocytes is accounted for by increased V_{max}. *Diabetologia* **30**, 426-430.

Oppenheimer, C. L., Pessin, J. E., Massague, J., Gitomer, W., and Czech, M. P. (1983). Insulin action rapidly modulates the apparent affinity of the insulin-like growth factor II receptor. *J. Biol. Chem.* **258**, 4824-4830.

Pershadsingh, H. A., Shade, D. L., Delfert, D. M., and McDonald, J. M. (1987). Chelation of intracellular calcium blocks insulin action in the adipocyte. *Proc. Natl. Acad. Sci. U.S.A.* **84**, 1025-1029.

Pessin, J. E., Mottola, C., Yu, K.-T., and Czech, M. P. (1985). Subunit structure and regulation of the insulin–receptor complex. *In* "Molecular Basis of Insulin Action" (M. P. Czech, ed.), pp. 3-30. Plenum, New York.

Pilkis, S. J., and Park, C. R. (1974). Mechanism of action of insulin. *Annu. Rev. Pharmacol.* **14**, 365-388.

Randle, P. J., and Morgan, H. E. (1962). Regulation of glucose uptake by muscle. *Vitam. Horm.* **20**, 199-249.

Randle, P. J., and Smith, G. H. (1958). Regulation of glucose uptake by muscle. *Biochem. J.* **70**, 490-500, 501-508.

Rennie, P., and Gliemann, J. (1981). Rapid down-regulation of insulin receptors in adipocytes: Artifact of the incubation buffer. *Biochem. Biophys. Res. Commun.* **102**, 824-831.

Rinaldini, L. M. (1959). An improved method for the isolation and quantitative cultivation of embryonic cells. *Exp. Cell Res.* **16**, 477-505.

Robinson, F. W., Blevins, T. L., Suzuki, K., and Kono, T. (1982). An improved method of reconstitution of adipocyte glucose transport activity. *Anal. Biochem.* **121**, 10-19.

Rodbell, M. (1964). Metabolism of isolated fat cells. *J. Biol. Chem.* **239**, 375-380.

Rodbell, M. (1966). Metabolism of isolated fat cells. II. The similar effects of phospholipase C and of insulin on glucose and amino acid metabolism. *J. Biol. Chem.* **241**, 130-139.

Rosenthal, J. W., and Fain, J. N. (1971). Insulin-like effect of clostridial phospholipase C, neuraminidase, and other bacterial factors on brown fat cells. *J. Biol. Chem.* **246**, 5888-5895.

Saggerson, E. D., Sooranna, S. R., and Evans, C. J. (1976). Insulin-like actions of nickel and other transition-metal ions in rat fat cells. *Biochem. J.* **154**, 349-357.

Saltiel, A. R. (1987). Insulin generates an enzyme modulator from hepatic plasma membranes: Regulation of cAMP phosphodiesterase, pyruvate dehydrogenase, and adenylate cyclase. *Endocrinology* **120**, 967–972.

Sasaki, K., Cripe, T. P., Koch, S. R., Andreone, T. L., Petersen, D. D., Beale, E. G., and Granner, D. K. (1984). Multihormonal regulation of phosphoenolpyruvate carboxykinase gene transcription. *J. Biol. Chem.* **259**, 15242–15251.

Shibata, Y., Flanagan, J. E., Smith, M. M., Robinson, F. W., and Kono, T. (1987). Sedimentation characteristics of vesicles associated with insulin-sensitive intracellular glucose transporter from rat adipocytes. *Biochim. Biophys. Acta* **902**, 154–158.

Simpson, I. A., and Cushman, S. W. (1986). Hormonal regulation of mammalian glucose transport. *Annu. Rev. Biochem.* **55**, 1059–1089.

Simpson, I. A., and Hedo. J. A. (1984). Insulin receptor phosphorylation may not be a prerequisite for acute insulin action. *Science* **223**, 1301–1304.

Smith, M. M., Robinson, F. W., Watanabe, T.. and Kono, T. (1984). Partial characterization of the glucose transport activity in the Golgi-rich fraction of fat cells. *Biochim. Biophys. Acta* **775**, 121–128.

Smith, R. M., and Jarett, L. (1983). Quantitative ultrastructural analysis of receptor-mediated insulin uptake into adipocytes. *J. Cell. Physiol.* **115**, 199–207.

Smith, U., Kuroda, M., and Simpson, I. A. (1984). Counter-regulation of insulin-stimulated glucose transport by catecholamines in the isolated rat adipose cell. *J. Biol. Chem.* **259**, 8758–8763.

Sonne, O., Gliemann, J., and Linde, S. (1981). Effect of pH on binding kinetics and biological effect of insulin in rat adipocytes. *J. Biol. Chem.* **256**, 6250–6254.

Stadie, W. C., Haugaard, N., and Vaughan, M. (1952). Studies of insulin binding with isotopically labeled insulin. *J. Biol. Chem.* **199**, 729–739.

Suzuki, K. (1987). Mechanism of glucose transport in adipocytes. *Folia Endocrinol. Jpn.* **63**, 389.

Suzuki, K., and Kono, T. (1979). Internalization of degradation of fat cell-bound insulin. *J. Biol. Chem.* **254**, 9786–9794.

Suzuki, K., and Kono, T. (1980). Evidence that insulin causes translocation of glucose transport activity to the plasma membrane from an intracellular storage site. *Proc. Natl. Acad. Sci. U.S.A.* **77**, 2542–2545.

Taylor, L. P., and Holman, G. D. (1981). Symmetrical kinetic parameters for 3-O-methyl-D-glucose transport in adipocytes in the presence and in the absence of insulin. *Biochim. Biophys. Acta* **642**, 325–335.

Terris, S., and Steiner, D. F. (1976). Retention and degradation of ^{125}I-insulin by perfused livers from diabetic rats. *J. Clin. Invest.* **57**, 885–896.

Toyoda, N., Robinson, F. W., Smith, M. M., Flanagan, J. E., and Kono, T. (1986). Apparent translocation of glucose transport activity in rat epididymal adipocytes by insulin-like effects of high pH or hyperosmolarity. *J. Biol. Chem.* **261**, 2117–2122.

Toyoda, N., Flanagan, J. E., and Kono, T. (1987). Reassessment of insulin effects on the V_{max} and K_m values of hexose transport in isolated rat epididymal adipocytes. *J. Biol. Chem.* **262**, 2737–2745.

Trischitta, V., Vigneri, R., Roth. R. A., and Goldfine, I. D. (1984). ATP and other nucleoside triphosphates inhibit the binding of insulin to its receptor. *Metabolism* **33**, 577–581.

Ueda, M., Robinson, F. W., Smith, M. M., and Kono, T. (1984). Effects of divalent cations on the regulation of insulin-sensitive glucose transport and cAMP phosphodiesterase in adipocytes. *J. Biol. Chem.* **259**, 9520–9525.

Ueda, M., Robinson, F. W., Smith, M. M., and Kono, T. (1985). Effects of monensin on insulin processing in adipocytes. *J. Biol. Chem.* **260**, 3941–3946.

Ullrich, A., Bell, J. R., Chen, E. Y., Herrera, R., Petruzzelli, L. M., Dull, T. J., Gray, A., Coussens, L., Liao, Y.-C., Tsubokawa, M., Mason, A., Seeburg, P. H., Grunfeld, C., Rosen, O. M., and Ramachandran, J. (1985). Human insulin receptor and its relationship to the tyrosine kinase family of oncogenes. *Nature (London)* **313**, 756–761.

Vallar, L., Biden, T. J., and Wollheim, C. B. (1987). Guanine nucleotides induce Ca^{2+}-independent insulin secretion from permeabilized RINm5F cells. *J. Biol. Chem.* **262**, 5049–5056.

Vega, F. V., and Kono, T. (1978). Effects of insulin on the uptake of D-galactose by isolated rat epididymal fat cells. *Biochim. Biophys. Acta* **512**, 221–222.

Vega, F. V., and Kono, T. (1979). Sugar transport in fat cells: Effects of mechanical agitation, cell-bound insulin, and temperature. *Arch. Biochem. Biophys.* **192**, 120–127.

Vega, F. V., Key, R. J., Jordan, J. E., and Kono, T. (1980). Reversal of insulin effects in fat cells may require energy for deactivation of glucose transport, but not for deactivation of phosphodiesterase. *Arch. Biochem. Biophys.* **203**, 167–173.

Vidaver, G. A. (1966). Inhibition of parallel flux and augmentation of counter flux shown by transport models not involving a mobile carrier. *J. Theor. Biol.* **10**, 301–306.

Villar-Palasi, C., and Larner, J. (1961). Insulin treatment and increased UDP-glycogen transglucosylase activity in muscle. *Arch. Biochem. Biophys.* **94**, 436–442.

Vinten, J. (1984). Accelerated net efflux of 3-O-methylglucose in isolated fat cells. *Biochim. Biophys. Acta* **772**, 244–250.

Vinten, J., Gliemann, J., and Østerlind, K. (1976). Exchange of 3-O-methylglucose in isolated fat cells. *J. Biol. Chem.* **251**, 794–800.

Wallberg-Henriksson, H., and Holloszy, J. O. (1985). Activation of glucose transport in diabetic muscle: Responses to contraction and insulin. *Am. J. Physiol.* **249**, C233–C237.

Wardzala, L. J., and Jeanrenaud, B. (1981). Potential mechanism of insulin action on glucose transport in the isolated rat diaphragm. *J. Biol. Chem.* **256**, 7090–7093.

Wardzala, L. J., Simpson, I. A., Rechler, M. M., and Cushman, S. W. (1984). Potential mechanism of the stimulatory action of insulin on insulin-like growth factor II binding to the isolated rat adipose cell. *J. Biol. Chem.* **259**, 8378–8383.

Watanabe, T., Smith, M. M., Robinson, F. W., and Kono, T. (1984). Insulin action on glucose transport in cardiac muscle. *J. Biol. Chem.* **259**, 13117–13122.

Weber, H. W., Chung, F.-Z., Day, K., and Appleman, M. M. (1987). Insulin stimulation of cAMP phosphodiesterase is independent from the G-protein pathways involved in adenylate cyclase regulation. *J. Cyclic Nucleotide Protein Phosphorylat. Res.* **11**, 345–354.

Wheeler, T. J., and Hinkle, P. C. (1985). The glucose transporter of mammalian cells. *Annu. Rev. Physiol.* **47**, 503–517.

Wheeler, T. J., Simpson, I. A., Sogin, D. C., Hinkle, P. C., and Cushman, S. W. (1982). Detection of the rat adipose cell glucose transporter with antibody against the human red cell glucose transporter. *Biochem. Biophys. Res. Commun.* **105**, 89–95.

Whitesell, R. R., and Abumrad, N. A. (1985). Increased affinity predominates in insulin stimulation of glucose transport in the adipocyte. *J. Biol. Chem.* **260**, 2894–2899.

Whitesell, R. R., and Gliemann, J. (1979). Kinetic parameters of transport of 3-O-methylglucose and glucose in adipocytes. *J. Biol. Chem.* **254**, 5276–5283.

Winegrad, A. I., and Renold, A. E. (1958). Studies on rat adipose tissue *in vitro*. *J. Biol. Chem.* **233**, 267–272.

Witters, L. A., Vater, C. A., and Lienhard, G. E. (1985). Phosphorylation of the glucose transporter *in vitro* and *in vivo* by protein kinase C. *Nature (London)* **315**, 777–778.

Wohltmann, H. J., and Narahara, H. T. (1967). Inability of anti-insulin serum to neutralize insulin after the hormone has become bound to muscle. *Biochim. Biophys. Acta* **135**, 173–175.

Yalow, R. S., and Berson. S. A. (1960). Immunoassay of endogenous plasma insulin in man. *J. Clin. Invest.* **39**, 1157–1175.

Zinman, B., and Hollenberg, C. H. (1974). Effect of insulin and lipolytic agents on rat adipocyte low K_m cAMP phosphodiesterase. *J. Biol. Chem.* **249**, 2182–2187.

NOTE ADDED IN PROOF. Several important observations were reported since the manuscript was submitted to the publisher.

G. E. Lienhard found that the anti-glucose transporter antibody, which was active to the erythrocyte transporter (see Section V), did not cross-react with the muscle transporter. (Orally presented at the Glucose Transport Symposium in the 72nd Federation Meeting held at Las Vegas, Nevada, on May 4, 1988.)

H. F. Lodish, B. Thorens, and Z.-Q. Cheng reported that the glucose transporter shown in Fig. 1 (in Section V) was a low-K_m transporter typically present in erythrocytes and certain other cell types, and that a different, high-K_m transporter exists in liver and several other tissues. (Orally presented at the Glucose Transport Symposium in the 72nd Federation Meeting held at Las Vegas, Nevada, on May 4, 1988.)

Blok *et al.* localized intracellular glucose transporters at the trans side of the Golgi apparatus in 3T3-L1 adipocytes by means of immunocytochemistry. [Blok, J. Gibbs, E. M., Lienhard, G. E., Slot, J. W., and Geuze, H. J. (1988). Insulin-induced translocation of glucose transporters from post-Golgi compartments to the plasma membrane of 3T3-L1 adipocytes. *J. Cell Biol.* **106**, 69–76.]

Calcium Channels

HARTMUT GLOSSMANN AND JÖRG STRIESSNIG

Institut für Biochemische Pharmakologie
A-6020 Innsbruck, Austria

I. INTRODUCTION

In this article we focus on voltage-dependent calcium channels in plasma membranes from mammalian electrically excitable cells. We will treat calcium channel drugs as structural and functional tools. No attempt is made to cover their clinical aspects. Some electrophysiological studies are presented but we do not focus on the role of calcium channels in the regulation of cellular activity. The vertebrate skeletal muscle calcium channel was discovered only recently (see Almers et al., 1985). Unexpectedly, progress with respect to purification, amino acid sequence data, and reconstitution was first achieved here. The physiological significance of these channels is unknown, but a surprisingly large body of evidence already suggests that polypeptides (which elsewhere serve as components of calcium channels) are important in the excitation–contraction coupling steps of vertebrate skeletal muscle. Another area of current interest is direct control of calcium channel function by neurotransmitter or hormone receptors and guanine nucleotide binding proteins. Ion and drug receptor binding sites, structural characterization of the skeletal muscle channel, modulation of channel function by drugs or extracellular signals, and reconstitution will therefore be our main themes. Calcium channels are among the Methuselahs of ion channels—perhaps older than the voltage-dependent sodium channel (Hille, 1984). The diversity as well as the complexity of the physiological control and pharmacological modulation of the calcium channel family only recently became apparent. Being pharmacologists our views are certainly biased, but we hope the reader will not quote Ezekiel, 13,3: "Woe to the foolish prophets who follow their own spirit and have seen nothing."

BACKGROUND

In early 1981 we were approached by the Bayer Company to characterize putative receptors for several 1,4-dihydropyridines. We worked with (±)-[^{3}H]nitrendipine first and chose a crude membrane preparation from guinea pig heart for initial binding studies. A Tris buffer (containing 150 mM NaCl and 1 mM Ca^{2+}) and a temperature of 37°C was selected. Nonspecific binding was defined as that not inhibited by 20 μM nitrendipine. Under these conditions the ligand labeled two sites with vastly different affinities and B_{max} values (B_{max} is the maximal number of binding sites.) In competitive inhibition studies high affinity binding was stereoselective but low affinity binding was not (Bellemann et al., 1981). Among the different unlabeled 1,4-dihydropyridines (tested under a secrecy agreement) one was highly selective for the high affinity (channel-linked) receptor and did not compete with (±)-[^{3}H]nitrendipine binding to the low affinity, high B_{max} sites. Two years later the structure and pharmacological activity of this "selective" 1,4-dihydropyridine (Bay K 8644) was revealed (Schramm et al., 1983), and by 1987 we had employed Bay K 8644 to differentiate channel-linked receptors in heart from (abundant) low affinity sites in photolabeling experiments with $(-)$-[^{3}H]azidopine (Ferry et al., 1987).

Having available probes potentially useful for such studies, we looked for negative controls as well (saturable binding sites were found by us in many tissues) to make the message airtight. Guinea pig skeletal muscle, human red blood cell ghosts, and highly purified *Electrophorus electricus* membranes were selected at tissues presumably lacking calcium channels. There had been no reports of significant pharmacological actions of 1,4-dihydropyridines on these tissues. To our surprise, two membranes (from skeletal muscle and the electric organ of *Electrophorus electricus*) showed the highest receptor density of all tissues investigated, at least with $(\pm)$-[^{3}H]nimodipine as radiolabel. We carefully avoided mentioning them in our first review (Glossmann et al., 1982), but decided to leave the human red blood cell ghost data in one of the tables. The ghost was overlooked and the richest source of discovered calcium channel drug receptors found anywhere (Fosset et al., 1983). Only years later was it found that it is the $(+)$ enantiomer from racemic [^{3}H]nimodipine that binds to the human erythrocyte membrane. That site is also a true pharmacological receptor, but for the nucleoside carrier (Striessnig et al., 1985). The binding of $(+)$-[^{3}H]nimodipine is even regulated allosterically by phenylalkylamines!

Since skeletal muscle is the richest source of channel drug receptors, we continued working on this tissue and published the first report on it in 1982 (Ferry and Glossmann, 1982b). It was a wise decision to continue with skeletal muscle from guinea pig instead of *Electrophorus electricus* since [^{3}H]nimodipine almost exclusively binds to nucleoside carriers in these latter membranes. We exemplify in Fig. 1 the hazard of relying solely on ligand binding.

One of the more specific ligands among the 1,4-dihydropyridine series is PN 200-110. The latter, a racemic compound in radiolabeled form (with very low specific activity), was given to us by Sandoz. Using a greater assay volume (1 ml) we succeeded, with guinea pig skeletal muscle membranes, in utilizing this ligand in calcium channel research (Ferry et al., 1983a). Later better and more novel tools were developed. With the help of the Goedecke Company we introduced $(+)$-cis-[^{3}H]diltiazem (Glossmann et al., 1983a) and with pharmacologists and chemists from Knoll AG developed $(-)$-[^{3}H]desmethoxyverapamil (Ferry et al., 1984a; Goll et al., 1984a) as well as the novel arylazide phenylalkylamine [N-methyl-^{3}H]LU 49888 (Striessnig et al., 1987). [^{3}H]Azidopine (Ferry et al., 1984b) is (as the phenylalkylamine aryla-

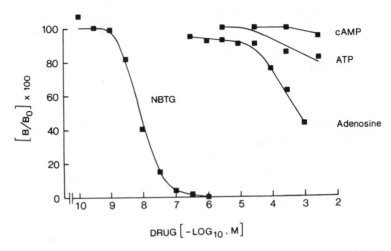

FIG. 1. Labeled calcium channel drugs do not bind only to calcium channels. A membrane preparation (0.08 mg of protein in 0.25 ml of 50 mM Tris–HCl buffer) from the electric organ of *Electrophorus electricus* (obtained from Drs. Prinz and Maelicke) was incubated at 25°C for 60 minutes with 2.6 nM ($\pm$)-[^{3}H]nimodipine. At the end of the incubation, membrane-bound ligand was separated from unbound ligand by (ice-cold) dilution and filtration as described (Glossmann and Ferry, 1985). B_0 is the "specific" binding (total bound ligand minus ligand bound in the presence of 3 μM unlabeled nimodipine), and B is specific binding in the presence of other ligands. The total binding per tube was 6990 $\pm$ 214 dpm; the nonspecific binding 527 $\pm$ 39 dpm. Nitrobenzylthioguanosine (NBTG), a potent nucleoside carrier transport inhibitor, competes with an IC$_{50}$ value of 8 nM at the nimodipine-labeled site. As adenosine (and inosine, not shown) also inhibits, ($\pm$)-[^{3}H]nimodipine labels mainly 1,4-dihydropyridine sites coupled to adenosine carriers and not calcium channel-linked receptors. (+)Nimodipine (IC$_{50}$ value 54 nM) was 8 times more potent than ($-$)nimodipine (IC$_{50}$ value 400 nM) in competitive inhibition studies, which is opposite to the stereoselectivity of the calcium channel but exactly the same as found for the nucleoside carrier on human red blood cell ghosts (Striessnig *et al.*, 1985).

zide) useful for identifying the drug receptor-carrying subunit of the L-type channel in several tissues and purified preparations, and chemists and pharmacologists from the Bayer Company were extremely helpful in this project.

The message is quite clear; the tools to characterize and isolate the L-type calcium channel came exclusively from drug companies. Nature apparently did not regard this ionic pore (with some exceptions) as an important target for toxins, and most of the ligands are available commercially to anyone. This contrasts with the situation for other ionic channels, where (some) tools became generally available only after the developers utilized them to advantage.

One or more subunits of the L-type calcium channels have now been cloned (Tanabe *et al.,* 1987; A. Schwartz, personal communication). Only 6 years passed from the first binding experiment to elucidation of the primary structure.

II. DIFFERENT TYPES OF CALCIUM CHANNELS

The plasma membrane of excitable cells contains several types of calcium channels. They are distinguished by voltage dependence, unitary conductance, selectivity, and, perhaps most importantly, by pharmacology. In many cells multiple channel types have been observed, but there are also some membranes (e.g., of the adrenal chromaffin cell) where only one type appears to exist.

The different types (termed L, T, and N) have been well characterized, especially in heart (Bean, 1985) and neuronal tissue. The L type (L = long lasting) is predominant in heart and smooth muscle cells; the L, T and N types are found in nerve cells (Bean, 1985; Bean *et al.,* 1986; Reuter *et al.,* 1986; Nilius *et al.,* 1986; McCleskey *et al.,* 1986, and references cited therein). T (transient) channels require a much more negative holding potential for activation by depolarizing voltage steps. At membrane voltages above -40 mV they are inactivated. In heart, and with Ba^{2+} as charge carrier, the single channel conductance of T is only one-third that of the L type (7.5 versus 25 pS) (Reuter *et al.,* 1986). The L type shows higher permeability for Ba^{2+} whereas the T type passes Ba^{2+} and Ca^{2+} equally well. The T channel opens very early at the beginning of a voltage step and inactivates rapidly, whereas the L channel shows slow activating and even slower inactivating behavior. In some instances the T-channel-mediated currents are referred to as "fast" or "tiny" Ca^{2+} currents and L-channel-mediated currents as "slow" and "large" currents. The N type (from neither L nor T) was first described in dorsal root ganglion neurons (Nowycky *et al.,* 1985a). The N and T types are insensitive to 1,4-dihydropyridine channel agonists and antagonists, whereas the L-type channel is activated by 1,4-dihydropyridine agonists and blocked by antagonists; the neuronal channel is the least sensitive (McCleskey *et al.,* 1986). Another interesting feature of the L-type channel (e.g., from heart) is its rapid disappearance from excised membrane patches (indicating the dependence of channel activity on intracellular metabolism) whereas the T channel survives.

A peptide toxin from the marine snail *Conus geographus,* ω-CgTx (ω-conotoxin GVIA), persistently blocks N and L channels in chick dorsal root ganglion cells and rat sympathetic neurons; in rat hippocampal cells, the T channel (when present) is only transiently blocked

(McCleskey *et al.*, 1986, 1987). L (or T) channels from muscle preparations (guinea pig ventricle, frog atrium or ventricle, chick myotubes, and rabbit ear artery smooth muscle) are not blocked. Thus, based on the results with this neurotoxin, the L-type channels are a subdividable set. Those in heart and in skeletal and smooth muscle are apparently insensitive whereas neuronal L *and* N channels are blocked. The blockade of both N and L channels in neurons suggests that there is a common structural component (toxin binding site) on both channel types. The L channel (1,4-dihydropyridine sensitive) is preferentially localized in neuronal cell bodies, whereas the ω-CgTx-sensitive N-type channel (1,4-dihydropyridine insensitive) appears to be largely confined to nerve terminals (Reynolds *et al.*, 1986a; Miller, 1987). Differences among gating behavior of L-type calcium channels in heart, chromaffin cells, or skeletal muscle exist (Hille, 1984; Cognard *et al.*, 1986a, and references cites therein).

Considering the multiple types of calcium channels with different conductances, activating and inactivating kinetics, drug and toxin sensitivity, and sensitivity to modulation (by neurotransmitter or hormone receptors either directly or via second messengers), one wonders if nature indeed created completely distinct polypeptide chains for L, T, and N channels and their respective subclasses. The complicated, intriguing mechanism by which selectivity and fast ion flux of the calcium channels is achieved suggests that at least this principle is conserved for all types within one or two polypeptide chains. The recent finding of diverse conductance levels in reconstituted highly purified calcium channel preparations (Glossmann *et al.*, 1987a; Hymel *et al.*, 1988a,b,c; Smith *et al.*, 1987) suggests that channel proteins associate to function as synchronously switching units in the membrane.

Currently we can characterize calcium channels biochemically only by specificity of drug binding. This must be kept in mind in discussions on channel "subtype" in the following sections even though the "L-type" designation was developed on electrophysiological criteria. Perhaps, by following one course one can uncover a prototype for all calcium channels.

III. L-TYPE CALCIUM CHANNELS

A. ELECTROPHYSIOLOGY

Calcium channels were initially studied by recording macroscopic currents in multicellular preparations. These studies were later extended to single cell preparations and to the investigation of elementary currents through single calcium channels employing the patch clamp technique (see Sakman and Neher, 1983). The principle of this technique is as follows: A membrane patch is drawn into the tiny mouth of a glass pipet (the internal diameter of the tip is around 2.5 μm). The close contact between the membrane and the pipet guarantees a high resistance ($>10^{10}$ ohm) between the interior of the pipet and the surrounding medium. This is termed a "gigaohmseal" or "gigaseal." The pipet can be used (after applying stronger negative pressure or current oscillations) to destroy the patch and measure whole cell currents. Cells may be dialyzed with a variety of solutions to decrease, e.g., the free internal Ca^{2+} concentration with EGTA. Such experimental conditions have allowed studies on the inactivation process of the calcium channels. Whereas whole cell currents represent the sum of many thousands of channels, the elementary currents in a membrane patch are believed to represent "single" channel activities. In turn, the pooled single channel data are then tested to describe the kinetics of all calcium channels evaluated from whole cell Ca^{2+} currents. We describe this briefly for a well studied system, namely, the L channel in heart cells, and discuss different models for calcium channel behavior.

1. *The Subset Model*

In single calcium channel recordings the amplitude of the elementary current depends on the membrane potential, the divalent charge carrier, and its concentration. Elementary currents of heart calcium channels with 10 mM Ca^{2+} in the external solution are of the order of 0.07 pA and are too small to be detected. With 90 mM Ba^{2+}, however, they amount to 1 pA when a voltage step from resting potential to +10 mV is applied to open the channel. A word of caution is necessary here. Although electrophysiology has reached the state of the art, especially with the patch clamp technique, which may be at its climax, some pharmacologists and biochemists feel that "electrotoxicology" would be a more appropriate term. Under many of the conditions used by electrophysiologists the biochemist would find no binding of labeled ligand to calcium channels in depolarized membrane fragments. Some batches of HEPES buffer contain impurities which reversibly inhibit the binding of phenylalkylamines or 1,4-dihydropyridines, and 100 mM Ba^{2+} completely blocks the binding of labeled phenylalkylamines to their channel-linked receptors (see Section V,B).

A single heart calcium channel (90 mM Ba^{2+} as charge carrier, depolarization every 2 seconds by 75 mV, duration of voltage step 0.3 seconds) displays two types of current records: sweeps without any single channel opening (blank sweeps) and traces with calcium channel activity. Here, at low time resolution, long periods of activity ("clusters") are interrupted by periods of quiescence. Clusters again consist of groups of openings (termed "bursts") separated by shut periods which are shorter than the quiescent periods between clusters. If the time resolution is very high, bursts are resolved into very short openings and closings. A histogram (vide infra) is a convenient way to derive the mean time constants for shut and open times. The number of components from the exponential distribution is related to the number of channel states. The mean lifetime of a given state is equal to the inverse of the sum of transition rates that lead away from their state (Trautwein and Cavalie, 1985). Blank sweeps are believed to reflect a condition wherein the calcium channel is unavailable for opening and the single channel has a clear tendency to open at the beginning of the clamp pulse, followed by long periods of silence. Averaging a whole series yields "the ensemble mean current." Averaging of a very large number of single Ca^{2+} currents provides a macro ensemble mean current virtually identical to the whole cell Ca^{2+} current of the heart, a very satisfactory result (Cavalie et al., 1986).

This type of investigation (with "step" depolarization and repolarization) introduces a bias as the repolarization artificially terminates shut events of the channel without knowing the duration of such events. To this end, "steady" depolarization is used, and histograms for mean open times and mean closed times are obtained. The important result from these experiments is that the distribution of the open times can be fitted with a single exponential function and one time constant of 0.8 msecond. Long openings were rare and observed in only 2 out of 71 experiments (Cavalie et al., 1986).

The shut time histogram reveals that the data can only be fitted by the sum of two exponential terms with two time constants (0.4 and 2.1 mseconds). There are indications that additional shut events of even longer duration exist, suggesting the existence of at least three distinct closed states. Cavalie et al. (1986) summarized their findings in a model, shown in Fig. 2, encompassing only two closed states sufficient to fit all the experimental data.

In this model for the behavior of the heart calcium channel, two subsets of states exist. One subset (Q) comprises the long-lived shut states of the channel. The occupancy of the channel in the Q state generates, e.g., groups of blank records on consecutive and identical depolarizations. The Q state is the inactivated state of the channel. In general, this process of inactivation is either nearly absent or enhanced by calcium or depolarization, or is regulated by both, depend-

A

B

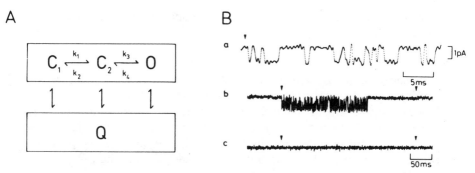

FIG. 2. The subset model of calcium channel function. (A) The two subsets are within boxes. C_1 and C_2 are the two closed states of the channel (there may be more), and O is the open, conducting state of the channel. The transition rates within this subset are fast. Subset Q comprises one or more long-lived shut states of the channel. Transitions between the two subsets are slow compared to those within upper subset (termed the B subset in the text). (B) The different transitions are exemplified with different time scales. In (a) behavior of a single heart calcium channel is shown. Immediately after depolarization (arrow) the channel opens (downward deflection); openings occur as bursts, and bursts are separated by silent periods corresponding to sojourn of the channel in C_1. The short closings within bursts correspond to sojourn in state C_2. After step depolarization (b) channel openings are grouped together as clusters of bursts which are spontaneously terminated although repolarization (arrow) has not occurred. Here the channel is in the inactivated state. In (c) the same channel cannot be opened despite depolarization (arrows), and a blank record is obtained. The model can easily incorporate the effects of channel activators or blockers and of dephosphorylation or phosphorylation: phosphorylation promotes transition from subset Q to subset B, Bay K 8644 favors the open state in subset B, etc. [From Cavalie et al. (1986), Pflügers Arch. 406, 241–258, with permission.]

ing on the system (see Horwitz, 1986, and references cited therein). In mammalian heart cells voltage-dependent inactivation and Ca^{2+}-dependent inactivation are observed. It is beyond the scope of this article to discuss the underlying mechanisms, but Ca^{2+}-dependent dephosphorylation is very likely one mechanism of inactivation, currently studied with purified, reconstituted calcium channels. In the inactivated Q state the channel is unavailable for opening.

The other subset of states (B) comprises channel states connected by fast transition rates. It includes the two closed states (C_1 and C_2) and the open state, O. The occupancy of the channel in C_2 produces short closings *during* bursts. The C_1 state represents closed periods *between* bursts. Thus, calcium channel behavior is characterized by "fast gating" within subset B and "slow gating" behavior between the two subsets. The prominent feature of the model is that the effects of calcium channel activators and blockers or modulation of channel behavior by phosphorylation and dephosphorylation can be easily integrated.

2. *The Mode Model*

In contrast to the model of calcium channel behavior derived by Trautwein and Cavalie (1985) and Cavalie *et al.* (1986), Hess and Tsien (1984) favor a "modal" behavior model of the cardiac calcium channel in the absence of drugs. In the model, shown in Fig. 3, the modes 1, 0, and 2 are differentiated by the pattern of channel activity in single channel recordings. In mode 0 (or null mode) the channel is unavailable for opening. in mode 1 brief openings are observed, and mode 2 is characterized by long lasting openings and very brief closings. The modal behavior hypothesis assumes that modes 1 and 2 are intrinsic forms of gating and that calcium channel activators such as Bay K 8644 favor mode 2 whereas a 1,4-dihydropyridine channel blocker stabilizes the channel in mode 0. The main difference between the subset and modal models is that the latter assumes mode 2 as a physiological

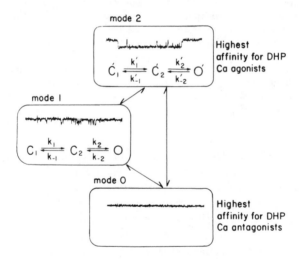

FIG. 3. The modal model of calcium channel function. The model is similar to the subset model with a major exception, namely, mode 2. Here it is assumed that very long opening times of the channel are a physiological set of states where sojourn in this mode is promoted by, e.g., 1, 4-dihydropyridine calcium channel agonists, and the transition to mode 0 is favored by calcium channel blockers. Rate constants among the modes (e.g., between mode 1 and 2 and mode 0) may be voltage dependent. The model illustrates that the inactivated (mode 0) state has the highest affinity for channel blockers. [From Hess and Tsien (1984), *Nature (London)* **311**, 538–544, with permission.]

set of states of the channel. The effects of β-adrenergic agonists are explained by modification of the rate constants in mode 1 and recruitment of (inactivated) channels from mode 0 to mode 1. Interestingly, with nitrendipine mixed effects were seen by Hess and Tsien (1984). Here an agonistlike effect (increase in the number of long openings) was accompanied by antagonist-promoted inactivation. This was interpreted (in pharmacological terms) as "partial" agonism. Mode 2 was also observed in chicken dorsal root ganglion cells, where the calcium channel agonist Bay K 8644 shifted the balance in favor of this subset of states (Nowycky et al., 1985b).

3. Extensions of the Modal Model

Kokubun et al. (1986) investigated calcium channels in adult rat heart cells with patch clamp techniques. They used the optical enantiomers of the benzoxadiazol 1,4-dihydropyridine 202-791 as tools. As outlined in Section IV,A, the $(+)$-(S) enantiomer is classified as a channel activator whereas the $(-)$-(R) enantiomer is a channel blocker. Findings with both enantiomers were interpreted within the mode model. The $(-)$-(R) enantiomer favored the 0 mode, the more depolarized the membrane was. However, at very low concentrations, (R) 202-791 increased the number of traces with long openings at negative holding potentials (promoting mode 2). $(+)$-(S) 202-791, which promoted mode 2 at negative holding potentials, had a clear blocking effect at holding potentials positive to -20 mV.

Use of the (S) and (R) enantiomers combined at resting membrane potentials increased activity of the calcium channel. This complicated interaction of the channel with the agonistic and antagonistic enantiomer, depending on holding potentials, was interpreted within an allosteric model supported by binding studies (see Section IV,F).

4. Blockade and Activation by Bay K 8644 May Have a Common Mechanism

The puzzling observation that the channel activators Bay K 8644 and $(+)$-(S)-202-791 can also block Ca^{2+} currents was investigated in more detail by Sanguinetti et al. (1986) with multicellular preparations (calf Purkinje fibers) and enzymatically dispersed single rat ventricle cells. They used a simple kinetic model for the calcium channel and examined how effects of Bay K 8644 at the macroscopic current level could be explained. For simplicity they assumed only three states of the channel: a resting state (R), an open (conducting) state (O), and

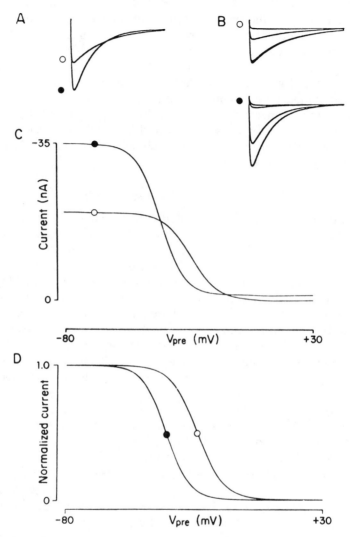

FIG. 4. Mechanism of action of 1,4-dihydropyridine channel activators—the rate constant sequential model. Here it is assumed that the channel has three states as in the subset model shown in Fig. 2, but for simplicity the two resting (closed) states are lumped together in one state, termed R. A transition from R to I (the inactivated state) is not allowed. Thus the channel can reach the resting state only by opening (state O); conversely, channels can only inactivate when opened. The effect of Bay K 8644 was assumed to be solely on the rate constant for leaving the open state to the resting state, namely, by decreasing it 10-fold. The rate constants for leaving the resting state and open state are voltage dependent. Thus, at −40 mV the rate constant for R → O is 0.00038, and at +20 mV it is 49.5 msecond^{-1} in the model calculation. In (A) the simulation of a membrane current without (open circle) and with Bay K 8644 is shown

an inactivated state (I). Voltage dependence was assigned only to the rate constants (K_{12} and K_{21}) between resting and open states:

$$R \underset{K_{21}}{\overset{K_{12}}{\rightleftharpoons}} O \underset{K_{32}}{\overset{K_{23}}{\rightleftharpoons}} I$$

In this sequential model (where no transition between R and I states is allowed) the mean open time is a function of $1/(K_{21} + K_{23})$. The mean open time is inversely proportional to the rate constant, K_{21}.

Sanguinetti et al. (1986) assumed that the only effect of the activating 1,4-dihydropyridine was to decrease K_{21} (e.g., by a factor 10). Simulation of calcium currents at different prepulses with or without Bay K 8644 shows that, for negative prepulses or holding potentials, currents are larger than in controls; at positive prepulses, however, they are smaller than controls. Thus, "the dualistic" action of the 1,4-dihydropyridine agonist can be, at the macroscopic current level, adequately explained by decreasing one of the rate constants for leaving the open state (Fig. 4). The model of Sanguinetti et al. (despite its shortcomings, also discussed in detail) is a very attractive one because of its simplicity.

A more complicated model that accounts for the stimulatory effects of 1,4-dihydropyridine blockers (e.g., nitrendipine) was suggested by Brown et al. (1986). As mentioned above, the "paradoxical" or dualistic effects of nitrendipine were observed by Hess and Tsien (1984) and later studied in greater detail with optically pure enantiomers of the compound 202-791 (Kokubun et al., 1986). In principle, Brown et al. (1986) assume either voltage-dependent binding or two distinct high affinity sites (mediating stimulatory and inhibitory effects) and postulate that the 1,4-dihydropyridines act on at least three states (resting, open, and inactivated). They studied the effects of (racemic) nitrendipine and (racemic) Bay K 8644 on whole cell and single channel

(voltage steps from -60 to -8 mV). In (B) currents are simulated from resting potentials of -60, -40, -20, and -8 mV in the absence (open circle) and presence of drug (filled circle). As the resting potentials become more positive the simulated current decreases. In (C) the inactivation curves obtained from simulated peak currents are plotted as a function of prepulse voltage. Note that there is crossing over of the two curves and that the activating 1,4-dihydropyridine blocks the peak current at more positive resting potentials. In (D) the normalized curves (with respect to maximum currents in the absence and presence of Bay K 8644) are shown. Note that these normalized curves do not reveal the opposite action of the activating 1,4-dihydropyridine at more positive holding potentials. [From Sanguinetti et al. (1986), J. Gen. Physiol. 88, 369–392, with permission.]

Ca^{2+} currents on single myocytes from guinea pig ventricle. Nitrendipine increased the whole cell current at negative holding potentials at -90 mV or more. At these holding potentials, the calcium channels are highly likely to be in the resting state. The concentration–response curve was well described with the two-site model (EC_{50} values 1 nM and 1.4 μM, respectively). At membrane potentials of -30 mV or less, nitrendipine inhibited according to a single-site model (IC_{50} value of 1.5 nM). At intermediate holding potentials mixed effects were seen. In contrast to the results of Sanguinetti et al. (1986), no inhibitory effects of Bay K 8644 were observed. When Bay K 8644 effects were studied at a holding potential of -30 mV the concentration–response curve was biphasic (EC_{50} values at 3 nM and 0.9 μM), but at holding potentials between -120 and -30 mV the results could be fitted with a single-site model. Brown et al. (1986) suggested that the stimulatory actions of the calcium channel blocker nitrendipine were produced by binding to a (nanomolar K_D) site on the resting state channel; the same site with similar affinity (at the conformationally distinct inactivated state) mediated inhibition.

A possible clue to the variable (and sometimes overlooked) "agonistic" effects of Ca^{2+} antagonists and "antagonistic" actions of the channel activators comes from whole cell patch clamp experiments with cultured dorsal root ganglion neurons (Scott and Dolphin, 1987). Here, GTPγS (a nonhydrolyzable analog of GTP) influenced the cellular response to gallopamil, nifedipine, and (+)-cis-diltiazem. Guanosine 5'-O-3-thiotriphosphate (GTPγS) causes persistent activation of guanine nucleotide binding proteins (G- or N-proteins) involved in signal transfer of hormone and neurotransmitter receptors. When the internally applied GTP analog was present at 0.5 mM, Ca^{2+} currents (recorded with Ba^{2+} as charge carrier) at low holding potentials (e.g., -80 mV) were greatly (and paradoxically) enhanced by the calcium channel blockers. Pretreatment with pertussis toxin [which ADP ribosylated the α chains of G_i (N_i) and G_o (N_o) and inactivated these GTP-binding proteins] prevented the nucleotide effect (see Section III,C). The results support an association of an activated GTP-binding protein (presumably G_i or G_o) with the resting state of the neuronal calcium channel. The resting state is favored by hyperpolarization and, in turn, facilitates the "agonistic" action of the channel blockers. As mentioned later (see Section III,C), there is some evidence (Yatani et al., 1987) for the direct regulation of cardiac calcium channels by another guanine nucleotide binding protein (N_s or G_s).

Thus, it seems that, next to the membrane potential, guanine nucleotide binding proteins (activated physiologically by hormone or neurotransmitter receptors), phosphorylation/dephosphorylation, and, last but not least, e.g., the steric configuration of a 1,4-dihydropyridine determine whether the channel will be more likely to be open or inactivated. The "two-subset" model of Cavalie et al. (1986), the schemes of Sanguinetti et al. (1986) and Brown et al. (1986), or the mode model (Hess and Tsien, 1984) discussed above are illustrative but still inadequate to account fully for the extremely complex physiological and drug-modulated behavior of L-type calcium channels.

5. The Action of Channel Drugs May Be Use or/and Voltage Dependent

Differences, sometimes by orders of magnitude, between dissociation constants for calcium channel drugs obtained with membranes and those found in classic experiments, pharmacological or electrophysiological, are an enigma. There are, however, vastly different conditions between electrophysiological and biochemical experiments. The conditions for the latter are almost always directed to facilitate high affinity binding. Divalent cations and chelators in the 0.1 M range (often employed by electrophysiologists) would drastically impair the phenylalkylamine or 1,4-dihydropyridine high affinity interaction. Also different are the predominantly use-dependent mechanisms (McDonald et al., 1984; Ehara and Kaufmann, 1978; Pelzer et al., 1982; Lee and Tsien, 1983) by which the phenylalkylamines and the benzothiazepine, (+)-cis-diltiazem, block the L-type calcium channel and the voltage-dependent mechanisms of 1,4-dihydropyridine effects (Sanguinetti and Kass, 1984; Bean, 1984; Cognard et al., 1986; Kokubun et al., 1986; Sanguinetti et al., 1986; Bean et al., 1986). These discrepancies have been at least partially resolved; blocking constants have been now observed in electrophysiological experiments that agree quite well with those obtained in equilibrium binding assays.

6. Opposite Action for Agonistic and Antagonistic 1,4-Dihydropyridines—Molecular Basis

The surprising finding that the (R)- and (S)-configurated enantiomers of chiral 1,4-dihydropyridines (lacking one ester group) such as Bay K 8644 or 202-791 have opposite actions on calcium channels (agonistic or antagonistic, depending on membrane potential) has puzzled pharmacologists and electrophysiologists for some time. A novel approach by Höltje and Marrer (1987) based on force field and quantum calculations has yielded a possible explanation. The conformational features of 1,4-dihydropyridines (Langs and Triggle, 1985) are best represented by the "boat model" (Langs and Triggle, 1984) wherein the 1,4-dihydropyridine ring exists in a flattened boat conformation with the phenyl substituent positioned on the bowsprit side above the boat in a flagpole orientation.

Höltje and Marrer (1987) examined the molecules oriented in such a way that the 1,4-dihydropyridine ring lay in the $X-Y$ plane and the aromatic system pointed in the direction of positive Z axis. Agonists carry the space-consuming ester groups on the "right" side of the ring; the non-ester groups are found on the "left" side. Antagonistic enantiomers present the ester substituents on the "left." In this area of space significant potential differences are revealed between channel activators and blockers: agonists show a strong negative molecular potential, antagonists, a positive potential.

Opposite electrostatic fields of the agonistic and antagonistic 1,4-dihydropyridines will therefore influence the potential of the receptor protein in different manners. The amino acid tryptophan was then used as a simplified receptor model, and the influence of both agonists and antagonists on the amino acid examined. It was found that the electrostatic potential of tryptophan is influenced directly by the agonistic or antagonistic 1,4-dihydropyridines. Thus agonists and antagonists within the 1,4-dihydropyridine series most likely induce opposite electrostatic potentials in the region of the receptor-carrying component of the calcium channel. As the receptor domain is intimately coupled to the Ca^{2+} binding sites (see Section V) and to the gating mechanism, 1,4-dihydropyridines may change the energy profile of the channel (see Section III,B).

B. MECHANISM OF ION PERMEATION

In this section we deal with ionic selectivity and permeation of calcium channels. It is well known that certain divalent cations, e.g., Ba^{2+} or Sr^{2+}, completely replacing Ca^{2+}, are able to carry current through the ionic pore. Other divalent cations (Cd^{2+}, Co^{2+}, Ni^{2+}) block Ca^{2+} currents, and, depending on the tissue, Mn^{2+} and Mg^{2+} may or may not pass (Hagiwara and Byerly, 1981).

Other relevant findings are that currents carried by Ba^{2+} are readily blocked by Ca^{2+} and that monovalent cations (such as Na^+ and K^+) are excluded in the presence of micromolar Ca^{2+}. Ca^{2+} currents increase as the external Ca^{2+} concentration is increased. The latter phenomenon shows half-maximal saturation with respect to $[Ca^{2+}]_e$ around 10–14 mM. The paradox of micromolar Ca^{2+} blocking monovalent cation fluxes and the saturation of Ca^{2+} currents with millimolar K_D values has puzzled electrophysiologists for years. Kostyuk *et al.* (1983) investigated calcium channels in isolated neurons from the mollusc, *Helix pomatia*. In Ca^{2+}-free solutions (e.g., with 0.1–1 mM EDTA or EGTA) Na^+ would carry current through nifedipine- or D-600-blockable channels. Divalent cations (IC_{50} values in parenthesis), namely, Ca^{2+} (0.2 μM), Sr^{2+} (3.5 μM), Ba^{2+} (14 μM) and Mg^{2+} (60 μM), blocked this Na^+ current. The series of relative permeabilities for monovalents without Ca^{2+} (i.e., with EDTA or EGTA) was $P_{Na}:P_{Li}:P_a:P_b = 1.0:1.04:0.44:0.21$, where a stands for hydrazinium and b for hydroxylammonium.

Kostyuk *et al.* (1983) summarized their findings in a model, wherein one external ion-selecting filter ($pK_{Ca}:pK_{Sr}:pK_{Ba}:pK_{Mg}$ = 6.6:5.5:4.8:4.2), when freed from Ca^{2+}, converts the channel to a monovalent ion-passing pore. Because in their experiments micromolar Ca^{2+} reduced Na^+ currents in a voltage-independent manner, this high affinity site was located near the external surface and not within the pore.

In addition to this regulatory high affinity Ca^{2+} binding site, another ion-selecting filter (one-third of the way down in the channel) was postulated which had a pK for Ca^{2+} around 2.6–3.6. This filter was assumed to be the site of action of the blocking divalent and trivalent (e.g., La^{3+}) cations and helped to explain the external Ca^{2+} dependence of the Ca^{2+} current with millimolar K_D values. Hess and Tsien (1984) tested the hypothesis of Kostyuk *et al.* (1983) of a one-ion binding site within the channel with voltage-clamped, internally dialyzed heart cells from guinea pigs. With mixtures of Ca^{2+} and Ba^{2+} and $[Ca^{2+}]_o + [Ba^{2+}]_o$ held constant, the total current was not a monotonic function of the mole fraction, $[Ba^{2+}]_o/([Ba^{2+}]_o + [Ca^{2+}]_o)$, as predicted by the one-ion binding site model. Instead, the measured current showed a clear minimum. Such anomalous mole fraction behavior suggests that the channel contains more than one binding site occupied by permeant ions moving in single file (Hille and Schwarz, 1978). The authors concluded that the anomalous mole fraction effect reflected stronger affinity of the channel for Ca^{2+} than for Ba^{2+}. They proposed a model wherein the calcium channel is a multiion single file pore with at least two binding sites within the pore.

The mechanism of calcium channel ion passage was investigated independently on single frog skeletal muscle fibers by Almers and McCleskey (1984). With an external solution containing virtually no Ca^{2+} (pCa 7.2) and 32 mM Na^+, they found currents which were blocked by micromolar concentrations of Ca^{2+}, very similar to the results of Kostyuk *et al.* (1983) or Hess and Tsien (1984). They termed this current I_{ns} (ns = nonselective). Nifedipine (IC_{50} 0.5 μM) blocked both I_{ns} and the Ca^{2+} current. (+)-*cis*-Diltiazem also inhibited I_{ns} and Ca^{2+} inward current with an identical IC_{50} value, namely, 80 μM. From this and other evidence the authors concluded that I_{ns} and the Ca^{2+} inward current were passing through the same (calcium) channel. Frog skeletal muscle calcium channels also displayed the anomalous mole fraction behavior. On varying the external solution composition (0–10 mM Ba^{2+} and 10–0 mM Ca^{2+}, keeping the total ion concentration at 10 mM), the current was smallest in mixtures of the two ions. The authors next addressed the question how the calcium channel might preferentially transport Ca^{2+}, an ion that it binds with highest affinity.

The dissociation rate constant, K_2, for Ca^{2+} from one binding site within the pore, calculated assuming a K_D of 0.7 μM and an association rate constant (K_1) of 10^9 M^{-1} second^{-1}, was 700 second^{-1}, many orders of magnitude lower than the observed single channel fluxes of Ca^{2+}, i.e., in the range of 3×10^5 ions second^{-1}. The theoretical flux through a single such high affinity binding site channel was not in line with physiological observations. However, were the affinity of the ion to the second binding site reduced by occupation of the first site, the high flux rate could be explained. Among other variables the repulsion factor between ions is highly dependent on the valency. For two divalent cations simultaneously occupying the two sites, McCleskey and Almers (1985) calculated that the probability of one Ca^{2+} leaving its site would be increased by 20,000-fold on repulsion by the second Ca^{2+}. Their illustrative model is shown in Figs. 5 and 6.

The anomalous mole fraction behavior, the nonselectivity of the calcium channel in the absence of calcium, and the high flux rate are well explained by the model. Since other divalents such as Co^{2+}, Cd^{2+}, Ni^{2+}, and Mn^{2+} blocked I_{ns} and the calcium inward current approximately equally, Almers and McCleskey concluded that these ions would not compete for the two high affinity binding sites within the pore. Instead, an additional, low affinity ion binding site at the external face of the channel was postulated.

Hess *et al.* (1986) and Lansman *et al.* (1986) used single channel and whole cell recordings to study ion permeation through calcium channels in isolated guinea pig ventricular cells. The majority of the experiments were performed with addition of the calcium channel activator Bay K 8644. Their results are in general agreement with those of McCleskey and Almers (1985) with a notable exception: the site of action of blocking ions (e.g., Cd^{2+} or Ca^{2+}). Whereas in skeletal muscle fibers an additional low affinity external cation binding site had to

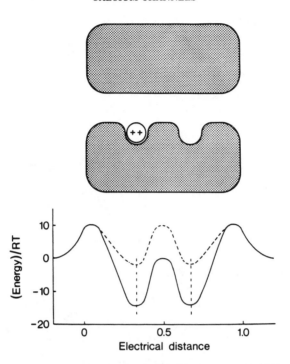

Fig. 5. Schematic view of the calcium channel. The top diagram depicts the channel with two ion binding sites, one of them complexed with a divalent cation; in the graph at bottom energy profiles (dashed line for Na$^+$, solid line for Ca^{2+}) are shown. In contrast to a channel where selectivity is governed by rejection (physicochemical obstacles at the mouths of the channel which sieve ions), the ion pore of the calcium channel is large (0.6-nm-diameter cations, such as tetramethylammonium, pass the skeletal muscle calcium channel; see McCleskey and Almers, 1985). The distance between the two ion binding sites was here assumed to be 1.05 nm, similar to troponin C. The energy profile (in J/mol, divided by RT) for an empty pore at zero membrane potential shows two (shallow) barriers at both ends and two deep (calcium) or shallow (sodium) wells. The abscissa gives the fraction of the transmembrane potential experienced at any given point. The channel is depicted as a symmetrical structure and can pass ions in both directions. [Reproduced (with minor modifications) from Almers *et al.* (1986), *Prog. Zool.* **33**, 61–73, with permission.]

be postulated for the blocking ions, Lansman *et al.* (1986) concluded that the block occurred at sites within the pore. Based on a careful analysis of reversal potentials and ion fluxes they reasoned that selectivity of the calcium channel could not be explained by rejection alone (for the selectivity by rejection hypothesis the selectivity filter is a critical narrowing of the pore). Instead, the ion with the highest affinity for the sites within the pore had the lowest mobility. The notable

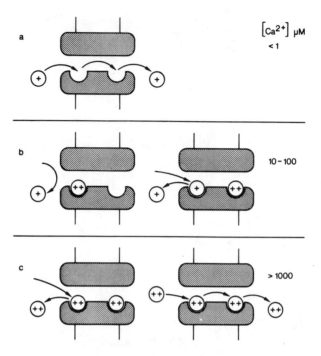

FIG. 6. How calcium channels pass ions. Calcium confers ion selectivity of ion transport of calcium channels by tight binding and high flux rates achieved by repulsion between two binding sites. Here the channel is depicted with permeant ions on the left (extracellular) side of the channel. In (a) Ca^{2+} is virtually absent, and a monovalent cation (e.g., Na^+) hopping from site to site is freely permeable. In (b) a (low) concentration of Ca^{2+} is present on the left side. Calcium is firmly bound and the monovalent ion is rejected or, alternatively, the second site (facing the cytosol) is occupied by Ca^{2+} and, although bound at the first site, Na^+ will not pass. This is a singly occupied pore where Ca^{2+} currents will be very low since Ca^{2+} may be moving back and forth between the sites but not escaping into the bulk fluid. In (c) Ca^{2+} is present at a concentration high enough to cause frequent double occupancy. Owing to electrostatic repulsion (shown on the left) Ca^{2+} finding the first site occupied will be rejected by the ion in the second site. In the other half of the cases (right side) the ion will escape to the cytoplasm. Flux is nearly proportional to the number of pores doubly occupied. [Reproduced (with minor modifications) from Almers *et al.* (1986), *Prog. Zool.* **33**, 61–73, with permission.]

exception was Mg^{2+}, which was a weak blocker and a poor permeator. This was attributed to the slowness of association between this cation and the pore, in agreement with the poor binding of this divalent cation to other Ca^{2+}-selective proteins, e.g., parvalbumin.

The classification of the ions as blockers or permeators of calcium channels derived by Lansman *et al.* (1986) is shown in Fig. 7. Although some discrepancies exist, the proposed mechanism of ion permeation

		Rapid Permeation	
		no	yes
Potent Block	yes	Cd La ultrastrong binding	Ba Sr Ca Mn strong binding
	no	Mg slow dehydra- tation	Li Na K Cs weak binding

FIG. 7. Ions may block or permeate the calcium channel. This diagram gives an overview of ions which block or pass the calcium channel. [From Lansman *et al.* (1986), *J. Gen. Physiol.* **88**, 321–347, with permission.]

through the calcium channel is supported by experiments with snail neuron (Byerley *et al.*, 1985), synaptosomal (Nelson, 1986) or skeletal muscle T-tubule calcium channels (Coronado and Affolter, 1986) incorporated into planar lipid bilayers, and mouse neoblastic G lymphocytes (Fukushima and Hagiwara, 1985).

Summary

The calcium channel appears to be unique among other ionic channels, as the physiological ion selectivity for Ca^{2+} is achieved by tight and selective binding of this divalent cation. High flux rates are achieved by repulsion of ions which dislodge each other by lowering the affinity. Ions move in succession through the pore. The properties of the Ca^{2+} binding sites resemble those commonly observed for high affinity Ca^{2+} binding proteins. The question of a common ancestor for the calcium channel and these proteins was raised (Lansman *et al.*, 1986). Amino acid sequence data have now revealed specific domains characteristic for Ca^{2+} binding sites on the cloned Ca^{2+} antagonist receptor protein (Tanabe *et al.*, 1987) similar to those on many Ca^{2+} binding proteins (Heizmann and Berchtold, 1987) or Ca^{2+}-dependent membrane binding proteins.

C. MODULATION OF FUNCTION

1. *β-Adrenergic Regulation of Cardiac Calcium Channels*

a. Electrophysiological Evidence. Evidence that the function of voltage-dependent calcium channels can be modulated by neurotransmitters or drugs was first obtained in cardiac muscle. The permeability of cardiac cell membranes to Ca^{2+} is significantly increased by catecholamines. This was first shown by ion flux studies and later by electrophysiological techniques. By means of the voltage clamp technique (for review, see Reuter, 1983) a catecholamine-induced increase

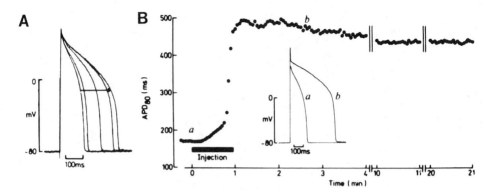

FIG. 8. Injection of catalytic subunit (CS) prolongs the action potential (AP) and increases its amplitude in isolated ventricular cells. (A) A microelectrode containing CS (9.6 mg/ml) was impaled into a myocyte, and CS was injected by pressure. The injection prolonged the AP from 130 to 315 mseconds. The arrow indicates the direction of change. (B) The same procedure as in (A) was used. The injection pressure was gradually increased from 2 to 5 bar during 60 seconds. Injection of CS prolonged the AP from 170 to 490 mseconds. The inset shows an AP before (a) and 1.5 minutes after (b) the injection of CS. A different cell from that used in (A) is shown. [From Osterrieder *et al.* (1982), *Nature (London)* **298**, 576–578, with permission.]

(higher level of the plateau and prolongation of the duration of the cardiac action potential) of the slow inward current largely carried by Ca^{2+} was demonstrated (Fig. 8). β-Adrenergic blockers antagonized the catecholamine effect. In patch clamp studies the nature of the catecholamine effect was extensively investigated. The size of elementary currents through single calcium channels was unaltered, but the probability of calcium channels entering the open state during depolarization was increased by β-adrenergic agonists, providing an increased mean current amplitude (Reuter, 1983; Cachelin *et al.*, 1983; Brum *et al.*, 1984). It should be emphasized that only cardiac L-type voltage-dependent calcium channels but not T-type channels are sensitive to β-adrenergic modulation.

Since the effect of catecholamines was mimicked by direct intracellular application of cAMP into cardiac fibers, the increase in calcium conductance appears to reflect receptor-controlled intermediate metabolic steps and not directly the consequence of adrenergic receptor occupation. Several studies have confirmed that β-adrenergic stimulation of adenylate cyclase (via the GTP-binding protein, G_s) leads to phosphorylation of the voltage-dependent calcium channel or a closely related regulatory protein, thereby altering channel function. Injection of the purified catalytic subunit (CS) of the cAMP-dependent protein kinase causes changes in the action potential identical to that caused by catecholamines (Osterrieder *et al.*, 1982; Brum *et al.*, 1983). The opposite effect is seen employing purified regulatory subunit (RS), which binds CS and thereby inhibits its phosphotransferase activity. Injection of RS causes depression of typical action potentials; this is reversible on addition of adrenaline to the bathing solution. The phosphorylation of voltage-dependent calcium channels does not seem to be necessary to make them available for opening during depolarization since injection of RS or inhibitors of protein kinase effects only small changes in calcium inward current without β-adrenergic stimulation (Osterrieder *et al.*, 1982). The contribution of other protein kinases to the regulation process is unlikely (Kameyama *et al.*, 1986).

Adrenergic receptor stimulation of voltage-dependent calcium channels is inhibited by muscarinic receptor stimulation, e.g., by acetylcholine. Muscarinic receptors in heart are negatively coupled to adenylate cyclase via G_i and inhibit adenylate cyclase activity. Certain reports (Breitwieser and Szabo, 1985; Hescheler *et al.*, 1986) provide convincing support for this mechanism. The antagonizing action of acetylcholine on action potentials is blocked by pertussis toxin. In contrast, Hartzell *et al.* (1986) suggested another pathway leading to a cAMP decrease. Their data point to a crucial role of the acetylcholine-induced cGMP increase leading to the activation of a cyclic nucleotide phosphodiesterase, a major receptor for cGMP in various cells hydrolyzing cAMP (Hartzell *et al.*, 1986). Their hypothesis is supported by the finding that cGMP has no effect on 8-bromo-cAMP-stimulated Ca^{2+} inward current. Accordingly, the phosphodiesterase inhibitor isobutylmethylxanthine, which inhibits the cGMP-stimulated phosphodiesterase activity, partially reduces or reverses the cAMP effect.

In contrast to cardiac calcium channels, K^+ conductance in cardiac atrial myocytes is increased by muscarinic agonists via a mechanism which does not appear to involve decreased levels of a second messenger (i.e., inhibition of adenylate cyclase activity). Direct coupling of this agonist effect to the potassium channel probably occurs via a pertussis toxin-sensitive G-protein termed G_k. Stimulation can be prevented by the toxin and is greatly facilitated by the nonhydrolyzable GTP analog GppNHp (5'-guanylimidodiphosphate) (Breitwieser and Szabo, 1985).

Recently, the involvement of G-proteins in the regulation of cardiac calcium channels has been reported (Yatani *et al.*, 1987). The guanosine triphosphate analog, GTPγS, prolonged the survival of calcium channels after excision from membrane patches, provided that isoproterenol or the calcium channel activator, Bay K 8644, was present in the bathing medium during the cell-attached mode. The involvement of local cAMP formation or protein kinase C was ruled out. Instead, by employing purified G_s (or its pure α subunit) preactivated with GTPγS, it was shown that the stimulatory effect was caused by a proximal, direct action of this G-protein. In contrast, G_k, which directly stimulates mammalian atrial potassium channels, and unactivated G_s were ineffective. Further studies are necessary to determine whether direct interaction of the G-protein with the calcium channel pore or modification of a channel-associated regulatory mechanism (e.g., phosphorylation–dephosphorylation) is responsible for this effect.

b. Biochemical Evidence. Phosphorylation of a voltage-dependent calcium channel-related protein has been implicated as the final step of a reaction cascade. Correlation of functional (e.g., Ca^{2+} uptake) and biochemical (phosphorylation of membrane proteins) evidence should help identify the protein substrate. Several groups have reported cAMP-dependent phosphorylation of low-molecular-weight proteins in cardiac membranes by endogenous kinases or purified cAMP-dependent protein kinase (Rinaldi *et al.*, 1981; Flockerzi *et al.*, 1983; Horne *et al.*, 1984). The difficulties and pitfalls of these studies become evident in the study of Horne *et al.* (1984). Nitrendipine and isoproterenol stimulated phosphorylation of a 42-kDa protein by an endogenous kinase. Simultaneous labeling of this polypeptide by a postulated irreversible affinity ligand for the 1,4-dihydropyridine receptor of voltage-dependent calcium channels, [³H]o-NCS-dihydropyridine, was taken as evidence for having phosphorylated a voltage-dependent calcium channel-related polypeptide. However, this ligand has now been proved to be a fully reversible ligand for voltage-dependent calcium channels (see Section VII,A). The physiological significance of this phosphorylated protein deserves further characterization.

The purification of skeletal muscle L-type calcium channels and reconstitution into artificial membranes provide a convenient system to study effects of cAMP-induced phosphorylation. The purified calcium channel protein consists of three to four "subunits" with molecular weights of 142,000–165,000 (α_1 and α_2 components are distinguished), 50,000–65,000 (β) and 30,000–35,000 (γ) (see Section VII,B). Phosphorylation of the α and β subunits has been claimed to be functionally important by different authors (Curtis and Catterall, 1985; Flockerzi *et al.*, 1986). Only the α_1 subunit has been identified unequivocally as a calcium channel component carrying the drug receptor (see Section VII,B). The role of the β subunit is still unclear. cAMP-dependent phosphorylation of purified and reconstituted L-type calcium channels from skeletal muscle alters its function in agreement with data obtained on cardiac voltage-dependent calcium channels, implicating an identical mechanism in the heart.

2. Neuronal Calcium Channel Function Is Modulated by Hormones and Neurotransmitters

Voltage-dependent calcium channels in endocrine cells and neurons allow Ca^{2+} to enter the cells and are important in the control of physiologic functions such as neuronal excitability and transmitter secretion (Miller, 1987). It is well established that Ca^{2+}-dependent action potentials are modulated by neurotransmitters in vertebrate neurons. It was hypothesized that modulation of calcium channels could be an important factor in the regulation of neurotransmitter release from presynaptic nerve terminals (Reuter, 1983). Calcium entry into the cell may be regulated either via direct modulation of calcium conductance (e.g., by interaction of an inhibitory or stimulatory agent with the channel itself or a channel-regulating mechanism) or by inhibition of potassium conductance responsible for repolarization. Thus membrane potential may be prevented from moving toward, or persisting as long, in the potential range favoring activation of calcium conductance. We discuss only studies in yielding strong evidence that voltage-dependent calcium channels rather than potassium channels are the target of neurotransmitter action. Modern electrophysiological techniques using pharmacological tools allow one to differentiate between these distinct targets. The patch clamp technique provides information about single channel currents and has been applied to the investigation of modulating effects of neurotransmitters on voltage-dependent calcium channel function (Marchetti et al., 1986). There is currently intensive research in this area. As outlined in Section II both L-type and T-type voltage-dependent calcium channels exist in heart, smooth muscle, and probably in skeletal muscle but together with N-type channels also in vertebrate neurons (Carbone and Lux, 1984a,b; Fedulova et al., 1985). The L-type channel is sensitive to 1,4-dihydropyridines (Nowycky et al., 1985a).

a. Several Neurotransmitters Exert Inhibitory Effects on Ca^{2+} Inward Currents in Vertebrate Neurons. The effects of diverse neurotransmitters on calcium channels are summarized in Table I. Catecholamines are the most widely investigated modulators of neuronal calcium currents in peripheral (e.g., dorsal root or sympathetic ganglion cells) or central neurons (e.g., locus coeruleus neurons). The mechanism responsible for this effect of catecholamines is not understood.

TABLE I

INHIBITION OF CALCIUM CHANNEL FUNCTION BY VARIOUS NEUROTRANSMITTERS AND DRUGS[a]

Neurotransmitter	Concentration	Cell type	Comment	Ref.[b]
Catecholamines	0.1–10 μM NA	Rat cervical ganglion	α-Adrenergic (10 μM phentolamine) but not β-adrenergic blockers antagonize effect	a
	10 μM NA	Rat cervical ganglion	Order of potency: A > l-NA > DA > isoproterenol; yohimbine but not prazosin antagonize effect	b
	100 μM NA	Embryonic chick DRG	Additive effects of NA and GABA	c
	100 μM A	Bullfrog sympathetic ganglion		d
	1–5 μM NA	Rat sympathetic ganglion		e
	0.01–10 μM NA, DA	Embryonic chick sensory neuron	Effects of NA, DA, and serotonin not additive; effect of all three amines blocked by haloperidol > yohimbine > phentolamine; no effect of clonidine; no antagonism by prazosin	f
	1 μM NA, 10 μM DA	Chick DRG	No effect of second messengers cAMP and cGMP; stabilizing effect of MgATP on calcium channel "run down"	g
	0.1–1 μM NA, 0.02–1 mM A	Nucleus locus coeruleus neurons	No antagonism by yohimbine, prazosin, or propranolol; limited effect of high concentrations phentolamine	h
	50 μM NA	Chick DRG	Pertussis toxin inhibits effect of NA and GABA	i
	10 μM NA and DA	Chick DRG, sympathetic ganglion	Differential effect of NA (and DA) on fast and slowly inactivating VDCCs; decreased opening probability rather than decreased single channel conductance shown for slowly	j

TABLE I (*Continued*)

Neurotransmitter	Concentration	Cell type	Comment	Ref.[b]
			inactivating current in patch clamp experiments	
Serotonin	0.01–10 μM serotonin	Embryonic chick sensory neurons		f
	10–100 μM serotonin	Bullfrog DRG	Effect not antagonized by methysergide and metergoline	k
	0.1 μM serotonin	Pituitary cell line	Effect inhibited by pertussis toxin and mimicked by GTPγS	u
Opioids	30 nM dynorphin A, 300 nM tifluadom	Cultured myenteric neurons	Effect on Ca^{2+} current only by κ-receptor but not by μ- and δ-receptor agonists; effect antagonized by naloxone; no effect by morphine	l
	1 μM dynorphin A	Mouse DRG	No effect by [leu]enkephalin; effect on N-type VDCC; inhibition reversed by naloxone (1 μM)	m
	1 μM DADLE	Neuroblastoma × glioma hybrid cells	Effect inhibited by pertussis toxin and restored after addition of GTP-binding proteins G_o and G_i	n
GABA$_B$ receptor agonists	100 μM GABA	Embryonic chick sensory neurons	Effect additive to NA	c
	1 μM–1 mM GABA	Guinea pig myenteric ganglia		o
	10–100 μM GABA	Chick sensory neurons	Reduction of both fast and slowly inactivating Ca^{2+} currents	p
	0.01–10 μM GABA	Embryonic chick sensory neurons	GABA effect mediated by a receptor system distinct from amine receptors	f
	50–100 μM baclofen	Rat DRG	Effect on fast and slowly inactivating Ca^{2+} currents	q
	50 μM GABA	Chick DRG	Pertussis toxin inhibits effect of NA and GABA	f

(*continued*)

TABLE I (Continued)

Neurotransmitter	Concentration	Cell type	Comment	Ref.[b]
Adenosine receptor agonists	50 nM 2-chloroadenosine	Rat DRG	Antagonized by IBMX and 8-PT	q
	1 mM adenosine, 1 μM l-PIA	Mouse DRG	Effect of several agonists did not correspond with relative potencies on adenosine A_I or A_{II} receptors	r
Muscarine	10–50 μM	Rat cervical ganglion		s
Prostaglandins	100–500 nM PGE$_1$	Rabbit cervical ganglion		t

[a] Abbreviations: NA, noradrenaline; A, adrenaline; DA, dopamine; PGE, prostaglandin E; GABA, γ-aminobutyric acid; VDCC, voltage-dependent calcium channel; DRG, dorsal root ganglion; DADLE, [D-Ala-D-Leu]enkephalin; IBMX, isobutylmethylxanthine; 8-PT, 8-phenyltheophylline.

[b] Key to references: a, Horn and McAffee (1980), J. Physiol. (London) 301, 191–204; b, McAffee et al. (1981), Fed. Proc. Am. Soc. Exp. Biol. (London) 40, 2246–2249; c, Dunlap and Fischbach (1981), J. Physiol (London) 317, 519–535; d, Koketsu and Akasu (1982), Jpn. J. Physiol. 32, 137–140; e, Galvan and Adams (1982), Brain Res. 244, 135–144; f, Canfield and Dunlap (1984), Br. J. Pharmacol. 82, 557–563; g, Forscher and Oxford (1985), J. Gen. Physiol. 85, 743–763; h, Williams and North (1985), Neuroscience 14, 103–109; i, Holz et al. (1986b), Nature (London) 319, 670–672; j, Marchetti et al. (1986), Pflügers Arch. 406, 104–111; k, Holz et al. (1986a), J. Neurosci. 6, 620–626; l, Cherubini and North (1985), Proc. Natl. Acad. Sci. U.S.A. 82, 1860–1863; m, MacDonald and Werz (1986), J. Physiol. (London) 377, 237–249, Gross and MacDonald (1987), Proc. Natl. Acad. Sci. U.S.A. 84, 5469–5473; n, Hescheler et al. (1987), Nature (London) 325, 445–447; o, Cherubini and North (1984), Br. J. Pharmacol. 82, 101–105; p, Deisz and Lux (1985), Neurosci. Lett. 56, 205–210; q, Dolphin et al. (1986), J. Physiol. (London) 373, 47–61, Scott and Dolphin (1986), Neurosci. Lett. 69, 59–64, Scott and Dolphin (1987a), Nature (London) 330, 760–762, Scott and Dolphin (1987b), J. Physiol. (London) 386, 1–17; r, MacDonald et al. (1986), J. Physiol. (London) 370, 75–90; s, Belluzzi et al. (1985), J. Physiol. (London) 358, 109–129; t, Mo et al. (1985), Brain Res. 334, 325–329; u, Lewis et al. (1986), Proc. Natl. Acad. Sci. U.S.A. 83, 9035–9039.

Data about the type of receptor that mediates the effect are also contradictory. There is some pharmacological evidence that the receptor is α_2-adrenergic in nature since inhibition of calcium-dependent potentials by noradrenaline in sympathetic ganglion cells is antagonized by yohimbine (1 μM); prazosin (10 μM) is without effect. Accordingly, clonidine, an α_2-adrenergic agonist, mimicked the effect of noradrenaline (McAfee et al., 1981). This is in contrast with other experiments wherein none of the agents, yohimbine, prazosin, phentolamine (Williams and North, 1985), or clonidine (Canfield and Dunlap, 1984), were effective. Moreover, Canfield and Dunlap (1984) found no additive effects with noradrenaline, dopamine, or serotonin [in contrast to γ-aminobutyric acid (GABA)] on calcium current inhibition. They postulated that their results reflected either the saturation of a common step removed from the initial drug–receptor interaction or the existence of a (novel) "single amine receptor," pharmacologically distinct from the classic receptors. The latter hypothesis was supported by the fact that the responses to dopamine, serotonin, and noradrenaline but not of GABA were inhibited with similar potency by serveral dopamine and serotonin antagonists.

Overall, these several studies do not allow conclusions about the nature of the catecholamine receptor mediating this effect. The concentrations of agonists necessary for inhibition of the Ca^{2+} current are considerably higher than those needed to activate the membrane potassium conductance. Activation of an α_2-receptor is responsible for the latter effect (Williams *et al.*, 1985). Therefore the potential role of catecholamines on neuronal calcium channels (compared to their effects on repolarization in the regulation of important physiological functions such as transmitter release and presynaptic inhibition) remains unknown. Similarly, as for catecholamines, novel classes of receptors for adenosine, GABA, and serotonin that might mediate transmitter-induced calcium current inhibition have been postulated (MacDonald *et al.*, 1986; Cherubini and North, 1984; Deisz and Lux, 1985; Holz *et al.*, 1986a).

So far the types of calcium channels inhibited by receptor agonists have not been unequivocally identified. Both a transient and slowly inactivating current were inhibited by GABA, noradrenaline, and dopamine (Deisz and Lux, 1985; Marchetti *et al.*, 1986) in avian dorsal root and sympathetic ganglion cells. Gross and MacDonald (1987) showed that the κ-opioid receptor agonist, dynorphin A, reduced the slow Ca^{2+} inward current by selectively affecting N channels. This effect was reversed by the opioid receptor antagonist naloxon. Inhibition of a transient (N-type) as well as a noninactivating (L-type) Ca^{2+} current by the $GABA_B$ receptor agonist baclofen was reported (vide infra) by Scott and Dolphin (1986, 1987b).

In contrast to many other investigators, Gray and Johnston (1987) reported *increased* rather than decreased activity of voltage-dependent calcium channels in hippocampal neurons induced by noradrenaline and β-adrenoceptor agonists. In whole-cell recordings the amplitude of a voltage-dependent Ca^{2+} inward current was increased by noradrenaline and (−)isoprenaline but not by clonidine and (+)isoprenaline, the biologically inactive enantiomer. This stimulation was most likely caused by a β-receptor-mediated intracellular increase of cAMP via stimulation of adenylate cyclase: the effect was mimicked by forskolin and the membrane-permeable cAMP-derivative, 8-bromo-cAMP. In single channel recordings an increase of the mean fractional open time by isoprenaline was demonstrated.

    b. Possible Molecular Mechanisms Involved in Calcium Channel Control—Novel Receptors and Role of GTP-Regulatory Proteins. With only preliminary characterization of the receptor systems involved, little is currently known about the coupling of receptor occupancy to modulation of voltage-dependent calcium channel function in vertebrate neuronal tissue. Perhaps mechanisms similar to those responsible for cardiac calcium channel regulation, namely, intracellular cyclic nucleotide mechanisms, are important in neurons. MgATP and cAMP retard calcium channel "rundown" (i.e., a decline of calcium conductance observed after removal or dilution of the cytoplasm) in vertebrate neurons (Kostyuk *et al.*, 1981; Forscher and Oxford, 1985). Until now, evidence for significant cAMP or cGMP-dependent processes has been found only in invertebrate neurons (Chad and Eckert, 1985; Pauperdin-Tritsch *et al.*, 1986).

    Forscher *et al.* (1986) investigated the nature of the noradrenaline-mediated decrease in Ca^{2+} currents in chick dorsal root ganglion cells. Employing the cell-attached patch clamp technique, they found that noradrenaline introduced into the cell bathing solution decreased currents outside the patch, whereas drug-free patch currents were not affected (Fig. 9). There was no significant alteration of intracellular cAMP content after exposure of the cells to noradrenaline, whereas isoproterenol and forskolin caused a 2- and 60-fold increase, respectively. Noradrenaline-mediated channel modulation was unaffected by this treatment. It was suggested that noradrenaline does not act through pathways which employ diffusible second messengers. Instead, the noradrenaline receptor appears to be tightly coupled to the channel possibly via another membrane-associated molecule.

    This hypothesis may be supported by recent findings that implicate a role for GTP-binding proteins as signal transducers in this process. Holz *et al.* (1986b) showed that preincubation of chick DRG neurons with pertussis toxin or intracellular administration of guanosine 5'-*O*-(2-thiodiphosphate), GDPβS, blocked the inhibitory action of noradrenaline and GABA on the Ca^{2+} current. Pertussis toxin and GDPβS are well-characterized inhibitors of the activation of GTP-binding proteins, which are identified as membrane transducing components mediating receptor effects on enzymes. The authors also confirmed the lack of effect of cAMP or cGMP. These results argue against a functional coupling of this GTP-binding protein to adenylate

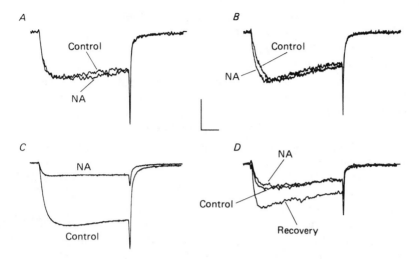

FIG. 9. Noradrenaline does not modulate channels in cell-attached membrane patches, whereas macroscopic currents outside the patch are strongly affected. (A) Patch currents recorded at a resting potential (r.p.) of +90 mV before (control) and after treatment with noradrenaline (NA) (2-minute exposure of the cell to 10 μM NA added to the bathing medium). V_h = r.p.; records are the average of five sweeps. (B) Patch currents recorded at r.p. +60 mV before and after a 2-minute exposure to 100 μM NA. V_h = r.p. − 50 mV. (C) The effect of 100 μM NA in the bathing medium on macroscopic calcium currents recorded at +10 mV from a cell in the same dish as (B). V_h = −50 mV. (D) In some patches currents increased upon washout; patch currents recorded at r.p. +60 mV before and after a 1-minute exposure to 10 mM NA. The recovery record was taken after an 11-minute wash in NA-free control solution. V_h = r.p. − 50 mV. Four different cells were used for A, B, C, and D. Calibrations: (A) 13 pA, 5 mseconds; (B) 37 pA, 10 mseconds; (C) 1.8 nA, 5 mseconds; (D) 25 pA, 5 mseconds. [From Forscher et al. (1986), J. Physiol. (London) 379, 131–144, with permission.]

cyclase and therefore suggest that G_o rather than G_i may be involved.

Scott and Dolphin (1986, 1987a,b) strongly support these findings. Internal perfusion of cultured rat dorsal root ganglion neurons with 0.5 mM GTPγS resulted in the differential inhibition of those channels underlying the transient portion (N type and possibly T type) of the Ca^{2+} current. The effect of GTPγS was abolished by pretreatment with pertussis toxin. Therefore, in the presence of GTPγS the remaining Ca^{2+} current was largely nonactivating, apparently carried by an L channel. The inhibitory effect of (−)baclofen on the Ca^{2+} inward current was increased by GTPγS but was reduced by GDPβS. (−)Baclofen is a potent agonist for γ-aminobutyric acid receptor type B (GABA$_B$). Thus, involvement of G-proteins in calcium channel regulation was shown for both components of the Ca^{2+} current. The transient component was inhibited by GTPγS whereas baclofen-induced inhibition of the noninactivating current was enhanced in the presence of GTPγS. The interaction of the latter current (carried by L channels) with G-proteins became evident when the effect of direct G-protein activation (via GTPγS) on channel regulation by drugs was studied (Scott and Dolphin, 1987b). Under control conditions 10 μM gallopamil (D 600) caused only a small and transient potentiation of this Ca^{2+} current followed by an inhibition. In the presence of GTPγS an immediate, more pronounced, and sustained potentiation of the maximum current was observed. The effect was inhibited by pertussis toxin pretreatment. Similar results were obtained with 30 μM diltiazem and 5 μM nifedipine (see also Section III,A). Taking into account earlier observations on the dualistic actions of calcium channel drugs (Brown et al., 1986; Kokubun et al., 1987), they explained these results by the stabilization of the resting state of the channel after G-protein activation, which potentiated the "agonistic" action of the channel blockers. Very similar to the $GABA_B$ receptor-mediated inhibition of Ca^{2+} currents, somatostatin blocks calcium channels via a G-protein (Lewis et al., 1986).

All these studies fit well with the results of Hescheler et al. (1987), who found that G_o is involved in the functional coupling of opiate receptors to neuronal calcium channels. They demonstrated that the inhibitory effect of the opioid [D-Ala-D-Leu]enkephalin (DADLE) on Ca^{2+} currents in neuroblastoma × glioma hybrid cells was almost completely inhibited by pretreatment with pertussis toxin. An effect of opiate-induced decrease in intracellular cAMP (Blume et al., 1979) was excluded. The effect was restored with intracellular application of N_i and N_o (see Fig. 10), the α subunit of the latter being about 10 times more potent than N_i. Thus N_o, which is abundant in neuronal tissue, could be an important candidate for the functional coupling of diverse receptors to neuronal calcium channels.

c. Is the Calcium Channel Regulated by Protein Kinase C? Recent attention has been focused on a possible role of protein kinase C. Hydrolysis of phosphatidylinositol phosphates by phospholipase C leads to two second messengers, namely, inositol trisphosphate (IP_3) and diacylglycerol (DAG). IP_3 releases Ca^{2+} from intracellular stores in several tissues. Diacylglycerol activates the ubiquitous enzyme protein kinase C in a Ca^{2+}- and phospholipid-dependent fashion. Synthetic, membrane-permeable analogs of DAG, such as 1,2-oleoylacetylglycerol (OAG), or tumor-promoting phorbol esters, like phorbol myristate acetate (PMA), 12-deoxyphorbol 13-isobutyrate (DBP), or 12-O-tetradecanoylphorbol-13-acetate (TPA), are also well-known di-

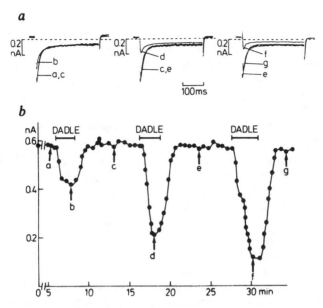

FIG. 10. Restoration of DADLE inhibition of the calcium inward current by intra-cellular application of G_i and G_o. Current traces (a) were recorded at the time points a–g indicated in the time course of the calcium inward current (b); test potentials were 0 mV. Pertussis toxin almost completely inhibits the inhibitory effect of DADLE on calcium currents. In the experiment illustrated (one of five with similar results), a pertussis toxin-pretreated cell was intracellularly infused with a mixture of G_i plus G_o, and 1 μM DADLE was added at different times indicated by the bars. The addition of G-proteins restores the inhibitory effect of DADLE. G-proteins were purified from membranes of porcine brain to 90% homogeneity (SDS–PAGE; Coomassie blue stain). The ratio of subunits α_i to α_o, to β–γ was $1:1:2.5$. Purified G-proteins were diluted to 15 nM each in pipet buffer supplemented with 0.5% bovine serum albumin. The control buffer and heated G-protein solutions had no effect on the calcium inward current under control conditions or in the presence of DADLE. [From Hescheler *et al.* (1987), *Nature (London)* **325**, 445–447, with permission.]

rect activators of this enzyme, thus providing important phar-macological tools (Hirasawa and Nishizuka, 1985).

In virtually all cell types exhibiting exocytosis, protein kinase C appears to be involved in stimulating the secretory process. The impor-tance of the synergistic action of protein kinase C activation and intra-cellular mobilization of Ca^{2+} has been described for several secretory systems (Hirasawa and Nishizuka, 1985). Agents that cause increased influx of Ca^{2+} through voltage-dependent calcium channels, such as the dinoflagellate toxin maitotoxin (see, however, Section IV,E) or the calcium channel agonist Bay K 8644 also potentiate phorbol ester- and phospholipase C-induced secretion in neuronal and peripheral tissues (Judd et al., 1986). On the other hand, protein kinase C activation seems to initiate a regulatory, negative feedback mechanism for agonist-induced phosphatidylinositol hydrolysis and Ca^{2+} mobilization, e.g., via thyrotropin releasing hormone (TRH), α_1-adrenergic, and muscarinic receptors (Drummond, 1985; Cooper et al., 1985; Vicentini et al., 1985).

The function of calcium channels is regulated by protein kinase C in neuronal tissue. Rane and Dunlap (1986) described reversible inhibition of dorsal root ganglion cell Ca^{2+} currents by OAG at similar concentrations reported for protein kinase C activation, e.g., in human platelets. DBP also caused inhibition, but effects of the two agents were not additive, consistent with the hypothesis that OAG and DBP exert their effect by means of a common mechanism. Using a different technique, Di Virgilio et al. (1986) obtained similar results with PMA in PC12 cells and in an insulin-secreting cell line, both of which contain voltage-dependent calcium channels. In addition, Messing et al. (1986) provided some biochemical evidence that protein kinase activation in PC12 cells may interfere with the function of voltage-dependent calcium channels. They observed parallel inhibition of K^+-stimulated $^{45}Ca^{2+}$ influx and of reversible binding of $(+)$-$[^3H]PN$ 200-110 in intact PC12 cells by PMA and DBP. The inhibitory constants were in the nanomolar range for both effects. Inhibition of reversible $(+)$-$[^3H]PN$ 200-110 binding was only slightly affected in a membrane preparation prepared from these cells but was restored by reconstituting the membranes with protein kinase C activity prepared from the cytosolic fraction. This suggests that the effect of phorbol esters on 1,4-dihydropyridine binding is mediated by this enzyme.

What are the consequences of protein kinase C modulation of Ca^{2+} influx for cellular function? R. J. Miller and co-workers provided the data to answer this question (Harris et al., 1986). Inhibition of K^+ depolarization-induced Ca^{2+} influx in PC12 cells by submicromolar concentrations of TPA develops simultaneously with augmentation of depolarization-evoked transmitter release, suggesting that these agents act directly on the exocytotic process. Thus, considering the synergistic action of Ca^{2+} and DAG, Ca^{2+} may act as a signal for exocytosis and, in addition, as a negative signal modulating its own influx.

In bag cell neurons from Aplysia, activation of protein kinase C by TPA increases the Ca^{2+} current (De Riemer et al., 1985). Preliminary reports indicate that this increase may be attributed to the activation of a second species of Ca^{2+} current (23 pS), in addition to the current

(10 pS) observed in the absence of protein kinase C activation (Strong *et al.*, 1986).

Regulation of Ca^{2+} currents by protein kinase C apparently plays an important role in smooth muscle cells. In studying voltage-dependent, L-type calcium channels of the aortic cell line A7r5, Galizzi *et al.* (1987) could demonstrate an attenuation of the (+)PN 200-110-sensitive $^{45}Ca^{2+}$ influx by diacylglycerol and phorbol esters. [Arg[8]]Vasopressin and bombesin, well-known activators of the polyphosphoinositide pathway, inhibited calcium channel activity to equal extents. These polypeptide hormones elicit smooth muscle contraction by liberation of Ca^{2+} from internal stores via an IP_3-mediated mechanism. Simultaneously they appear to inhibit entry of extracellular Ca^{2+} via voltage-dependent calcium channels through protein kinase C activation.

3. *Summary*

Several neurotransmitters inhibit Ca^{2+} currents through voltage-dependent calcium channels in neuronal cells. Two different pathways are suggested. First, G-proteins, most likely G_i or G_o, interact directly with the channel in a manner very similar to adenylate cyclase regulation. The second pathway is a regulatory cascade, involving protein kinase C. Further studies will show if the enzyme directly affects channel function by calcium channel phosphorylation or acts more indirectly. Differential effects of neurotransmitters on the different types of calcium channels described in neuronal tissue have been observed and could be of use in understanding their individual importance for particular neuronal functions.

IV. Tools to Characterize the L-Type Calcium Channel

A. 1,4-Dihydropyridines

The prototype 1,4-dihydropyridine, nifedipine, discovered by Bossert and Vater (1971), has been modified in numerous analog structures. (For reviews, also covering structure–activity relationships, see Meyer *et al.*, 1985; Triggle and Swamy, 1983.) Only a few have been introduced as radiolabeled ligands for calcium channel research. The great majority of the nifedipine analogs are chiral, mostly due to nonidentical ester groups or nonidentical 2,6-substituents (Meyer *et al.*, 1985). Optically pure enantiomers of the chiral molecules are very valuable in differentiating between calcium channel-linked receptors and binding sites unrelated to calcium channels. The specific activities vary between 20 and 160 Ci/mmol for tritium-labeled compounds. The most widely used label is the optically pure $(+)$-[^{3}H]PN 200-110 which offers reasonable stability in aqueous solutions, high specific activity, and high affinity for the inactivated state of the channel which is predominant in (depolarized) membrane fragments or solubilized preparations. Another advantage is that this benzoxadiazol 1,4-dihydropyridine shows almost no interaction with binding sites not linked to calcium channels. The highest specific activity ligands available are $(\pm)$-[^{125}I]iodipine (Ferry and Glossmann, 1984) and $(-)$-[^{125}I]iodipine with specific activities of 2200 Ci/mmol. They are valuable for rapid autoradiography and detection of minute amounts of calcium channel-linked receptors (Glossmann and Ferry, 1985).

The 1,4-dihydropyridines are unique in that some congeners are represented by optical antipodes that show opposite pharmacological effects (see Schramm et al., 1983, 1986; Spedding, 1985). One set of antipodes increase contractility of the heart, constrict smooth muscle, and release neurotransmitters; these are termed "calcium channel agonists" or "calcium channel activators." The best characterized are Bay K 8644 and 202-791. This class of compound is distinguished from the 1,4-dihydropyridine channel blockers (or Ca^{2+} antagonists) and contain only one ester in the 1,4-dihydropyridine ring. The optical antipodes $(+)$-(S) 202-791 and $(-)$-(S) Bay K 8644 behave as activators whereas $(-)$-(R) 202-791 and $(+)$-(R) Bay K 8644 are typical channel blockers (Uematsu et al., 1986; Hof et al., 1985; Franckowiack et al., 1985; Zernig et al., 1986). Likewise, the optical enantiomers of Bay 6653 (H 160/51) show opposing actions (Gjörstrop et al., 1986). Both enantiomers of 202-791 are available as radiolabels with high specific activity (135 Ci/mmol). Only the labeled $(-)$-(R) 202-791 enantiomer was found to bind with reasonable affinity to, e.g., cardiac membranes (K_D 2 nM); the $(+)$-(S) 202-791 ligand did not bind to any measurable extent to (depolarized) membrane fragments (Vaghy et al., 1987a). In competition experiments the unlabeled "agonistic" enantiomer showed a K_i of 304 nM for cardiac membrane receptors (Vaghy et al., 1987a) and 1080 nM for the guinea pig skeletal muscle 1,4-dihydropyridine receptor (Striessnig et al., 1985). The agonistic enantiomer, although apparently useless for investigation of channel drug receptors in membrane fragments, may be of value for intact, polarized cells. The 1,4-dihydropyridines discriminate in a tissue-specific manner among isoreceptors by means of their dissociation constants (see Section IV,G).

All 1,4-dihydropyridines tested so far show lower affinity for the skeletal muscle isochannel 1,4-dihydropyridine receptor than, e.g., for that of the heart using identical incubation conditions and membrane-bound channels. This does not exclude the possibility that compounds exist with preferential affinity for the skeletal muscle receptor. Perhaps it is appropriate here to mention that compounds made available for academic research are selected out of many, and they show little systemic toxicity and often high potency on smooth muscle preparations. Calcium channel drugs that are highly neurotoxic or that impair skeletal muscle function may exist but will probably (it is hoped) be forever kept in the vaults of the pharmaceutical industry. The structures of some 1,4-dihydropyridines are shown in Figs. 11a and 11b.

B. PHENYLALKYLAMINES

Compared to the 1,4-dihydropyridines much less is published about the structure–activity relationships of the phenylalkylamines (see, e.g., Mannhold et al., 1986, 1987; Goll et al., 1986). The radiolabeled phenylalkylamines (see Fig. 12) show (in contrast to the available radiolabeled 1,4-dihydropyridines) a pK_a around 9 (e.g., the pK_a of verapamil is 8.7) and exist at pH 7.4 almost entirely in charged form. $(\pm)$-[^{3}H]Verapamil was the first useful ligand in this series but has been replaced by $(-)$-[^{3}H]desmethoxyverapamil [$(-)$D 888, devapamil] and [N-methyl-^{3}H]LU 49888. K_D values of these ligands are around 2 nM [approximately 10- to 20-fold higher affinity compared to $(\pm)$vera- pamil]; the compounds are optically pure enantiomers. Similar to $(\pm)$verapamil, radiolabeled methoxyverapamil (D 600, gallopamil) is a racemate. The general usefulness of tritiated racemic gallopamil as a channel-specific ligand (with the exception of highly purified heart membranes; Ehrlich et al., 1986), like that of $(\pm)$-[^{3}H]bepridil, is not proved; these ligands are not discussed here.

C. BENZOTHIAZEPINES AND RELATED COMPOUNDS

The structure of the benzothiazepine diltiazem is shown in Fig. 13. This compound contains two asymmetric carbon atoms, and four diastereoisomers exist. $(+)$-cis-Diltiazem is the enantiomer potent in calcium channel-blocking activity. $(+)$-cis-Diltiazem is the only labeled ligand from a structurally diverse class of compounds which seem to ineract more or less selectively with the benzothiazepine receptor of the L-type calcium channel. Next to fostedil (KB 944) (see Linn et al., 1983), trans-diclofurime (Spedding et al., 1987; Mir and Spedding, 1987) has been classified as a $(+)$-cis-diltiazem-like compound, based on radioligand binding studies. Another interesting structure, MDL 12,330 A (a lactamimide) shows similar properties to $(+)$-cis-diltiazem in radioligand binding studies with $(\pm)$-[^{3}H]nitrendipine (Lee et al., 1985), but its selectivity is not well characterized. Finally,

a

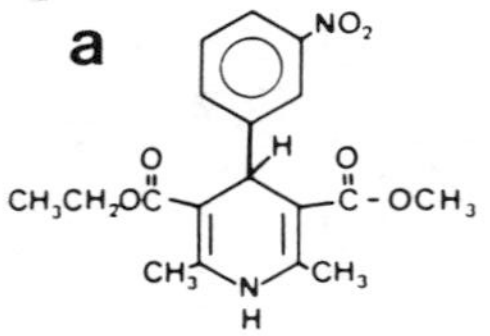

NITRENDIPINE

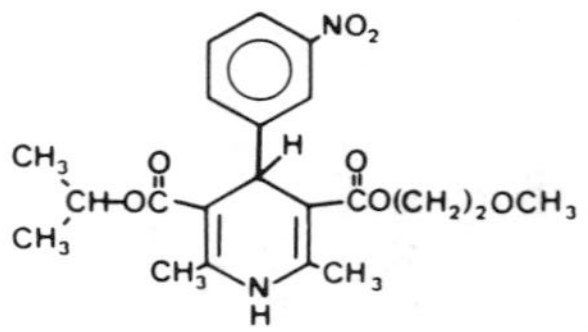

NIMODIPINE

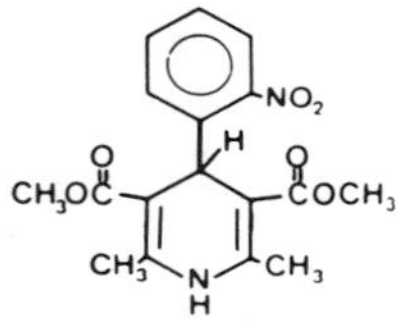

NIFEDIPINE

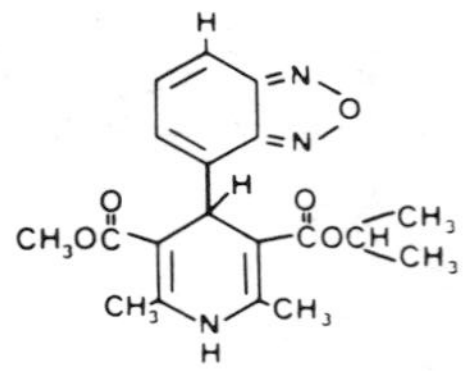

PN 200-110

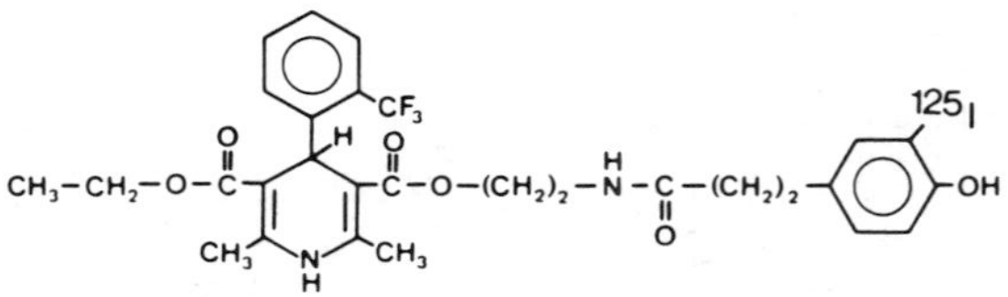

IODIPINE

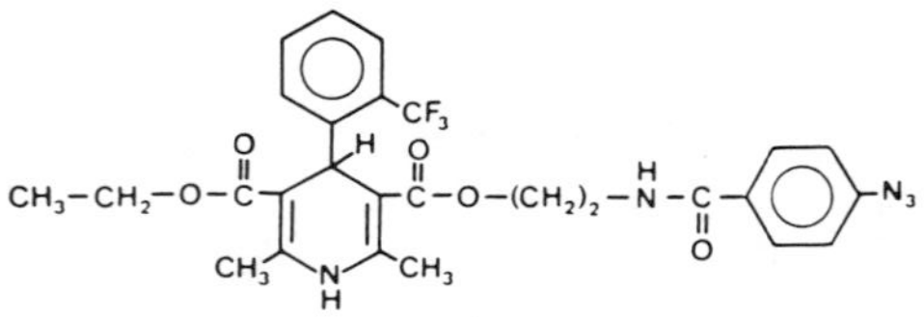

AZIDOPINE

FIG. 11. 1,4-Dihydropyridines. (a) 1,4-Dihydropyridine channel blockers (Ca^{2+} antagonists) which are used as radiolabels. With the exception of nifedipine the structures are chiral. The (+) enantiomer of nimodipine binds selectively to the nucleoside carrier (see Fig. 1), the (−) enantiomer with high affinity to the inactivated state of the L-type calcium channel. [^{125}I]Iodipine is a high affinity, high specific activity (2200 Ci/mmol) ligand and [^{3}H]azidopine a high affinity photoaffinity ligand. (b) Chiral 1,4-dihydropyridines, where one enantiomer is a channel blocker and the other a channel activator. Bay K 8644 and 202-791 are well characterized. (±) Bay K 8644 and (*R*) and (*S*) 202-791 are available in radiolabeled form.

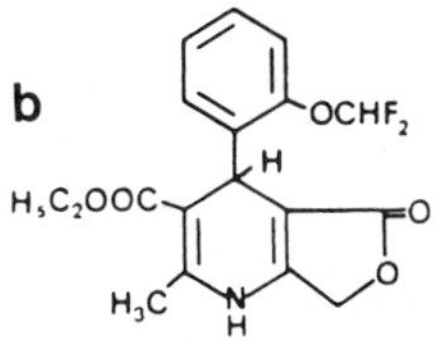

CGP 28392 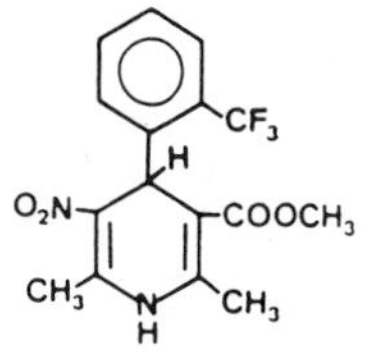 BAY K 8644 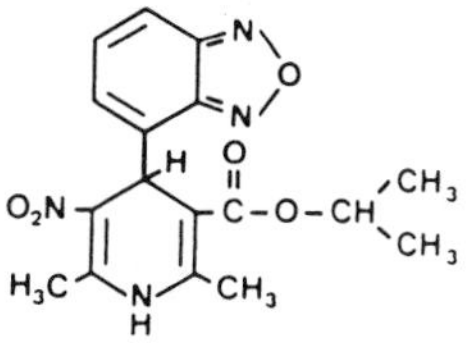 202-791

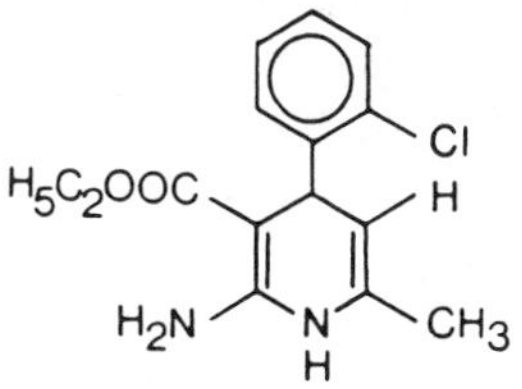

BAY F 6653 = H 160/51 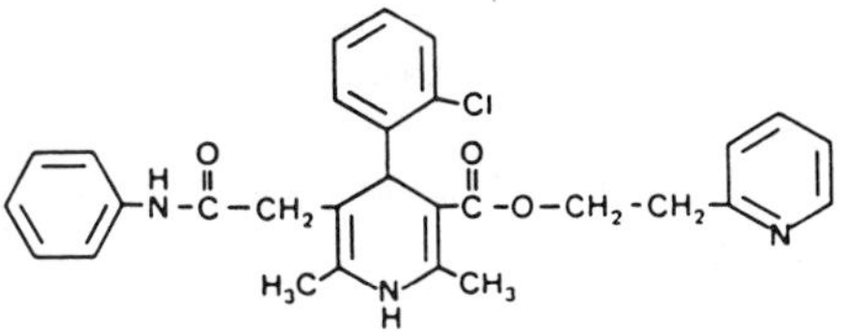 YC-170

FIG. 11-continued

(+)tetrandrine, an alkaloid from *Stephania tetrandra* and long known as an antianginal and antiarrhythmic agent in Chinese folk medicine, binds selectively to the benzothiazepine domain of the calcium channel (King *et al.*, 1988a).

D. DIPHENYLBUTYLPIPERIDINES AND RELATED COMPOUNDS

Diphenylbutylpiperidines (which include [³H]fluspirilene) and the benzothiazinone and [³H]HOE 166 (the latter being optically pure), interact with sites apparently distinct from other known drug receptor sites (Fig. 14). [³H]Fluspirilene (a notoriously hydrophobic, almost insoluble compound) appeared to display a K_D of 0.1 nM for the skeletal muscle isochannel in rabbit T-tubule membranes, whereas K_D values for nerve, cardiac, and smooth muscle membranes were 35, 50, and 50 nM (Galizzi *et al.*, 1986a). Thus, [³H]fluspirilene seems to be unique in showing 500-fold selectivity for skeletal muscle L-type calcium channels versus heart and neuronal channels. In competition studies with unlabeled fluspirilene and its congeners (penfluridol, pimozide, and clopimozide) the IC_{50} values in brain, smooth muscle, and heart membranes were reported to be 1 to 2 orders of magnitude higher than in skeletal muscle (Qar *et al.*, 1987). We have not found such high isochannel selectivity in binding inhibition experiments with

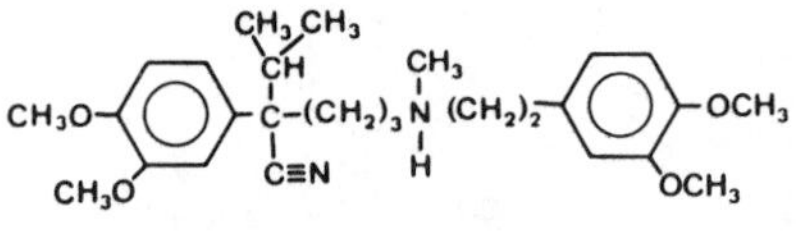

(±)VERAPAMIL

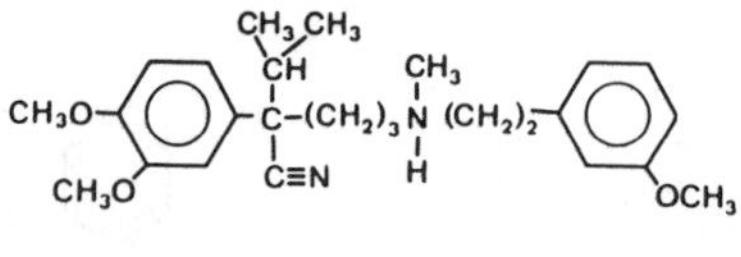

(-)DESMETHOXYVERAPAMIL

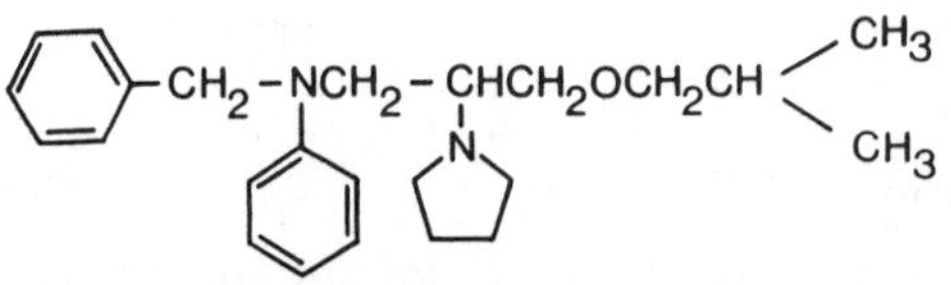

BEPRIDIL

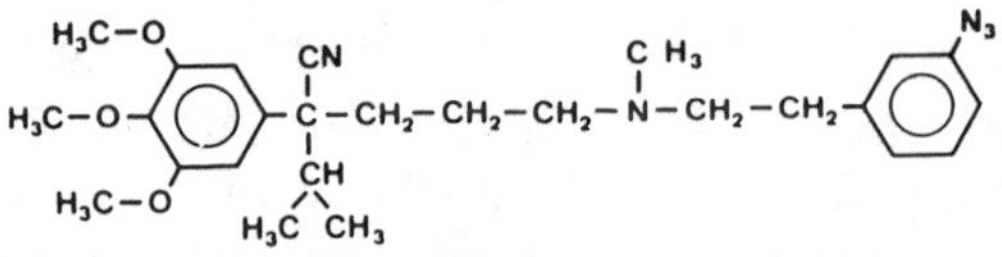

LU 49888

Fig. 12. Phenylalkylamines and related compounds. The structures of verapamil, desmethoxyverapamil, bepridil, and LU 49888 are shown. [³H]Verapamil is available as the racemate; desmethoxyverapamil and LU 49888 are used as the optically pure (−) enantiomers in tritiated form for structural characterization (and photoaffinity labeling) of the phenylalkylamine receptors. (±)-[³H]Bepridil is not well characterized but is claimed to bind to the phenylalkylamine receptor.

(−)-[³H]desmethoxyverapamil and unlabeled pimozide or fluspirilene (H. Glossmann and J. Striessnig, unpublished experiments). King *et al.* (1988b) obtained a K_D value for [³H]fluspirilene of 0.6 nM (B_{max} 1.5 pmol/mg protein) in highly purified porcine cardiac membranes and confirmed this dissociation constant with kinetic data. Binding is

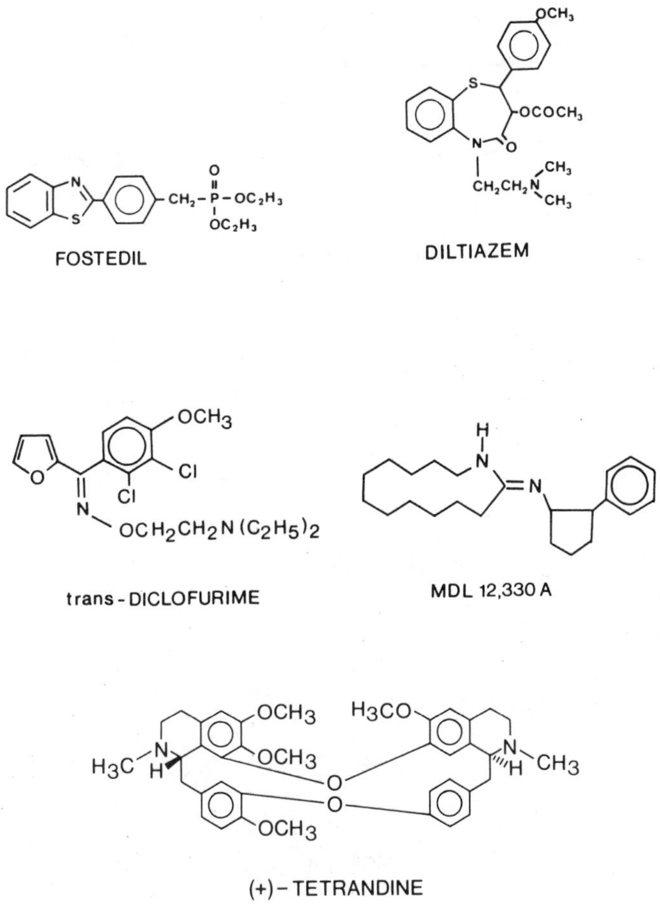

FOSTEDIL

DILTIAZEM

trans-DICLOFURIME

MDL 12,330 A

(+)-TETRANDINE

FIG. 13. Benzothiazepines and compounds claimed to bind at the benzothiazepine-selective receptor. Of the four diastereoisomeric benzothiazepine structures only (+)-cis-diltiazem is a calcium channel blocker and available in tritiated form for structural characterization. A variety of other drugs are claimed to bind more or less selectively to the benzothiazepine-selective receptor of the calcium channel, and their structures are shown.

stimulated by cations which block calcium channels (e.g., Cd^{2+}) whereas permeant ions (e.g., Ca^{2+}) inhibit.

These results argue strongly against the hypothesis of Galizzi et al. (1986) that fluspirilene possesses extreme isochannel selectivity; methodological problems (e.g., membrane concentration dependence of IC_{50} values and/or loss of the hydrophobic drug on glassware or plastic) are the most likely explanations for the apparent high affinity to skeletal muscle channels. [^{3}H]HOE 166 displays nanomolar dissocia-

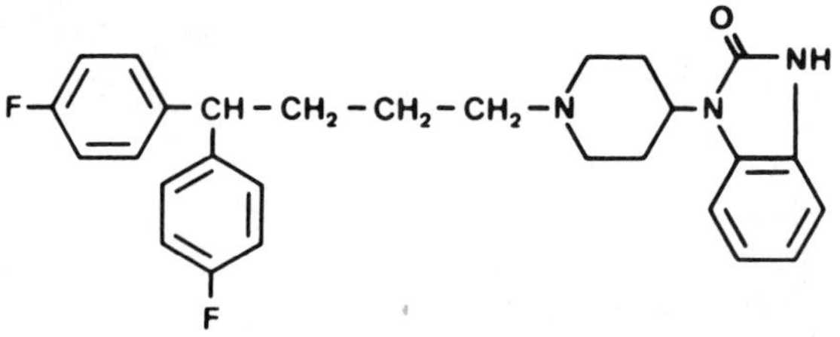

PIMOZIDE

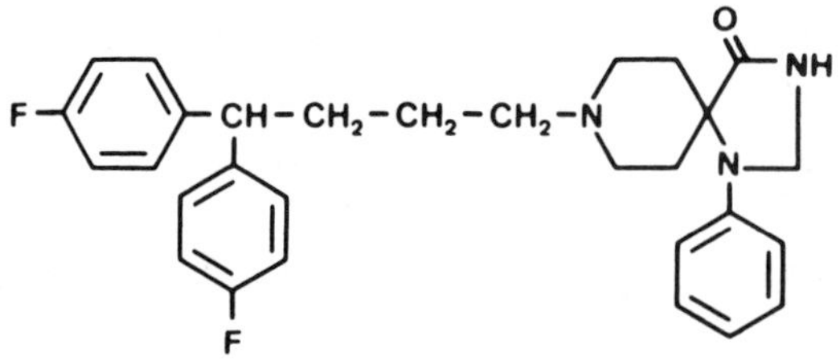

FLUSPIRILENE

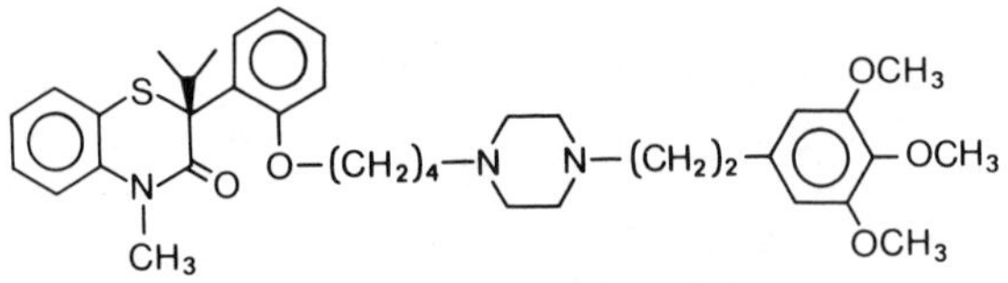

HOE 166

FIG. 14. Diphenylbutylpiperidines and benzothiazinones. Pimozide and fluspirilene are suggested to interact with a receptor on the L-type calcium channel which is distinct from the receptors defined by 1,4-dihydropyridines, (+)-cis-diltiazem, and phenylalkylamines. [³H]Fluspirilene is available for structural research. HOE 166 [(R)−(+)−3,4-dihydro-2-isopropyl-4-methyl-2-[2-[4-[4-[2[(3,4,5-trimethoxyphenyl)ethyl]piperazinyl]-butoxy]-phenyl]-2H[1,4-benzothiazine-3-one dihydrochloride] is also shown.

tion constants for heart, brain, and skeletal muscle calcium channels and has been characterized extensively by our group (Striessnig et al., 1988a).

So far no overt agonists among the other classes of calcium channel drugs have been described. The observation that (±)-trans-diltiazem is a vasoconstrictor (Nagao et al., 1972) has apparently been overlooked, and our suggestion that the optical enantiomers of the phenylalkyl-amines may also give agonistlike actions has never been tested. To this end dose–response curves for (+)verapamil (in pharmacological experiments) must be analyzed with (−)verapamil as in radioligand binding studies (see, e.g., Glossmann and Ferry, 1985; Ferry et al., 1985a).

E. Toxins

1. ω-Conotoxin GVIA (ω-CgTx)

Naturally occurring toxins have not been such critical tools in calcium channel research as they have been in nicotinic receptor or sodium channel research. The only well-characterized toxin suitable for structural research is ω-CgTx. This is a 27-amino acid polypeptide isolated from the venom of Conus geographus (Olivera et al., 1985). The synthetic toxin, which is now commercially available, cannot be distinguished from the natural toxin in functional tests (Rivier et al., 1987). ω-CgTx contains three tyrosine residues and can easily be iodinated (Fig. 15). ^{125}I-ω-CgTx labels saturable sites in membrane fragments of neuronal origin (Cruz and Olivera, 1986; Abe et al., 1986; Knaus et al., 1987; Wagner and Snowman, 1987). Binding occurs in a quasi-irreversible manner (apparent half-saturation 1.5–60 pM). Sites with low affinity (apparent half-saturation 0.5 nM) have also been found (Abe et al., 1986; Cruz and Olivera, 1986). Binding of the toxin is inhibited by submillimolar concentrations of divalent cations and La^{3+} (Wagner and Snowman, 1987).

^{125}I-ω-CgTx recognizes mainly N-type calcium channels distinct from L-type calcium channels. First, in rat and guinea pig brain (Knaus et al., 1987; Wagner and Snowman, 1987) the density of sites for ^{125}I-ω-CgTx is nearly one order of magnitude higher than for L-type calcium channel-selective drugs (e.g., 1,4-dihydropyridines; see Section IV,G). Second, binding is not modulated by 1,4-dihydropyridines, phenylalkylamines, or benzothiazepines. Third, ^{125}I-ω-CgTx binding is abolished in the presence of neurotoxic aminoglycoside antibiotics, which inhibit the Ca^{2+} influx through N-type calcium channels responsible for neurotransmitter release. The clinical use of these aminoglycosides may be associated with impairment of neu-

Cys-Lys-Ser-Hyp-Gly-Ser-Ser-Cys-Ser-Hyp-Thr-Ser-Tyr-Asn-
Cys-Cys-Arg-Ser-Cys-Asn-Hyp-Tyr-Thr-Lys-Arg-Cys-Tyr-NH₂

FIG. 15. Amino acid sequence of ω-CgTx GVIA. The neuronal calcium channel toxin is basic and highly cross-linked by disulfide bridges, as are most other toxins from Conus geographus venom. Note the presence of hydroxyproline and the amidated carboxy-terminal end. The major iodination product is monoiodinated at Tyr[22] [underlined; compare with Cruz et al. (1987), Biochemistry 26, 820–824].

romuscular transmission, causing such symptoms as increased muscular weakness, respiratory depression, and general flaccid paralysis especially in patients with myasthenia gravis or in association with anesthesia (Knaus et al., 1987; Wagner et al., 1987). The ability of several aminoglycosides to inhibit binding of ^{125}I-ω-CgTx (Table II) correlates well with their toxicity as reflected by the maximal therapeutic levels (Caputy et al., 1981; Martindale, 1982). Interaction of aminoglycosides with L-type calcium channel-linked drug receptors was not observed. Aminoglycosides are the first examples ("lead structures") for "organic" N-type calcium channel blockers.

Abe and Saisu (1987) synthesized an arylazido ^{125}I-ω-CgTx derivative as a photolabel. Three polypeptides with apparent molecular masses of 310, 240, and 34 kDa were specifically photolabeled in rat synaptic plasma membranes by this probe. Using a similar approach, we photolabeled three polypeptides with apparent molecular masses of 260, 195, and 45 kDa in guinea pig cerebral cortex (Fig. 16). Interestingly, the two larger polypeptides have the same mass as those reported to carry high affinity drug receptors for the phenylalkylamine [N-methyl-^{3}H]LU 49888 in guinea pig hippocampus (Striessnig et al., 1988b). In the same preparation only the 195-kDa polypeptide is labeled by (−)-[^{3}H]azidopine.

Preliminary attempts to clone the genes for a 1,4-dihydropyridine-insensitive but ω-CgTx-sensitive calcium channel observed in *Torpedo* electric lobes (Yeager et al., 1987) have been reported (Umbach and Gundersen, 1987). When *Xenopus laevis* oocytes were injected with poly(A)$^+$ RNA from the electric lobe of *Torpedo californica*, expression of this type of calcium channel in addition to those observed in untreated oocytes resulted.

2. Other Toxins

Maitotoxin and atrotoxin (Hamilton et al., 1985) as well as other toxins are neither structurally nor functionally well characterized. A polypeptide toxin (molecular weight 19,000) from the coral *Goniopora*, which appears to be a calcium channel activator (Qar et al., 1986), interacts weakly with the 1,4-dihydropyridine receptor in skeletal muscle T-tubule membranes. Its usefulness for structural research has not been established.

F. L-TYPE CALCIUM CHANNEL DRUG RECEPTOR SITES

Certain 1,4-dihydropyridines (e.g., nifedipine, nitrendipine), phenylalkylamines (e.g., verapamil, gallopamil), and the benzothiazepine

TABLE II
Effects of Antibiotics on N-Type Channel (^{125}I-ω-Conotoxin GVIA) and L-Type Channel Ligand Binding[a]

Drug	^{125}I-ω-Conotoxin GVIA			$(+)$-[^{3}H]PN 200-110, IC$_{50}$ (μmol/liter)	$(-)$-[^{3}H]Desmethoxy-verapamil, IC$_{50}$ (μmol/liter)	MTL (μmol/liter)
	IC$_{50}$ (μmol/liter)	nH	Maximum inhibition (% control)			
ω-Conotoxin GVIA	2.1×10^{-5} ± 0.15×10^{-5}	2.03 ± 0.25	100	n.d.[b]	n.d.	n.d.
Neomycin	5.2 ± 0.5	1.33 ± 0.19	100	>100	>1000	42.1
Gentamycin	15.3 ± 2.4	1.18 ± 0.20	100	>100	>1000	18.7
Tobramycin	19.1 ± 1.3	1.16 ± 0.08	100	>100	>1000	21.2
Streptomycin	28.3 ± 7.2	1.67 ± 0.56	100	>1000	>1000	34.5
Amikacin	71.9 ± 9.1	1.14 ± 0.14	100	>1000	>1000	48.6
Kanamycin	161.1 ± 20.2	1.53 ± 0.26	100	>1000	>1000	68.9
Polymyxin B	6.6 ± 0.3	3.16 ± 0.29	100	5.3 ± 1.1, 78% inhibition (1 mmol/liter)	3.2 ± 1.4, 81% inhibition (1 mmol/liter)	n.d.
Benzylpenicillin	n.e.[c] (1 mmol/liter)		0	>100	n.e. (1 mmol/liter)	550.5
Cephalothin	n.e. (1 mmol/liter)		0	n.e. (1 mmol/liter)	n.e. (1 mmol/liter)	n.d.
Erythromycin	n.e. (0.1 mmol/liter)		0	>100	>100	68.2
Tetracyclin	n.e. (1 mmol/liter)		0	>100	>100	62.3
Chloramphenicol	n.e. (1 mmol/liter)		0	>1000	>1000	108.3
Lincomycin	n.e. (1 mmol/liter)		0	n.e. (1 mmol/liter)	n.e. (1 mmol/liter)	n.d.

[a] Experiments were performed with guinea pig cerebral cortex membranes. Note that the IC$_{50}$ values of aminoglycosides for inhibition of N-type channel ligand binding are fairly well correlated to the maximal therapeutic level (MTL). The aminoglycosides do not inhibit L-type channel radioligand binding. Polymyxin B (a cationic detergent) inhibits binding of all ligands, presumably by general membrane perturbation. From Knaus *et al.* (1987), *Nauyn–Schmiedeberg's Arch. Pharmacol.* **336**, 583–586, with permission.

[b] n.d., Not determined.

[c] n.e., No effect up to the concentration given.

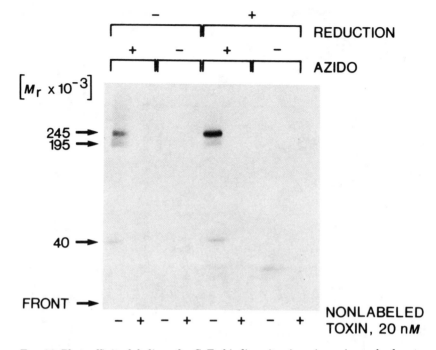

FIG. 16. Photoaffinity labeling of ω-CgTx binding sites in guinea pig cerebral cortex membranes. ^{125}I-ω-CgTx (2000 Ci/mmol) was reacted with an excess of N-hydroxysuccinimidyl-aziodobenzoate for 60 minutes on ice in the dark. The reaction was quenched by dilution in 50 mM Tris–HCl, pH 7.4. An aliquot of photolabel (~145,000 cpm, azido +) or of underivatized (azido −) ^{125}I-ω-CgTx was incubated with 0.5 mg of guinea pig cerebral cortex membrane protein in the absence or presence of 20 nM unlabeled ω-CgTx at 25°C. After 25 minutes the membranes were transferred to petri dishes and irradiated for 30 minutes with UV light. The irradiated samples were centrifuged, and the pellets were solubilized in electrophoresis sample buffer and separated on 5–15% polyacrylamide gels under reducing (in the presence of 10 mM dithiothreitol) or nonreducing conditions (10 mM N-ethylmaleimide). Radioactive bands were visualized on Kodak XAR film.

($+$)-*cis*-diltiazem are highly specific blockers of (L-type) calcium channels (for review, see Fleckenstein, 1983; Godfraind *et al.*, 1986). The action and binding of chiral molecules are stereoselective and are often observed (especially for 1,4-dihydropyridines) at nanomolar or subnanomolar concentrations. The sites where these compounds bind on the channel are termed "receptors" (by pharmacological criteria), whether or not endogenous ligands exist. A surprising feature of the (so far known) calcium channel drug receptors is that they are reciprocally allostericly coupled among themselves (and to divalent cation binding sites).

There is agreement that the 1,4-dihydropyridine receptor is distinct from that for the phenylalkylamines and the benzothiazepine (+)-*cis*-diltiazem. Controversy exists with respect to the phenylalkylamine and benzothiazepine sites. Galizzi *et al.* (1986b) demonstrated pure competitive interaction among (+)-*cis*-diltiazem, (−)desmethoxyverapamil, and (±)bepridil in skeletal muscle T-tubule membranes, supporting the "unitary mechanism of calcium antagonist action" (Murphy *et al.*, 1983). On the other hand, Garcia *et al.* (1986), Reynolds *et al.* (1986b), and Balwierczak *et al.* (1987) interpret their experimental findings with the assumption of three distinct (instead of two) receptor sites, supporting our early working model (Glossmann *et al.*, 1984a).

In addition to equilibrium binding studies, dissociation experiments are often used to discriminate between pure competitive or allosteric inhibitors. An example is shown in Fig. 17. In the model (which covers all observations made in radioligand binding studies with membranes or purified channels) three sites (termed 1, 2, and 3 for the 1,4-dihydropyridine, the phenylalkylamine, and the benzothiazepine receptor, respectively) are symbolized by closely adjacent circles, connected by bidirectional arrows (Fig. 18). The plus or minus signs indicate positive or negative heterotropic allosteric interactions observed in ligand binding studies. Interactions (which are reciprocal) between receptor sites 2 or 3 with receptor site 1 are positive or negative, depending on temperature, ligand(s), and other factors. For example, with purified guinea pig skeletal muscle calcium channels, the phenylalkylamine, (−)desmethoxyverapamil, stimulates 1,4-dihydropyridine binding; in particulate membranes, however, there is allosteric inhibition (Striessnig *et al.*, 1986b). Interactions between receptor sites 2 and 3 are always negative.

An additional feature of the model is that each site can exist in a low or high affinity state, depending on occupation of the adjacent sites, temperature, ions, pH, or lipids and on the radioligand employed to characterize the site (Glossmann *et al.*, 1985a,b). This is shown schematically in Fig. 19. The skeletal muscle T-tubule calcium channel 1,4-dihydropyridine receptor saturated in equilibrium binding studies at 37°C with structurally different radiolabeled compounds displays different B_{max} values. In the first approximation the B_{max} is inversely correlated to the K_D of the respective ligand. For instance, the tritium-labeled 1,4-dihydropyridine Bay K 8644 (K_D 1.8 nM) labels fewer than 10% of the sites (at 25 or 37°C) compared with (+)-[³H]PN 200-110 (K_D 0.2–0.7 nM) (Glossmann *et al.*, 1985a–c; Ildefonse *et al.*, 1985). Apparently, ligands stabilize different proportions of sites in high and low affinity states. Based on these observations a spectrum (ranging from overt agonists, to dualists, to pure antagonists) within the 1,4-di-

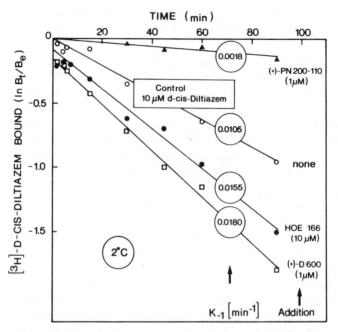

FIG. 17. Dissociation experiments to discriminate simple competitive from other (e.g., allosteric) inhibition. Allosteric inhibition may be complete and often cannot be easily discriminated from competitive inhibition. To this end the receptor is complexed with a labeled ligand, and, after equilibrium is reached, the forward reaction is blocked with the unlabeled ligand at a concentration identical to that used to define nonspecific binding. In this experiment with guinea pig skeletal muscle T-tubule membranes, the receptor site 3 was labeled with (+)-*cis*-[³H]diltiazem at 2°C. After equilibrium was reached, (+)-*cis*-diltiazem (10 μM) was added (time 0 on the graph) with or without additions as indicated. When the 1,4-dihydropyridine (+)PN 200–110 was added, the off-rate is greatly reduced, although at this temperature equilibrium binding of diltiazem is inhibited. Note that 1 μM (+)D 600 and 10 μM HOE 166 increase the dissociation rate constant, K_{-1}. A pure competitive inhibitor cannot increase the off-rate, hence the mechanism of inhibition of equilibrium binding of (+)-*cis*-[³H]diltiazem by HOE 166 or (+)D 600 must be more complex [as is, of course that by (+)PN 200-110].

hydropyridines was postulated (Glossmann *et al.*, 1984b). Low affinity states are often not detected with dilution–filtration technology as dissociation constants (as a rule of thumb) are proportional to the dissociation rate constant. The label trapped in the low affinity state rapidly dissociates on dilution, and only ligand stabilized with high affinity is recovered on a glass fiber filter. The low and high affinity states, induced by overt agonists, could possibly be observed in drug competition experiments with a potent 1,4-dihydropyridine antagonist. Our efforts to prove this assumption gave a negative result.

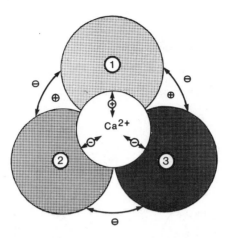

Fig. 18. The allosteric interaction model of the L-type calcium channel drug receptor sites. The receptors (1 stands for 1,4-dihydropyridine-selective, 2 for phenylalkylamine-selective, and 3 for benzothiazepine-selective sites) interact with each other by reciprocal allosteric coupling mechanisms and with divalent cation binding sites, indicated by Ca^{2+} in the center circle. The plus or minus signs indicate whether positive or negative heterotropic allosteric effects have been observed in *in vitro* radioligand binding experiments. Note that receptor site 1 is positively coupled to the divalent cation binding sites and that (depending on temperature, ligands, and other factors) allosteric interactions between receptor 1 and receptors 2 and 3 may be positive (stimulation) or negative (inhibition). Two of the receptors (1 and 2) have been shown to reside on one polypeptide chain of the isolated purified calcium channel from skeletal muscle.

With (+)-*cis*-diltiazem added (to saturate receptor site 3) to guinea pig skeletal muscle T-tubule membranes, (±)-[^{3}H]nimodipine recognizes twice as many receptors at 37°C than without the allosteric regulator. [The occupation of receptor site 3 also alters the rate constants (K_{+1}, K_{-1}) as well, but the K_D for nimodipine for this isochannel is only marginally decreased.] The purified guinea pig skeletal muscle calcium channel, when labeled with either (−)-[^{3}H]azidopine or (+)-[^{3}H]PN 200-110 at 25°C, shows a dramatic increase in B_{max} by (+)-*cis*-diltiazem or (−)desmethoxyverapamil, although with respect to the maximal number of receptors (+)-*cis*-diltiazem has little effect at this temperature on either maximal (−)-[^{3}H]azidopine or (+)PN 200-110 labeling in the intact membrane. This indicates that the allosteric conversion constant (governing the equilibrium between high and low affinity states) is not only a function of temperature, as usually observed with membranes. Thus, for the channel in intact membranes nimodipine is a "dualist;" (−)azidopine and (+)PN 200-110 are almost pure "antagonists," but for the isolated channel the latter two ligands behave as nimodipine does for the membrane-bound structure.

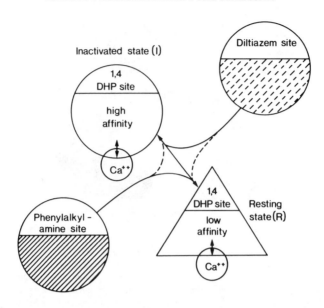

FIG. 19. The drug receptor sites exist in low and high affinity states. This dual existence is exemplified for the receptor site 1. In the absence of divalent cations (cation site empty or filled with monovalents), no high affinity binding can be discovered in *in vitro* ligand binding experiments with radiolabeled 1,4-dihydropyridine channel blockers. With Ca^{2+} bound, as shown, the receptor can exist in the low affinity or high affinity state. The distribution of receptors in these states is determined by the structure of the ligand and by the temperature. For example, a high K_D ligand [like [^{3}H]Bay K 8644] will stabilize only a fraction of channels in the high affinity state at 37°C in skeletal muscle T-tubule membranes. Conversely, a low K_D ligand [like (+)PN 200-110] can label most of the receptors as it stabilizes only a few percent of the channels in the low affinity state. Occupancy of the adjacent receptor sites leads (in this conceptual model) to alterations of the allosteric conversion constant governing the equilibrium between low and high affinity states. To bridge the gap between electrophysiology and biochemistry the high affinity state for channel blockers is tentatively assumed to be equivalent to the inactivated state (I) or, within the subset model, to the sojourn in subset Q, whereas the low affinity state for blockers is assumed to be equivalent to the "resting state" (or subset B).

Thus B_{max} values of (and stoichiometries between) receptors should be regarded with some caution.

In the center of the model are the divalent cation sites, which are also connected by bidirectional arrows to the drug receptors. The 1,4-dihydropyridine receptor is positively coupled and receptor sites 2 and 3 are negatively coupled to divalent cation sites. These will be discussed in more detail in Section V.

Although a vast amount of kinetic and equilibrium binding data has been published, kinetic analysis of the receptor–ligand interactions of the calcium channel is at a very primitive stage as compared to knowledge acquired for nicotinic channels (see, e.g., Covarrubias *et al.,* 1986). In a few instances the allosteric interactions, predicted by *in vitro* binding experiments, have been confirmed in pharmacological experiments. For example, the temperature-dependent stimulation of 1,4-dihydropyridine binding (to receptor site 1) by (+)-*cis*-diltiazem (acting on receptor 3) is reflected in a (temperature-dependent) 30-fold shift (at 37°C) to the left of a 1,4-dihydropyridine (nimodipine) concentration–response curve by subthreshold concentrations of diltiazem determined by negative inotropic responses in perfused rat hearts (De Pover *et al.,* 1983). This (+)-*cis*-diltiazem potentiation also has been studied extensively by Garcia *et al.* (1986). (+)-*cis*-Diltiazem increased (at 37°C) only the B_{max} of receptor site 1 [labeled by (±)-[^{3}H]nimodipine] in (depolarized) guinea pig heart membranes (Glossmann and Ferry, 1985). Shifts of the dose–response curve to the left indicate that (+)-*cis*-diltiazem increased the probability of the channel existing in the inactivated state; the apparent dissociation constant in intact cells depended on the state, the inactivated channel having the highest affinity (see Section III,A).

The states (high and low affinity) of the receptors observed *in vitro* could be compared to the states through which the channel cycles in the intact cell membrane. Whereas voltage governs the states of the *in situ* channel transiently, drugs apparently stabilize analogous conformations more or less permanently *in vitro.*

The working three-site model does not exclude further sites on L-type calcium channels for drugs and toxins. There is some evidence that [^{3}H]HOE 166 or [^{3}H]fluspirilene label a site distinct from that recognized by 1,4-dihydropyridines, phenylalkylamines, and the benzothiazepine (+)-*cis*-diltiazem. The model does not account for homotropic allosteric interactions (and cooperativity among identical sites), but it does allow for 1,4-dihydropyridine receptor (and receptor 2 or 3) stabilization in different states and explains even biphasic competitive inhibition curves (e.g., agonists versus radiolabeled antagonists at 37°C). Homotropic allosteric interactions have not been reported in radioligand experiments with (depolarized) membrane fragments, but cooperative effects with 1,4-dihydropyridines are found in intact cells (Kokubun *et al.,* 1986). It is beyond the scope of this article to discuss this elegant study with isolated rat heart cells in detail. In essence the authors suggest that two distinct high affinity 1,4-dihydropyridine binding sites exist on L-type calcium channels, where blockers and activators can interact. Voltage dependence on both binding affinity and homotropic cooperativity is postulated. Reconstitution experiments with purified calcium channel components (Glossmann *et al.*, 1987a; Hymel *et al.*, 1988b) indeed give hints that more than one 1,4-dihydropyridine receptor-carrying polypeptide is necessary to form a voltage-dependent calcium channel. Kokubun *et al.* (1986) postulated two distinct but coupled sites (perhaps on the same polypeptide chain); better structural data (i.e., obtained by covalent labeling) than currently available are needed to refute or confirm their hypothesis.

G. SUBTYPES OF L-TYPE CALCIUM CHANNELS—BIOCHEMICAL EVIDENCE FOR ISOCHANNELS

A striking difference in equilibrium dissociation constants for 1,4-dihydropyridine receptors is found between skeletal muscle T-tubule channels and heart calcium channels (Ferry and Glossmann, 1983; Glossmann *et al.*, 1984a,b; Glossmann and Ferry, 1985). All heart calcium channel 1,4-dihydropyridine receptor sites exhibit almost identical dissociation constants (0.25 nM) for ($\pm$)-[^{3}H]nimodipine at 37°C, whereas in skeletal muscle T-tubule channels the K_D is around 1.5 nM and in brain membranes, approximately 0.6 nM (Ferry and Glossmann, 1982a; Glossmann and Ferry, 1985). The existence of isoreceptors (as biochemical evidence for the existence of further subtypes of L channels) is a distinct possibility, especially if one takes into account the tissue- but not species-specific effects of the allosteric regulator (+)-*cis*-diltiazem on 1,4-dihydropyridine binding (Ferry and Glossmann, 1983). In brain membranes the allosteric regulator (at 37°C) decreases the K_D for (−)-[^{3}H]nimodipine (Ferry and Glossmann, 1982a). In skeletal muscle the main effect [at 37°C and with ($\pm$)-[^{3}H]nimodipine as ligand] is an increase in B_{max}, whereas in heart there is no change in K_D but a more or less pronounced increase in B_{max} (the rate constants are changed in every case). Data in favor of this hypothesis are summarized in Table III. Additional support comes from the pH profile of 1,4-dihydropyridine binding, the ability of heparin to inhibit 1,4-dihydropyridine binding mainly to skeletal T-tubule membranes (but not to brain membranes), and a variety of other criteria including chelator sensitivity (Glossmann *et al.*, 1984a,b, 1985a).

Utilizing equilibrium dissociation constants one finds little if any discrimination between phenylalkylamine or benzothiazepine receptors in skeletal muscle, heart, or brain. The gating kinetics of skeletal muscle calcium channels are also different from those in heart (see Hille, 1984; and references cited by Cognard *et al.*, 1986a). It is tempting to speculate that tissue-specific differences in the 1,4-dihydro-pyridine receptor and differences in gating kinetics have a common denominator (e.g., differences in primary structure, posttranslational modification). In any event the available data are best explained by the hypothesis that the L-type channels labeled at the 1,4-di-hydropyridine site are a heterogeneous and subdividable set. In analogy to isoenzymes we term the subsets "isochannels." It should be noted that one isochannel, namely, the neuronal L channel, is persistently blocked by ω-CgTx (Cruz et al., 1987).

V. DIVALENT CATION BINDING SITES OF THE CALCIUM CHANNEL

A. THE 1,4-DIHYDROPYRIDINE-SELECTIVE SITE

The binding of labeled 1,4-dihydropyridines to calcium channel-linked receptor sites is dependent on divalent cations. Pretreatment of crude or purified membrane fractions with millimolar concentrations of EDTA, EGTA, or CDTA reduces or blocks high affinity interaction with the dihydropyridine ligands; the notable exception (see Fig. 20) is the particulate (membrane-bound) calcium channel from skeletal muscle (Glossmann et al., 1982; Luchowski et al., 1984; Gould et al., 1982; Glossmann and Ferry, 1983a, 1985). The rank order of chelation sensitivity is brain = aortic membranes > heart >> skeletal muscle. Ileal membranes are sensitive if pretreated with 10 mM EDTA; there is little effect if EDTA is simultaneously added with the ligand. Addition of divalent cations reversed the inhibition (Table IV). Saturation analysis revealed that the effect of the chelators was solely by reduction of B_{max} (Gould et al., 1982; Luchowski et al., 1984; Glossmann and Ferry, 1983). Restoration of binding by Ca^{2+} or Mg^{2+} is inhibited by the trivalent cation La^{3+} (at 100 μM) (Gould et al., 1982; Glossmann et al., 1982; Glossmann and Ferry, 1983a). Differential sensitivity among tissues cannot be explained by varying contents of membrane-bound Ca^{2+}. Temperature, time of exposure to and concentration of chelators, order of addition (ligand and chelator added simultaneously or pretreatment with chelator followed by ligand), and the tissue source itself are all important variables in these experiments.

Kinetics of chelator effects in guinea pig brain membranes showed that addition of EDTA (5 mM) to preformed channel complexes with a labeled 1,4-dihydropyridine [($\pm$)-[^{3}H]-nimodipine] led to an apparent monophasic dissociation of the ligand. At 25°C K_{-1} was 0.026 min-

TABLE III

BIOCHEMICAL EVIDENCE FOR ISORECEPTORS

A. 1,4-Dihydropyridine receptor

Tissue	Species	Ligand	K_D (nM)	T	Effect of (+)-cis-diltiazem	pH Profile	Ref.[a]
Skeletal muscle	Guinea pig	[³H]Nimodipine	1.5	37°C	Increase in B_{max}, small decrease in K_D	Sigmoidal	a, b
Heart	Many	[³H]Nimodipine	0.25	37°C	Increase in B_{max}, no change in K_D	Bell shaped	a, c, d
Brain	Guinea pig	[³H]Nimodipine	0.6	37°C	Decrease in K_D, no change in B_{max}	Bell shaped	a, e

B. Phenylalkylamine receptor[b]

Tissue	Species	K_D (nM)	Ref.[a]
Skeletal muscle	Rabbit, guinea pig	1.5; 2.2	f, g
Heart	Cat, bovine	2.5; 1.4	h, i
Brain	Guinea pig	1.6	j

C. Benzothiazepine receptor[c]

Tissue	Species	K_D (nM)	Comments	Ref.[a]
Skeletal muscle	Guinea pig, rabbit	39; 50	1,4-Dihydropyridinne antagonists increase B_{max} at 30°C (depending on intrinsic activity)	k, g
Brain	Rat	50	1,4-Dihydropyridine antagonists decrease K_D at 37°C (depending on intrinsic activity)	l
Heart	Porcine, canine	80 (40); 58	1,4-Dihydropyridines decrease K_D at 37°C (depending on intrinsic activity)	m, n

[a] Key to references: a, Glossmann and Ferry (1985), *Methods Enzymol.* **109**, 513–550, Ferry and Glossmann, *Br. J. Pharmacol.* **78**, 81P; b, Glossmann *et al.* (1984), *J. Cardiovasc. Pharmacol.* **6**, S608–S621; c, DePover *et al.* (1983), *Biochem. Biophys. Res. Commun.* **114**, 922–929; d, Ferry *et al.* (1985a), *Br. J. Pharmacol.* **84**, 811–824; e, Ferry and Glossmann (1982), *Naunyn–Schmiedeberg's Arch. Pharmacol.* **321**, 80–83; f, Goll *et al.* (1984a), *FEBS Lett.* **176**, 371–377; g, Galizzi *et al.* (1986b), *J. Biol. Chem.* **261**, 1393–1397; h, Goll *et al.* (1986), *Naunyn–Schmiedeberg's Arch. Pharmacol.* **334**, 303–312; i, Ruth *et al.* (1985), *Eur. J. Biochem.* **150**, 313–322; j, Ferry *et al.* (1984a), *Naunyn–Schmiedeberg's Arch. Pharmacol.* **327**, 183–187; k, Glossmann *et al.* (1983a), *FEBS Lett.* **160**, 226–232; l, Schoemaker and Langer (1985), *Eur. J. Pharmacol.* **111**, 273–277; m, Balwierzak *et al.* (1987), *Mol. Pharmacol.* **31**, 175–179; n, Garcia *et al.* (1986), *J. Biol. Chem.* **261**, 8146–8157.

[b] Labeled with (−)-[³H]desmethoxyverapamil.

[c] Labeled with (+)-*cis*-[³H]diltiazem.

TABLE IV

CHELATOR SENSITIVITY OF 1,4-DIHYDROPYRIDINE BINDING TO CALCIUM CHANNEL RECEPTORS

Tissue	Species	Incubation conditions	Ligand	Results	Comment	Ref.[a]
Skeletal muscle (crude membranes)	Guinea pig	Chelators present with ligand at 25°C	$(\pm)$-[³H]Nitrendipine	Stimulation (20%)	Ligand added together with chelator	a
Skeletal muscle (microsomes)	Guinea pig	Preincubation with EDTA at 37°C	$(\pm)$-[³H]Nimodipine	15% inhibition at 10 mM	Ligand added after chelator	b
Skeletal muscle (T-tubule membranes)	Rabbit	Chelator (EGTA) present at 10°C	$(\pm)$-[³H]Nitrendipine	No effect	Ligand added with chelator	c
Skeletal muscle (T-tubule membranes)	Rabbit	EDTA (100 μM) inhibits, EGTA and (OH) EDTA do not inhibit	$(\pm)$-[³H]PN 200-110	50% inhibition	Effect not caused by Mg^{2+} removal; EGTA ineffective	d
Skeletal muscle (solubilized)	Guinea pig	Chelators present with ligand at 37°C	$(\pm)$-[³H]Nimodipine	>80% reduction of binding by EDTA, CDTA, EGTA ($K_{0.5}$ = 20 μM)	$(+)$-cis-Diltiazem decreased sensitivity to chelators	e
Heart (crude membranes)	Guinea pig	Chelator present with ligand at 25°C	$(\pm)$-[³H]Nitrendipine	25% inhibition at 1 mM EDTA	Ligand added with chelator	a
Heart (crude membrane)	Rabbit	Chelator present with ligand at 25°C	$(\pm)$-[³H]Nitrendipine	No inhibition at 1 mM EDTA	Ligand added with chelator	f
Heart (crude membranes)	Rabbit	Chelator present during preparation and incubation	$(\pm)$-[³H]Nitrendipine	74% reduction of B_{max} when pretreated with 10 mM EDTA	Ligand added after chelator	f
Heart (membranes	Bovine	EGTA (1 mM) added during incubation	$(\pm)$-[³H]Nimodipine	100% inhibition	Ligand added with chelator	g

Tissue	Species	Conditions	Ligand	Effect	Comment	Ref.
Heart (purified membrane)	Chick	Chelator EDTA present at 25°C	(±)-[^{3}H]Nitrendipine or (+)-[^{3}H]PN 200-100	EDTA converts 1,4-DHP receptors to low affinity	Mg^{2+} and Ca^{2+} can reverse the inhibition	h
Aortic membranes	Calf	Chelator present with ligand	(±)-[^{3}H]Nitrendipine	85% reduction of B_{max} by 1 mM EDTA	Ligand added with chelator	f
Ileal membranes	Guinea pig	Chelator present with ligand	(±)-[^{3}H]Nitrendipine	25% inhibition (B_{max}) by 1 mM EDTA	Ligand added with chelator	f
Ileal membranes	Guinea pig	Chelator present with ligand	(±)-[^{3}H]Nitrendipine	60% inhibition by 1 mM EDTA		a
Ileal membranes	Guinea pig	Chelator present during preparation and incubation	(±)-[^{3}H]Nitrendipine	80% reduction of B_{max} by pretreatment with 10 mM EDTA	Ligand added after chelator	f
Brain membranes	Guinea pig	Chelators present with ligand at 25°C	(±)-[^{3}H]Nitrendipine	60% inhibition by 1 mM EDTA	Ligand added with chelator	a
Brain membranes	Guinea pig	Pretreatment with 5 mM EDTA at 37°C, wash with Mg^{2+}-free buffer	(±)-[^{3}H]Nimodipine	>95% inhibition by pretreatment	Ligand added without chelator	i
Brain membranes	Rat	Pretreatment with EDTA, EGTA at 0°C; incubation at 25°C	(±)-[^{3}H]Nitrendipine	80% reduction by washing with EDTA/EGTA	Ligand added with 10 µM EGTA	j

[a] Key to references: a, Gould et al. (1983b), Mol. Pharmacol. 25, 235–241; b, Glossmann et al. (1985a), Arzneim. Forsch. 35, 1917–1935; c, Fosset et al. (1983), J. Biol. Chem. 258, 6086–6092; d, Galizzi et al. 1985), Biochem. Biophys. Res. Commun. 132, 49–55; e, Glossmann and Ferry (1983b), Naunyn–Schmiedeberg's Arch. Pharmacol. 323, 279–291; f, Luchowski et al. (1984), J. Pharmacol. Exp. Ther. 230, 607–613; g, Ruth et al. (1985), Eur. J. Biochem. 150, 313–322; h, Ptasienski et al. (1985), Biochem. Biophys. Res. Commun. 129, 910–917; i, Glossmann and Ferry (1985), Methods in Enzymology, Vol. 109, pp. 513–550, Academic Press, Orlando, Florida; j, Gould et al. (1982), Proc. Natl. Acad. Sci. U.S.A. 79, 3656–3660.

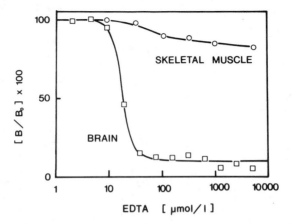

FIG. 20. Differential (tissue-specific) sensitivity of calcium channels with respect to divalent cation regulation. Membranes from guinea pig cerebral cortex (brain) and skeletal muscle T-tubules were treated at 37°C with increasing concentrations of EDTA, and receptor 1 was probed with ($\pm$)-[³H]nimodipine. Binding of the labeled ligand was almost completely inhibited in the brain, whereas inhibition was marginal in particulate skeletal muscle. [From Glossmann *et al.* (1985a), *Arzneim. Forsch.* **35**, 1917–1935, with permission.]

ute^{-1}; at 30°C, 0.076 minute^{-1}. With the positive allosteric regulator of 1,4-dihydropyridine binding, (+)-*cis*-diltiazem, the dissociation rate constant was lowered to 0.009 minute^{-1} at 30°C. These results indicated that the removal of the divalent cation(s) was highly temperature dependent and that (+)-*cis*-diltiazem stabilized the complex between the 1,4-dihydropyridine receptor, the divalent cation(s), and the calcium channel (Fig. 21). Removal of the divalent cation from brain membrane calcium channels is highly temperature dependent. Guinea pig brain membranes pretreated with 5–10 mM EDTA at 0°C and subsequently washed in Ca^{2+}-free (but not chelator-containing) buffer, showed binding identical to that of control membranes. Such chelator preincubations at 37°C reduced ($\pm$)-[³H]nimodipine binding by over 90% (Ferry and Glossmann 1983a, 1985). This suggests that sidedness of the membranes (e.g., availability of the channel-bound Ca^{2+} to the chelators) could not play a significant role. Instead, raising the temperature appeared to decrease the affinity of the channel for Ca^{2+} or to shift the equilibrium between two conformations of the channel where one conformation allows Ca^{2+} to leave. In experiments with purified calcium channels from guinea pig skeletal muscle we have found a similar temperature dependence (J. Striessnig, unpublished).

The decrease in B_{max} in the different particulate channel preparations is explained by conversion of a high affinity state of the 1,4-dihydropyridine receptor to a very low affinity state (Glossmann and Ferry, 1985; Glossmann et al., 1985a). It was postulated that the high affinity complex of labeled 1,4-dihydropyridines with the channel is a *ternary* complex $Ch \cdot Ca^{2+} \cdot DHP$ where Ch is the channel and DHP stands for a 1,4-dihydropyridine channel blocker. Considering the coupled equilibrium equations:

$$K_a = \frac{[Ch][Ca^{2+}]}{[Ch \cdot Ca^{2+}]} \qquad (1)$$

$$K_b = \frac{[Ch \cdot Ca^{2+}][DHP]}{[Ch \cdot Ca^{2+} \cdot DHP]} \qquad (2)$$

$$K_c = \frac{[Ca^{2+}][Ch \cdot DHP]}{[Ch \cdot Ca^{2+} \cdot DHP]} \qquad (3)$$

$$K_d = \frac{[Ch][DHP]}{[Ch \cdot DHP]} \qquad (4)$$

one finds $K_a K_b = K_c K_d$. The equilibrium constant K_d must be very high since no binding to the cation-free channel is found in filtration assays with the usual concentrations of labeled ligands. A reasonable assumption is that $K_d = 100 K_b$. It follows that $K_a = 100 K_c$. Thus, the 1,4-dihydropyridine must stabilize the binding of Ca^{2+} as Ca^{2+} stabilizes the binding of the 1,4-dihydropyridine.

The complete reversibility of the chelator effect by readdition of divalent cations allowed tests of ion selectivity for binding sites of the channel in particulate brain membranes. These "refilling" experiments revealed a complex interaction between the divalent cation binding sites and the 1,4-dihydropyridine receptor (see Fig. 22). Divalent cations recognized as calcium channel blockers (Ni^{2+}, Zn^{2+}, Co^{2+}) showed biphasic refilling curves; Sr^{2+} and Ba^{2+} refilled with Hill slopes between 0.3 and 0.5, whereas Ca^{2+}, Mn^{2+}, and Mg^{2+} gave Hill slopes between 1.5 and 3.0. Positive as well as negative cooperative effects were found, suggesting more than one cation binding site coupled to the 1,4-dihydropyridine receptor (Glossmann and Ferry, 1983a). The ions differed with respect to maximal refilling potency, Ca^{2+} and Sr^{2+} being nearly indistinguishable. A plot of the refilling potency, normalized for Ca^{2+} (=100%), versus the crystal radius is shown in Fig. 23. Similar data have been found for rat brain (Gould et al., 1982) and guinea pig ileum membranes (Luchowski et al., 1984), indicating that the divalent cation binding sites of the calcium chan-

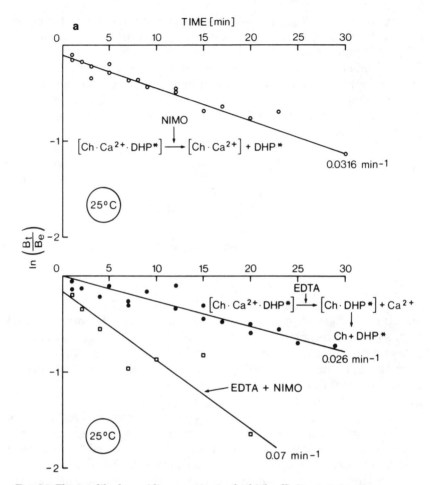

FIG. 21. The 1,4-dihydropyridine receptor in the high affinity state is a ternary complex. (a) Top: Guinea pig brain membranes were labeled at receptor 1 of the calcium channel (Ch) with (±)-[³H]nimodipine. At equilibrium association of labeled ligand (DHP*) was blocked by adding a large excess of unlabeled Ca^{2+} antagonist. Bottom: The conversion of the ternary complex to the (very) low affinity (Ch·DHP*) state was induced by addition of 5 mM EDTA. This low affinity state is unstable and will release the labeled ligand. When both blockade of the forward reaction of DHP* and removal of the divalent cation are induced at time zero, the high affinity complex dissociated with a rate constant approximately equal to the sum of the individual dissociation rate constants. (b) The allosteric regulator (+)-cis-diltiazem stabilizes the ternary complex of a 1,4-dihydropyridine with the receptor site 1 and divalent cations. Here 10 μM (+)-cis-diltiazem was present throughout the incubation, and the off-rates are slowed down considerably in the presence of the allosteric regulator. For this subtype of L-channel receptor 1 the effect of (+)-cis-diltiazem on the binding of a 1,4-dihydropyridine is mainly on the dissociation constant. The latter is decreased (at 37°C) by a factor of 3. [From Glossmann et al. (1985a), Arzneim. Forsch. 35, 1917–1935, with permission.]

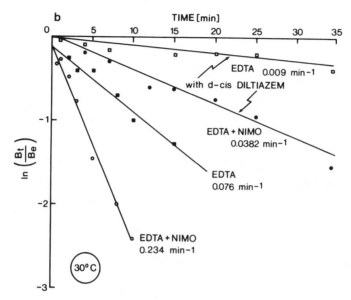

FIG. 21-*continued*

nels linked to the 1,4-dihydropyridine receptors have very similar properties.

In guinea pig brain membranes the $K_{0.5}$ values (total added ion concentration necessary to recover 50% of the respective maximal response) have been determined in Tris–Cl buffer. The rank order of ions giving monophasic refilling isotherms was $Ca^{2+} > Mn^{2+} > Mg^{2+} > Sr^{2+} > Ba^{2+} >> Ca^{2+}$. The rank order is not identical with the relative affinities of the divalents for heart calcium channels derived by Lansman *et al.* (1986): $Cd^{2+} > Ca^{2+} = Sr^{2+} > Ba^{2+} > Mg^{2+}$ (vide infra).

The effect of the positive allosteric modulator of 1,4-dihydropyridine binding, (+)-*cis*-diltiazem, on the $K_{0.5}$ values is shown in Table V. It is interesting that Sr^{2+} and Ba^{2+} not only gave Hill slopes below 1 for refilling but also displayed the highest decrease with respect to $K_{0.5}$ value. Since the increase in affinity of $(\pm)$-[^{3}H]nimodipine by 10 μM (+)-*cis*-diltiazem for the guinea pig brain calcium channel 1,4-dihydropyridine receptor is 3-fold (K_D decreases from 0.6 to 0.2 nM; Ferry and Glossmann, 1982) the results strongly argue that (+)-*cis*-diltiazem affected 1,4-dihydropyridine binding in native (i.e., not refilled) membranes by increasing the affinity of the (already) bound divalent cation(s), in line with dissociation experiments shown in Fig. 21.

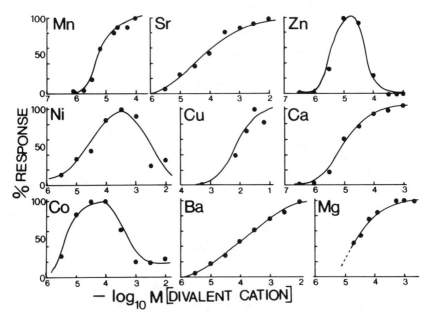

Fig. 22. Divalent cation requirement of the 1,4-dihydropyridine receptor. Here the guinea pig brain calcium channel was completely depleted of divalent cations by pretreatment with EDTA at 37°C. Under the conditions employed no high affinity binding of $(\pm)$-[³H]nimodipine was found. By reintroducing divalent cations (after carefully washing the membranes free of EDTA) high affinity binding is recovered. This recovery is for Ca^{2+} a concentration-dependent increase in B_{max}, i.e., the number of receptors in the high affinity state. The figure shows the refilling curves which are normalized with respect to Ca^{2+} (=100% recovery of high affinity binding). Note that ions which block the channel have biphasic refilling curves; ions which permeate easily (Ba^{2+}, Sr^{2+}) have apparent Hill coefficients less than 1.0. [From Glossmann and Ferry (1985), *Methods in Enzymology*, Vol. 109, pp. 513–550, Academic Press, Orlando, Florida.]

B. The Phenylalkylamine-Selective Site

Monovalent and divalent cations inhibit receptor binding of labeled phenylalkylamines (Table VI). In skeletal muscle microsomes from guinea pigs $(\pm)$-[³H]verapamil binding is inhibited in the order Mn^{2+} > Ca^{2+} > Mg^{2+}. The $K_{0.5}$ values are in the low millimolar range (Goll *et al.*, 1984b). Similar findings were reported for the rabbit T-tubule membrane (Galizzi *et al.*, 1984a). The latter authors investigated the mechanism of inhibition of $(\pm)$-[³H]verapamil binding and found that Ca^{2+} increased the K_D (from 27 to 55 nM) and decreased the B_{max}

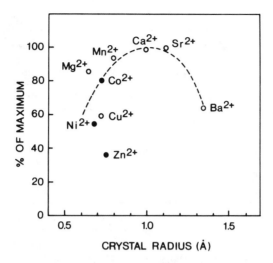

FIG. 23. Refilling potency of the calcium channel divalent cation sites may be related to the crystal radius. When the ion binding sites of the guinea pig brain calcium channel are depleted of divalents by pretreatment with EDTA, divalent cations are able to recover the high affinity binding. However, the ability for maximum recovery differs for the different cations. In this graph the maximum recovery has been normalized to that seen with Ca^{2+}. There is a correlation between the crystal radius and the maximum recovery. The relationship does not hold, however, for Zn^{2+}, Ni^{2+}, or Co^{2+} (filled circles), which have nearly identical crystal radii but differ considerably with respect to maximal recovery.

(from 50 to 33 pmol/mg protein) as $[Ca^{2+}]$ increased from 0 to 0.72 mM. Thus Ca^{2+} appeared to be a mixed-type inhibitor whereas Mn^{2+} was a pure noncompetitive blocker (reduction of B_{max}, no change of K_D). Similar findings with optically pure $(-)$-[^{3}H]desmethoxy-verapamil have been reported for rabbit skeletal muscle microsomes, rat brain membranes, and guinea pig hippocampus membranes (Glossmann et al., 1985b).

The question of divalent cation inhibition of phenylalkylamine binding was reinvestigated by Galizzi et al. (1985) employing $(-)$-[^{3}H]desmethoxyverapamil. They found that Tris (50 mM) shifted the apparent affinity of certain ions for the blocking divalent cation binding site by 100-fold. Substitution of Tris–Cl by HEPES also increased the selectivity of T-tubule membranes for divalent cations. Under these conditions the $K_{0.5}$ value for Ca^{2+} was 5 μM, and Mg^{2+} was over 30 times less effective as a blocker. Similar to the results obtained with $(\pm)$-[^{3}H]verapamil, Galizzi et al. (1985) found that the

TABLE V

(+)-cis-DILTIAZEM INCREASES THE AFFINITY
OF THE CALCIUM CHANNEL FOR DIVALENT CATIONS[a]

Ion	Control	With (+)-cis-diltiazem
Ca^{2+}	14.5 ± 8.6	6.9 ± 6.1
Mg^{2+}	43.0 ± 14.1	19.4 ± 4.6[b]
Mn^{2+}	25.2 ± 12.2	10.3 ± 8.3
Sr^{2+}	99.0 ± 18.5	14.2 ± 5.2[b]
Ba^{2+}	267.0 ± 126.2	51.2 ± 38.1[b]
Ni^{2+}	16.4 ± 10.0	9.5 ± 4.2
Co^{2+}	14.9 ± 13.5	5.9 ± 5.4
Cu^{2+}	6306 ± 2582	8528 ± 3175

[a] Refilling of divalent cation binding sites linked to 1,4-dihydropyridine receptors of guinea pig brain calcium channels was determined. For each ion three to four complete dose–response curves were measured in the absence or presence of 10 μM (+)-cis-diltiazem. The data were fitted to the general dose–response equation and the ED_{50} values (total concentration of ion yielding 50% of the maximum recovery for the high affinity state of the 1,4-dihydropyridine receptor) determined. The ligand employed was (±)-[³H]nimodipine, the temperature 37°C. ED_{50} values are given in μM. Note that (+)-cis-diltiazem increases the apparent affinity of several cations to reconstitue the high affinity state.
[b] Statistically significant difference ($p < 0.05$).

divalent cation-free conformation of the receptor bound (−)-[³H]desmethoxyverapamil with high affinity and that saturation of the Ca^{2+} coordination site by Ca^{2+} led to a decrease of the affinity of the labeled ligand by at most a factor of 5 (K_D without Ca^{2+} 1.8 nM, with 35 μM Ca^{2+} 6.3 nM). At saturating Ca^{2+} concentrations B_{max} decreased 31%. These findings were explained by assuming two states (or populations) of the (−)-[³H]desmethoxyverapamil sites: one where Ca^{2+} modulated affinity (69% of all sites) and the other (31%) where Ca^{2+} decreased affinity (at least by a factor of 50) to such an extent that B_{max} decreased. However, another study, also performed in HEPES buffer, gave results identical to those in Tris buffer (see Table VI); in our laboratory we did not find a dramatic effect of HEPES on cation sensitivity with partially purified skeletal muscle T-tubule preparations.

TABLE VI

INHIBITION OF THE PHENYLALKYLAMINE-SELECTIVE SITE BY DIVALENT CATIONS

Tissue	Species	Assay conditions	T	Ligand	Results	Ref.[a]
Skeletal muscle (T-tubule membranes)	Rabbit	20 mM tris–HCl buffer	10°C	(±)-[3H]Verapamil	$Ca^{2+} = Mn^{2+} > Mg^{2+} > Sr^{2+} > Ba^{2+} \gg Co^{2+} > Ni^{2+}$ ($K_{0.5}$: $0.3 = 0.3 > 0.4 > 1.3 > 1.7 \gg 3 > 8$ mM)	a
Skeletal muscle (T-tubule membranes)	Rabbit	10 mM HEPES	25°C	(−)-[3H]Desmethoxyverapamil	$Ca^{2+} > Sr^{2+} > Ba^{2+} > Mg^{2+}$ ($K_{0.5}$: $5 > 25 > 50 > 170$ µM)	b
Brain (hippocampus membranes)	Guinea pig	50 mM Tris–HCl buffer	25°C	(−)-[3H]Desmethoxyverapamil	$Cd^{2+} > Zn^{2+} > Ca^{2+} \gg Mg^{2+}$ ($K_{0.5}$: 0.01–1 mM)	c
Skeletal muscle (microsomes), EDTA pre-washed	Rabbit	50 mM HEPES	22–24°C	(−)-[3H]Desmethoxyverapamil	$Cd^{2+} = Hg^{2+} > Mn^{2+} > Ca^{2+} > Co^{2+} > Ba^{2+}$ ($K_{0.5}$: 0.03–10 mM)	d
Skeletal muscle (microsomes)	Guinea pig	50 mM tris–HCl	2°C	(±)-[3H]Verapamil	$Mn^{2+} > Ca^{2+} > Mg^{2+}$ ($K_{0.5}$: $0.1 > 0.3 > 1$ mM)	e
Brain (forebrain minus thalamus and hypothalamus)	Rat	50 mM HEPES	22–24°C	(−)-[3H]Desmethoxyverapamil	Stimulation at low ion concentrations (0.1 mM); inhibition: $Cd^{2+} > La^{3+} > Ca^{2+} > Mn^{2+} = Ba^{2+} > Co^{2+}$	d

[a] Key to references: a, Galizzi et al. (1984a), Eur. J. Biochem. 144, 211–215; b, Galizzi et al. (1985), Biochem. Biophys. Res. Commun. 132, 49–55; c, Glossmann et al. (1985b), J. Cardiovasc. Pharmacol. 7, S20–S30; d, Reynolds et al. (1986b), J. Pharmacol. Exp. Ther. 237, 731–738; e, Goll et al. (1984b), Eur. J. Biochem. 141, 177–186.

C. The Benzothiazepine-Selective Site

Balwierczak and Schwartz (1985) reported that $(+)$-cis-[^{3}H]diltiazem binding to dog heart membranes was inhibited by Ca^{2+}. The $K_{0.5}$ value was 0.3 mM, and with 1 mM Ca^{2+} added the K_D for the ligand increased from 72.6 to 182.5 nM without changing B_{max} (2.4 pmol/mg protein). In guinea pig skeletal muscle T-tubule membranes, $(+)$-cis-[^{3}H]diltiazem binding was inhibited by cations in the order Cd^{2+} $> Mn^{2+} > Ca^{2+} > Mg^{2+} >> K^+ > Na^+$ (Glossmann et al., 1985c). Again, as seen with $(\pm)$-[^{3}H]-verapamil, inhibition constants were in the high micromolar to millimolar range.

Similar values were reported for porcine heart membranes, where 50% inhibition of $(+)$-d-cis-[^{3}H]diltiazem binding was found at 10 mM Mg^{2+}, 200 mM Na^+, or 400 mM Na^+ (Garcia et al., 1986). In contrast, Galizzi et al. (1985) found that in HEPES buffer Ca^{2+} at 5 μM inhibited $(+)$-cis-[^{3}H]dilitiazem binding to rabbit skeletal muscle T-tubule membranes.

Summary

The 1,4-dihydropyridine receptor of the calcium channel is reciprocally allosterically coupled in a positive manner to multiple (at least two) high affinity Ca^{2+} binding sites. The interaction is readily apparent in brain, less so in heart and some smooth muscle preparations, and not at all in particulate membranes from skeletal muscle. With calcium channels solubilized from skeletal muscle the dependence of high affinity 1,4-dihydropyridine binding on divalents is also apparent and is maintained throughout purification. This offers the opportunity of investigating directly the interaction of radiolabeled divalent cations with the purified channel components and the influence of channel activators or blockers on the binding parameters. Binding of compounds selective for the phenylalkylamine or benzothiazepine receptors is inhibited by divalent cations in particulate as well in purified channel preparations (from skeletal muscle). It appears that, on occupation by ligands, the respective drug receptor domains alter the interaction of the divalent cation sites with their ligands. This is supported by molecular analysis of agonistic and antagonistic enantiomers of 1,4-dihydropyridines (see Section III,A,6). The tight coupling suggests that the drug receptor domains are close to the divalent cation binding sites, perhaps on the same polypeptide chain. Unfortunately, no comprehensive model incorporating biochemical and electrophysiological data is available to fully explain the functional implications for channel blockade and activation.

VI. ROLE OF CALCIUM CHANNELS IN VERTEBRATE SKELETAL MUSCLE

A. EXCITATION–CONTRACTION COUPLING

1. *Structural and Functional Aspects*

Contraction of *invertebrate* skeletal muscles is highly dependent on extracellular Ca^{2+}. It is appropriate to note that the first calcium action potential was recorded in muscle fibers of crab legs by Fatt and Katz (1953), later to be clearly identified as a calcium spike (Fatt and Ginsborg, 1958). Influx of Ca^{2+} in arthropod skeletal muscles is mediated by voltage-sensitive calcium channels (Ashcroft and Stanfield, 1982; Gilly and Scheuer, 1984) which in scorpion muscle have sufficient capacity to raise total fiber Ca^{2+} at a rate of 6 μM/msecond (see Scheuer and Gilly, 1986). *Vertebrate* skeletal muscles, however, are virtually insensitive to reduction in extracellular Ca^{2+}; hence the major source of the Ca^{2+} needed for contraction must come from intracellular stores.

The mechanism by which relaxation of skeletal muscle occurs (the energized sarcoplasmic Ca^{2+} pump lowers the intrafiber free Ca^{2+} concentration) is known in almost every detail. In contrast, the events leading to Ca^{2+} release are still not understood. There is, however, increasing evidence that voltage-dependent surface membrane calcium channels and Ca^{2+}-release channels in the sarcoplasmic reticulum cooperate intimately in this process. Before focusing on voltage-dependent calcium channels and their functional role in vertebrate skeletal muscle, we describe structural features important in this context, discuss the composition and properties of the Ca^{2+}-release channel, and give a brief review of current theories of excitation–contraction coupling.

Mammalian skeletal muscle fibers are up to 0.5 m long and have diameters of 0.04–0.1 mm (Eisenberg, 1983). A surface action potential must activate the contractile elements in the depth of the fiber almost simultaneously with those near the surface. Signal propagation radially from the surface is mediated by a specialized structure of the sarcolemma termed the transverse-tubule or the T system. The T system forms a complex 3-dimensional network (being electrically and structurally continuous with the plasmalemma) within the fiber and makes specific contacts with specialized elements of the sarcoplasmic reticulum (terminal cisternae). At these contacts the T-tubule membrane is termed "junctional;" other parts not associated with sarcoplasmic reticulum are termed "free" (Peachey and Franzini-Armstrong, 1983). The fractional surface of transverse tubules that is apposed by terminal cisternae is 67%. The surface area (per unit volume of fiber) of the transverse tubule is 0.22 μm^{-1} ($\mu m^2/\mu m^3$) in frog sartorius muscle (Mobley and Eisenberg, 1975) or 0.3 μm^{-1} (Peachey, 1965). This corresponds to 2.2–3 × 10^3 cm^2 surface area/cm^3 of fiber volume.

Where the membranes of the cisternae and the T-tubules meet, so-called feet (T-SR feet) and (less numerous) pillars link both membranes. The average center-to-center repeat distance of the feet is 28.5 nm, and the space between feet varies between 12.5 and 20.0 nm. They extend approximately 10 nm from the surface of the terminal cisternae membrane; the gap spacing of the triad junction is around 12 nm (Mitchell et al., 1983). The feet were always suspected to represent a structural element for signal transmission across the junction, although their exact functional activity was obscure. A purely mechanical role (to maintain the transverse tubule and sarcoplasmic membrane at a fixed distance) could therefore not be excluded.

Franzini-Armstrong and Nunzi (1983) deduced a four-subunit structure of these feet in fish muscle. A similar 4-fold symmetry structure was later identified on isolated heavy sarcoplasmic reticulum vesicles from rat skeletal muscle (Ferguson et al., 1984). Clusters of four particles, organized in parallel rows, in the opposing junctional T-tubule membrane were also observed.

Recently the Ca^{2+}-release channel was isolated from sarcoplasmic (triad) membrane fractions after solubilization with either CHAPS or digitonin (Imagawa et al., 1987b; Inui et al., 1987a; Lai et al., 1988). Purification was aided by the highly specific interaction of the plant alkaloid ryanodine with this channel. This alkaloid modulates channel function by locking it in the "open state" (Inui et al., 1987a). Tritium-labeled ryanodine binds with nanomolar dissociation constants to the sarcoplasmic channel structure. Binding is stimulated by ATP and requires micromolar free Ca^{2+}. As the dissociation of ryanodine is extremely slow, prelabeling (in the presence of the nonhydrolyzable ATP analog AMP-PCP) allows purification from solubilized (triad-enriched) membranes, even in a single step (sucrose gradient centrifugation). The receptor migrates as a single peak with an apparent sedimentation coefficient of 30 S (Lai et al., 1988). A monoclonal antibody affinity column retains the ryanodine receptor from which it can be eluted by 0.5 M NaSCN (Imagawa et al., 1987b). Whatever the purification method, there is agreement that subunits of 360–450 kDa carry the ryanodine receptor (and regulatory sites for ATP and Ca^{2+}).

Electron micrographic studies of the purified Ca^{2+}-release channel show characteristics typical of the foot structure, including the 4-fold symmetry recognized earlier in fixed muscle fibers or in isolated sarcoplasmic reticulum vesicles (Inui et al., 1987a; Lai et al., 1988). Thus, Ca^{2+}-release channels, ryanodine receptors, and feet are synonymous terms representing the same structure. The volume of an isolated foot structure was estimated to be 5.8×10^{-18} cm^3 (calculated as a $21 \times 21 \times 12$ nm cube plus four cylindrical pillars anchoring the foot structure in the membrane with 5 nm diameter and 7 nm length) or 5.4×10^{-18} cm^3 ($26 \times 26 \times 8$ nm) by Inui et al. (1987a) and Lai et al. (1988), respectively. With a protein density of 0.73 cm^3/g, 4500–5000 kDa of densely packed protein would fit into this structure. Whereas Lai et al. (1988), judging from electron micrographs of negatively stained Ca^{2+}-release channel complexes, suggest a minimum of four 400 kDa subunits in a four-leaf clover structure, Inui et al. (1987b) propose a more densely packed structure with 12 subunits (e.g., 3 subunits in each "leaf"). Lai et al. (1988) suggested that a pore (1–2 nm diameter) is at the center of the ryanodine receptor complex with the four subunits surrounding it.

Reconstitution of the purified polypeptides in lipid bilayers yielded Ca^{2+}-release channels. Depending on the purification method, they either possessed properties similar to those of the native channel (Hymel et al., 1988a; Lai et al., 1988) or behaved kinetically and pharmacologically different (Imagawa et al., 1987b). Interestingly, in reconstitution experiments, subconductance levels are observed: namely, 20, 40, 65, 100, 130, 180, 290 pS (Lai et al., 1988) or 38, 15, 30, 60 pS (Hymel et al., 1988a). Although various explanations have been offered for this phenomenon, the model of Hymel et al. (1988a) prescribing a cooperative aggregate, termed "oligomeric channel," consisting of, e.g., 16 "monochannels" is very attractive. As virtually identical findings (i.e., cooperative channel aggregates) are reported for the reconstituted 1,4-dihydropyridine-sensitive calcium channel from T-tubule membranes (Hymel et al., 1988b; see section VII,C), it is proposed (Hymel et al., 1988c) that both channels are organized as similarly sized oligomers bridging the junctional space between the sarcoplasmic reticulum and the T-tubule. It is tempting to speculate that the particles which cluster in groups of four in the junctional T-tubule membrane (see above) represent the 1,4-dihydropyridine-sensitive channel. In contrast to the ryanodine-sensitive Ca^{2+}-release channel from sarcoplasmic reticulum, ultrastructural data on the purified L-type calcium channel from skeletal muscle are not available.

The most common form of the association of the T-tubules with the sarcoplasmic reticulum is a triadic structure where two cisternal elements flank a single T-tubule. In invertebrate muscles the corresponding structure is a dyad (one cisternal element and one T-tubule). In mammalian muscle two triads are found in each sarcomere. The key role of the triad in excitation–contraction coupling was discovered by Huxley and collaborators (see Huxley, 1971) in an ingenious series of experiments. They used a very fine (1 μm diameter) pipet to locally depolarize the skeletal muscle fibers. Local contractions could be elicited only at certain, anatomically defined "hot spots," later to be identified as triads.

Since that time the mechanism by which the action potential propagated along the T-tubule leads to Ca^{2+} release from the terminal cisternae in vertebrate skeletal muscle has been under intensive investigation. The sequence of events linking the initial excitatory event to the final mechanical response has been termed excitation–contraction coupling by Sandow (1952, 1965). In general three different hypotheses have been proposed, the electrical hypothesis, the mechanical hypothesis, and the chemical hypothesis. Any hypothesis must account for the fact that there is a minimum latency period of 1–5 mseconds between the maximum of the electrical potential and the start of Ca^{2+} release from the terminal cisternae (Frank, 1980; Volpe et al., 1986a); it must also explain the refractory state and mechanical activation in the absence of ionic conductance changes.

a. The Electrical Hypothesis. The electrical hypothesis (termed "ionic current coupling mechanism") is based on the assumption that there is electrical continuity between the T-tubule membrane and the terminal cisternae via conductance channels (opened on depolarization) which in turn pass electric current into the cisternae and lead to Ca^{2+} release (Mathias et al., 1980). There is little evidence to support this mechanism.

b. The Mechanical Hypothesis. In the charge movement hypothesis it is proposed that molecules extend across the T-SR gap and charged groups are contained in the membrane of the T-tubules. Being sensors of potentials, the charged groups can physically move, according to the hypothesis, by tens of angstroms. The nonlinear voltage-dependent charge movement in skeletal muscle, first described by Schneider and Chandler (1973), is similar to gating currents (Hille, 1984) but two orders of magnitude slower than those of the sodium channel (Schneider and Chandler, 1973). (For reviews of gating currents and charge movement, see Almers, 1978; Schneider, 1981.) Charge movements become discernible when ionic currents are blocked and linear components of capacity are subtracted. The records are composed of two phases: Q_{on} is observed at the onset of depolarization. and Q_{off} follows at the termination.

In the literature the charge movement hypothesis is often referred to as the "rigid rod model" or "remote control model" because in one of the (hypothetical) examples depicted by Chandler et al. (1976a) the charged complex was connected by a "rigid rod" to a plug. The channel of the sarcoplasmic reticulum, which controls Ca^{2+} release, was here assumed to be mechanically plugged when the charged complex was in the resting position; on activation the plug is removed and Ca^{2+} is released. The model can also explain the refractory state. It has been recently shown that under certain experimental conditions (and assumptions) the charge movement is linearly correlated to the peak rate of Ca^{2+} release from the sarcoplasmic reticulum (Melzer et al., 1986). Others (see, e.g., Lamb, 1986a–c) have observed that the charge movement phases have different components which can be discriminated by their sensitivity to drugs (vide infra).

c. The Chemical Hypothesis. In the chemical hypothesis a mechanism is postulated by which a trigger substance is released or formed in the triadic junction, diffuses across the gap, and turns on the Ca^{2+} release mechanism. For the chemical hypothesis it is worthwhile to quantitate the release (or rate of formation) of a putative trigger from the myoplasmic surface of the T-tubule membrane. The volume in 1 cm³ of muscle where a local concentration of 10 μM of a trigger substance is required in the 20-nm gap (separating the myoplasmic surface of the T-tubule membrane from the terminal cisternae) is calculated to be 4.4×10^{-3} cm³ (given 2.2×10^3 cm² T-tubule surface/cm³ of muscle). Thus, 2.6×10^{12} molecules must exist in this restricted area. This corresponds to a surprisingly small number of 120 molecules/μm² of T-tubule membrane which have to be released or formed within 1–2 mseconds. So far two chemical messengers have been advocated, namely, inositol 1,4,5-trisphosphate and Ca^{2+}. The entry of Ca^{2+} via voltage-dependent calcium channels into the gap is not considered to be relevant for the twitch response (see Frank, 1980; Volpe et al., 1986a). One reason is that the kinetics of the channel are extremely slow, the time constant for activation being in the range of 150 mseconds, and the activation threshold is high (−30 mV). This does not, however, exclude the possibility that these channels are important for contractures (vide infra).

Recently a fast-activated inward Ca^{2+} current in twitch muscle fibers of the frog, *Rana montezume*. was found. This current was activated at -60 mV, and the time constant for activation was 5 mseconds (Cota and Stefani, 1986). The current was blocked by Cd^{2+} (and 5 μM gallopamil) and disappeared as a function of time on exposure to hypertonic recording solution (0.35 M sucrose). The authors concluded that these fast-activated channels could immediately open after the sodium channels and partially account for the Ca^{2+} influx by an action potential. This flux (around 0.2–1.3 pmol/cm^2 surface area) is an order of magnitude higher than that through the slow-activated calcium channels (see references cited by Cota and Stefani, 1986).

The suggested source of Ca^{2+} for the action potential-evoked contraction is the intracellular surface of the T-tubule membrane (see Frank, 1980, and references cited therein). Here it is assumed that Ca^{2+} is released on depolarization and activates the calcium channel of the terminal cisternae. Evidence also in favor of Ca^{2+} being (either solely or in part) the trigger has been obtained with mechanically skinned frog skeletal muscle fibers. These fibers (termed Natori type) have sealed-off T-tubules which form closed compartments and have an intact excitation–contraction coupling system. Dissipation of T-tubule K^+ and Na^+ gradients (with monensin or gramicidin D) evokes rapid force development and $^{45}Ca^{2+}$ efflux from the cisternae. With the Na^+,K^+-ATPase pump (known to be preferentially localized in the T-tubule membrane) blocked by digitoxin (a hydrophobic cardiac glycoside which, in contrast to ouabain, penetrates cell membranes) the ionophores were ineffective. Since pretreatment with 5 mM EGTA completely abolishes monensin-stimulated $^{45}Ca^{2+}$ efflux, it appears that Ca^{2+} released by T-tubule depolarization is essential in excitation–contraction coupling (Volpe and Stephenson, 1986).

In contrast to mechanically skinned fibers, in chemically skinned fibers T-tubule–cisternal functions become altered with leaky membranes and hence can be used to investigate the role of Ca^{2+} and other putative chemical transmitters on Ca^{2+} release and tension development (Volpe *et al.*, 1986b). With such preparations it can be shown that Ca^{2+} is important for release of Ca^{2+} from the cisternae by controlling the rate of Ca^{2+} efflux through a Ca^{2+}-sensitive calcium channel (Meissner, 1984; Volpe *et al.*, 1986b; Fabiato, 1985). The free Ca^{2+} concentration required is surprisingly low (around 3 μM). As mentioned above this (ryanodine-modulated) Ca^{2+}-sensitive release channel has been purified and reconstituted.

Inositol 1,4,5-trisphosphate (IP$_3$) was recently suggested to be an alternative to Ca^{2+} as a messenger across the gap. Volpe *et al.* (1985)

showed that IP_3 promotes Ca^{2+} release from isolated sarcoplasmic reticulum fragments from rabbit fast twitch muscles. These authors suggested that P_3-sensitive channels exist on terminal cisternal membranes which (perhaps in concert with Ca^{2+} released by them) are responsible for the Ca^{2+} efflux needed for contraction. In chemically skinned muscle fibers IP_3 elicits tension development in a dose-dependent manner. The possible role of IP_3 in excitation–contraction coupling was underlined by experiments with mechanically and chemically skinned skeletal muscle fibers from the semitendinosus muscle of the frog, *Rana esculenta* (Vergara *et al.*, 1985). Here inhibitors of IP_3 formation (e.g., neomycin) blocked excitation–contraction coupling, putative inhibitors of P_3-phosphatase (e.g., low Mg^{2+}, Cd^{2+}, Zn^{2+}) potentiated the effects of externally applied IP_3, and electrical stimulation of the [^{3}H]inositol-prelabeled muscles increased the myoplasmic concentration of radioactive inositol phosphates. The authors suggested that a voltage-dependent cleavage mechanism of phosphatidylinositol 4,5-bisphosphate in the T-tubule membrane is responsible for excitation–contraction coupling.

T-tubule membranes contain a significant percentage of phosphatidylinositol phosphates (4–5% of total phospholipid), and enzymes that phosphorylate phosphatidylinositol to phosphatidyl 4-monophosphate and phosphatidylinositol 4,5-bisphosphate have now been found in rabbit and frog T-tubules (Varsanyi *et al.*, 1986; Hidalgo *et al.*, 1986). Two groups, however, could not reproduce the effects of IP_3 on either tension development (Lea *et al.*, 1986) or Ca^{2+} release (Scherer and Ferguson, 1985) in skinned muscle fibers or sarcoplasmic reticulum microsomes, respectively. This casts serious doubts on the hypothesis of IP_3 being the messenger. In addition, the rate of formation appears to be too slow (Volpe *et al.*, 1986a).

Another role of IP_3 was suggested by Thieleczek and Heilmeyer (1986), who found for chemically skinned fibers that 10 μM IP_3 increased the Ca^{2+} sensitivity of the steady-state isomeric force development in high Ca^{2+}-buffered solutions by approximately 2-fold. The effect was slowly reversible and concentration dependent. The authors excluded possible Ca^{2+} release mechanisms; hence, modulation of one or more components of the contractile apparatus was suggested.

2. Calcium Channel Drugs and Excitation–Contraction Coupling

Here we describe in more detail the results summarized in Table VII. With few exceptions most of the data has been obtained with frog and mature mammalian muscles under a wide range of experimental conditions. Contractures are muscle shortenings or tension develop-

TABLE VII

EFFECTS OF CALCIUM CHANNEL DRUGS ON EXCITATION–CONTRACTION COUPLING STEPS IN SKELETAL MUSCLE

Drug class	Tissue	Species	T	Method	Results	Constants[a]	Comments (conclusions)	Ref.[b]
Phenylalkylamines	Gastrocnemius (slow muscle) fibers	*Leptodactylus ocellatus*	22–23°C	Contractures by 40 mM K$^+$	(−)Verapamil = (−)gallopamil > (+)verapamil = (+)gallopamil reversibly inhibited contractions	8 μM	Apparent use-dependence of effect	a
	Extensor longus digiti IV (toe)	*Rana pipiens*	20°C	Contractures by 123 mM K$^+$	(±)Verapamil = (±)gallopamil completely inhibited contractures	30–50 nM		b
				Twitch	No effect on twitch response			
				Contractures by 20 mM K$^+$	Gallopamil increased contractures	0.1 μM		
	Tibialis anterior fibers	*Rana temporaria*	7°C	Contracture or twitch	(±)Gallopamil paralyzed the fiber after a single K$^+$ contracture; paralysis could be reversed by raising the temperature to 22°C	30 μM	Gallopamil binds to a site in the T-tubule membrane, similar to a Ca^{2+} channel	c
	Semitendinosus fibers	*Rana temporaria*	5°C	Charge movement	Charge movement blocked under identical conditions where paralysis by (±)gallopamil is observed	30 μM	Gallopamil blocks the movement of a rigid rod	d
	Lumbricalis digitus IV	*Rana temporaria*	6–7°C	Contractures under voltage clamp conditions	(±)Gallopamil caused paralysis of force only in the depolarized state; potential-dependent binding of gallopamil	5–100 μM	Effects of gallopamil are seen when Ca^{2+} channels are blocked with Cd^{2+}	e
	Semitendinosus (mechanically skinned)	Not given	Not given	Contractures by K$^+$	(±)Gallopamil blocked contractions but not in reprimed fibers	10 μM	Gallopamil stabilizes the inactivated force	f

	Tissue	Species	Temp.	Parameter	Result	Concentration	Comments	Ref.
	Skeletal muscle	Rabbit	20°C	Charge movement	(±)Gallopamil decreased charge movement but did not block contraction	30 μM	(Part of the) charge movement is a Ca^{2+} gating current	g
Benzothiazepines	Skeletal muscle fibers	Frog (?)	22°C	Twitch, contractures	(+)-cis-Diltiazem potentiated the force by up to 80%	1 μM		i
	Extensor digitorum	Mouse and rat	22°C	Twitch	(+)-cis-Diltiazem increased the twitch amplitude by 42.2%; (−)-cis-diltiazem >10 times less effective	EC_{50} for (+)-cis-diltiazem: 10–20 nM		
				Mechanical threshold potential	(+)-cis-Diltiazem decreased threshold	0.5–1 μM (+)-cis-diltiazem		
	Semitendinosus single fibers	Rana catesbiana	10°C	Charge movement	(+)-cis-Diltiazem increased charge movement	0.25–0.5 mM	Diltiazem shifts the voltage dependence of the charge movement to more negative values	n
1,4-Dihydropyridines	Semitendinosus (mechanically skinned)	Not given (frog?)	Not given	Contractures by K^+	(±)Nitrendipine blocked contractures	10 μM	Nitrendipine blocks (in contrast to gallopamil) reprimed fibers	f
	Skeletal muscle fibers	Rabbit	22°C	Charge movement	Nifedipine blocked a fraction of the charge movement	2–10 μM	Nifedipine may also affect the contraction; part of charge movement is a Ca^{2+} gating current	j

(continued)

TABLE VII
(Continued)

Drug class	Tissue	Species	T	Method	Results	Constant[a]	Comments (conclusions)	Ref.[b]
	Skeletal muscle fibers	Frog	11°C	Charge movement Ca²⁺ transients	Nifedipine affected charge movement in the presence of low external Ca²⁺, inhibited Ca²⁺ transients	10 nM to 0.5 μM	Intramembrane charge movement is the gating current of the Ca²⁺ channel	k
	Semitendinosus fibers	*Rana esculenta*	10°C	Twitch	Nifedipine partially inhibited the tension Bay K 8644 increased the tension	10 μM 0.1 μM	Inward 1,4-DHP-sensitive currents are responsible for the second (slow) phase of contracture	l
	Short toe muscles	*Rana temporaria*	6–7°C	Contractures under voltage clamp conditions	Nifedipine shifted the rheobase by −20 mV; no paralysis as seen with gallopamil	1–3 μM	Nifedipine prolongs the contraction plateau	m
	Semitendinosus single fibers	*Rana catesbiana*	10°C	Charge movement	Nitrendipine inhibited the quantity of charge movement	10(5) μM	Inhibition of charge movement without inhibition of Ca²⁺ current	n

[a] Unless otherwise noted, IC$_{50}$ values are given.

[b] Key to references: a, Kaumann and Uchitel (1976), *Naunyn–Schmiedebergs Arch. Pharmacol.* **292**, 21–27; b, Frank (1984), *Can. J. Physiol. Pharmacol.* **62**, 374–378; c, Eisenberg *et al.* (1983), *J. Physiol. (London)* **341**, 495–505; d, Hui *et al.* (1983), *Proc. Natl. Acad. Sci. U.S.A.* **81**, 2582–2585; e, Berwe *et al.* (1987), *J. Physiol. (London)* **385**, 693–707; f, Fill and Best (1986), *Biophys. J.* **49**, 13a; g, Lamb (1986a), *Biophys. J.* **49**, 12a; h, Gonzales-Serratos *et al.* (1982), *Nature (London)* **298**, 292–294; i, Walsh *et al.* (1984), *Biochem. Biophys. Res. Commun.* **122**, 1091–1096; j, Lamb (1986b), *J. Physiol (London)* **376**, 85–100; k, Rios *et al.* (1986), *Biophys. J.* **49**, 13a, Rios and Brum (1987), *Nature (London)* **325**, 717–720; l, Ildefonse *et al.* (1985), *Biochem. Biophys. Res. Commun.* **129**, 904–909; m, Neuhaus (1986), *J. Physiol. (London)* **378**, 128 P; n, Walsh *et al.* (1987), *Pflüger's Arch.* **409**, 217–219.

ments produced by means other than action potentials; twitches or tetani initiated by the latter are termed contractions.

Kaumann and Uchitel (1976) investigated the effects of the optical isomers of verapamil and gallopamil on K^+-induced contractures in slow muscle fibers of the South American frog *Leptodactylus ocellatus* at 20–23°C. They observed that both drugs inhibited the contractures in a concentration-dependent manner and had similar IC_{50} values. The respective (−) isomers were 4–5 times more potent than the (+) isomers. IC_{50} values for (−)gallopamil and (−)verapamil were around 8 μM. Interestingly the phenylalkylamines were more effective when the muscles were repeatedly challenged by exposure to 40 mM K^+. The effects were completely reversible.

Frank (1984) tested (racemic) verapamil and gallopamil on K^+-induced contractures in extensor longus digiti IV (toe) muscles from the frog, *Rana pipiens*. He observed that with 20 mM K^+ (in choline–Ringer solution) gallopamil (at 0.1 μM) increased the amplitude of contractures. Complete dose–response curves for verapamil and gallopamil were recorded for contractures induced by 123 mM K^+. Both drugs completely inhibited at 1 μM; 20% inhibition was observed at 10 nM (IC_{50} for both drugs, 30–50 nM). Although gallopamil was slightly more potent than verapamil these differences were not significant. Most importantly, Frank (1984) observed that it took 2 hours to achieve equilibrium for the drugs. He reasoned that, as the phenylalkylamines are nearly fully protonated at pH 7.2 [pK_a of gallopamil (D 600), 8.5], the long time was necessary to establish a steady-state concentration, because only the uncharged molecules can penetrate membranes.

In contrast to the K^+-induced contracture, the twitch response (i.e., induced by electrical stimulation) was not changed by the drugs, except at high concentrations (50 μM) where a potentiation was seen. Recovery from the inhibitory effects of the phenylalkylamines was variable and incomplete. The results fit well with the hypothesis (Frank, 1980) that twitch responses are mediated by Ca^{2+} released as "trigger," whereas K^+-induced contractures required Ca^{2+} influx via Ca^{2+}-selective channels. However, the stimulation of contractures by gallopamil (at low concentrations of drug and with 20 mM K^+) remained unexplained.

Eisenberg *et al.* (1983) investigated the effects of racemic gallopamil (30 μM) in single fibers from the tibialis anterior muscle of the frog, *Rana temporaria*. Fibers exposed to the drug at 7°C give a single K^+ contracture after which they become paralyzed. Neither a twitch nor a K^+ response could be elicited. However, paralyzed fibers warmed to 22°C recover and show both twitch and K^+-induced contractures.

Fibers treated at 22°C are not paralyzed at all. The authors explained their findings by postulating that gallopamil binds to a site in the T-tubule membrane which is chemically similar to a calcium channel without being part of a channel directly involved in current flow.

In a subsequent paper Hui *et al.* (1983) investigated the influence of gallopamil on charge movement. Fibers presoaked with gallopamil at 5°C did not differ in nonlinear current responses from those of untreated fibers. Only when K^+ depolarization preceded the experiment was charge movement abolished, as was seen with the contracture earlier. Thus, as for the paralysis, three conditions had to be met (low temperature, D 600 present, and prior depolarization) to block the charge movement. It was suggested that gallopamil blocks the movement of a rigid rod which links T-tubule membrane depolarization to Ca^{2+} release from the sarcoplasmic reticulum.

The experiments of Eisenberg *et al.* (1983) were extended by Berwe *et al.* (1987). Force development of small bundles of the lumbricalis digitus IV muscle of the hind limb of the frog, *Rana temporaria,* was measured under voltage clamp conditions at 7°C. Fibers depolarized from a holding potential of −90 to 0 mV with 5 μM gallopamil added produced only one contracture. Repolarization to −90 mV (after spontaneous relaxation) and subsequent depolarization yielded negligible force development. Hyperpolarization to −120 or −150 mV restored the response (as did elevated temperature in the experiments by Eisenberg *et al.,* 1983). At concentrations between 5 and 100 μM gallopamil was without effect as long as the fibers were held at negative membrane potentials. Paralysis of force developed only in the depolarized state. The authors concluded that the action of gallopamil is voltage dependent.

In order to explain their results within the context of the charge movement hypothesis, Berwe *et al.* (1987) proposed the following model. There is a potential sensor in T-tubule membranes that exists in the resting state, R, at negative membrane potentials. On depolarization it converts to the active state, A (which initiates release of Ca^{2+} from the sarcoplasmic reticulum), and subsequently to an inactive state, I. Here the release becomes blocked. It is assumed that gallopamil blocked by binding with high affinity to the I state and thereby stabilized it (in I_0). The parallelism with different states of the channels is obvious:

$$R \leftrightarrow A \leftrightarrow I \underset{\text{gallopamil}}{\overset{}{\leftrightarrows}} I_0$$

In order to test the postulated potential-dependent binding of gallopamil the potential dependence of force restoration was investigated.

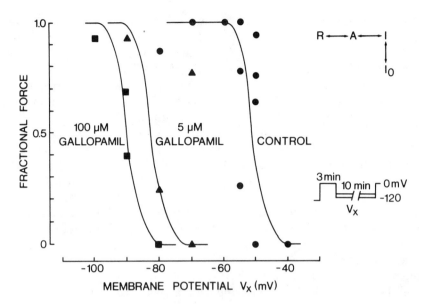

FIG. 24. Effects of gallopamil on excitation–contraction coupling in skeletal muscle. In frog skeletal muscles mechanical refractoriness can be induced by a large depolarization. Then, depending on duration and potential during a conditioning pulse (indicated by V_x), force may be restored by a second depolarizing step. When the conditioning prepulse is such that the membrane potential is held at −40 mV for 10 minutes, no restoration is seen. Full restoration under control conditions is observed between −70 and −50 mV. In the presence of 5 μM (±)gallopamil the force–restoration curve is shifted to the left; increasing the concentration by a factor of 20 (100 μM) leads to a further shift to the left. (From Berwe et al. (1987), J. Physiol. **385**, 693–707, with permission.]

To this end the force was inactivated by a large (3-minute) depolarization to 0 mV, followed by a conditioning pulse of 10 minutes' duration. The membrane potential was varied during the conditioning period, followed by a second depolarization. Fibers kept at −40 mV during the conditioning period did not show restoration of force; full force was restored by holding potentials of −70 to −60 mV (transition potential in the absence of drugs, −51 mV). With 5 μM gallopamil the force–restoration curve is shifted along the voltage axis by 30 mV to more negative values (transition potential in the presence of 5 μM gallopamil, −83 mV); 100 μM gallopamil shifts the curve to −90 mV (see Fig. 24).

Thus, gallopamil retarded further the restoration of force. These results are similar to the action of certain antiarrhythmic drugs on the sodium channel (Hondeghem and Katzung, 1977; Bean et al., 1983) and to the effect of 1,4-dihydropyridines on the voltage dependence of calcium channel availability (Sanguinetti and Kass, 1984) and prove the voltage dependence of binding of gallopamil to the potential sensor. Berwe et al. (1987) investigated next whether calcium channel blockade would change the gallopamil effects. They used 2 mM Cd^{2+} (a concentration which is 4 times the half-block concentration for Ca^{2+} currents) and still found the paralysis induced by gallopamil. Their results also explain why force restoration was not observed by Eisenberg et al. (1983) in experiments at reduced resting potentials whereas McCleskey (1985) observed complete recovery from gallopamil block after 7–23 hours with a holding potential of −100 mV.

Berwe et al. (1987) concluded that paralysis is not a direct consequence of a blocked slow inward Ca^{2+} current. Gallopamil (at high concentrations) induces a negative shift in the threshold for activation of force (5–10 mV) first reported by Dörrscheid-Käfer (1977). The additional increase in force was also observed by Berwe et al. (1987) under certain experimental conditions. They suggested that gallopamil can also bind to the active state (A) of the potential sensor, stabilizing it in A_0. The following scheme was proposed:

$$R \longleftrightarrow A \longleftrightarrow I$$
$$\text{gallopamil} \longrightarrow \updownarrow \qquad \updownarrow \longleftarrow \text{gallopamil}$$
$$A_0 \qquad I_0$$

Again, there is striking analogy to the action of 1,4-dihydropyridines (e.g., the enantiomers of 202-791) which can block or activate calcium channels, depending on holding potential (Kokubun et al., 1986).

(+)-cis-Diltiazem blocks slow Ca^{2+} currents (20–24°C) in isolated cut frog muscle fibers with an IC_{50} value of about 60 nM; complete block develops at 0.3 µM (Gonzales-Serratos et al., 1982). These results were obtained with test pulses every 4–5 minutes from a holding potential of −100 mV. Contractility studies with (+)-cis-diltiazem (at 1 µM) indicated that this calcium channel blocker potentiated the force up to 80% over controls. Both relaxation time and duration of the twitch were prolonged. The effect declined, with a half-time of 10 minutes, after removal of the drug. A similar potentiation was seen with sustained K^+ depolarization.

The effect of (+)-cis-diltiazem on mammalian skeletal muscle was investigated in more detail by Walsh et al. (1984). Extensor digitorus longus muscle preparations (10–20 fibers) from mice or rats were electrically stimulated (0.5-msecond duration impulses to provide three twitches at 5-second intervals) at 22°C. (+)-cis-Diltiazem produced twitch potentiation. The half-time for development of maximal potentiation at 0.1 µM (+)-cis-diltiazem was 3 minutes. The twitch amplitude increase was 42.2% (maximum) at 0.1 μM and 12% at 5 nM, suggesting an EC$_{50}$ value of 10–20 nM. At higher drug concentrations (1 μM) the percent increase was less than at 0.1 μM (30%). The diastereoisomer $(-)$-cis-diltiazem was approximately 10 times less effective and increased tension to a maximal percentage of only 35.0%. The authors also measured the mechanical threshold potential under conditions where sodium channels are blocked with tetrodotoxin. In this analysis the membrane potential needed for a just visible contraction is plotted against the pulse duration of the stimulus. Typically, as pulse duration is increased, less positive internal potentials are needed from a given holding potential to elicit the contraction. The threshold potential reaches a constant ("rheobasic") value, which is useful to quantify drug-induced changes. At 0.5 μM, $(+)$-cis-diltiazem decreased (i.e., to more negative potentials) the mechanical threshold base by 10.3 mV and at 1 μM, by 15.7 mV. At 50 nM a small, but not statistically significant decrease in the rheobase was found.

Ildefonse et $al.$ (1985) investigated the effects of nifedipine and Bay K 8644 on Ca^{2+} currents and tension development in single twitch fibers of the semitendinosus muscle of the frog, $Rana$ $esculenta$, with 1.8 mM Ca^{2+} at 17°C. They kept the holding potential at -90 mV and measured tension development and currents for depolarization steps to -30, -20, and -10 mV. They observed that tension developed in two phases, a rapid and a slow phase. The time course of the second, slower phase appeared to correlate with measured inward Ca^{2+} current. The greater the voltage jump, however, the earlier the second phase of tension developed so that at jumps from -90 to -10 mV the two phases were no longer distinct. Nifedipine (10 μM) greatly reduced the Ca^{2+} current (IC$_{50}$ value 0.2 μM), and tension development was partly inhibited. Bay K 8644 (0.1 μM) increased the Ca^{2+} current for voltage jumps to -30 mV; simultaneously the peak of the slower component of tension was increased and accelerated.

Fill and Best (1986) investigated the effects of gallopamil and nitrendipine on mechanically skinned fibers from semitendinosus muscle. Immediately after contracture (induced by ionic substitution) fibers entered a refractory state and required a recovery period ("reprime") before another contracture could be elicitated. Whereas 10 μM nitrendipine produced a time-dependent block of contracture (50% block at 0.5 minute, complete block after 2 minutes) which persisted throughout the recovery period and after repriming, 10 μM gallopamil was most effective when the fibers were in the inactivated state but was ineffective on fully reprimed fibers. The latter finding is in good agreement with the results of Berwe et $al.$ (1987).

Lamb (1986b,c) in experiments with rabbit skeletal muscle fibers (22°C) found that a component (50% of the maximum) of the charge movement was suppressed by 2–10 μM nifedipine. Charge moved by depolarizing to potentials more negative than -60 mV was, however, unaffected by the drug. Some fibers did not contract after nifedipine treatment, others did. Lamb concluded that in the noncontracting fibers the normal release mechanism for Ca^{2+} was disrupted and that, as observed in the second, slow phase of contractions in frog by Ildefonse et al. (1985), contraction was dependent on influx of Ca^{2+} by the 1,4-dihydropyridine-sensitive calcium channel.

Neuhaus (1986) observed with frog muscle fibers that the threshold for force activation was shifted from -50 to -70 mV by 1–3 μM nifedipine. This is similar to the findings reported by Walsh et al. (1984) with (+)-cis-diltiazem. When voltage steps from -90 to -30 mV were applied, the plateau of force was prolonged and the Ca^{2+} inward current was blocked by nifedipine. Nifedipine inactivated by high intensity UV irradiation produced neither blockade of Ca^{2+} currents nor plateau prolongation. Cd^{2+} (2 mM) produced a similar effect. Neuhaus suggested that the slow inward Ca^{2+} current accelerated the inactivation of Ca^{2+} release from the sarcoplasmic reticulum.

Walsh et al. (1987) investigated the effects of (+)-cis-diltiazem and nitrendipine on the charge movement and calcium currents in bullfrog semitendinosus muscle fibers. Nitrendipine (10 μM) inhibited Q_{on} from 15.3 to 4.8 nC/μF. There was no blockade of Ca^{2+} currents by nitrendipine under these conditions (see Section VI,B). In contrast, high concentrations of (+)-cis-diltiazem (500 μM) blocked the Ca^{2+} current but increased the charge movement; Q_{on} increased from 10.9 to 14.4 nC/μF and Q_{off} from 17.4 to 28 nC/μF under the influence of 250 μM (+)-cis-diltiazem. The voltage dependence of the charge movement as well as the maximum of the charge moved was changed by (+)-cis-diltiazem (see Fig. 25). The authors suggested that sites that bind calcium channel blockers are important in excitation–contraction coupling.

Rios and Brum (1987) investigated in great detail the effects of nifedipine on increases in myoplasmic Ca^{2+} (termed Ca^{2+} transients) associated with pulse depolarization of single fibers of frog semitendinosus and the charge movement. They observed that at holding potentials of -70 mV nifedipine (0.5 μM) caused a 70% reduction of the Ca^{2+} release flux; however, at holding potentials of -10 mV there was almost no reduction. Nifedipine did not block T-tubule membrane Ca^{2+} currents. Nifedipine at concentrations of 10 nM, 0.1 μM, and 0.5 μM reduced the charge movement by 36, 62, and 67% when a test pulse

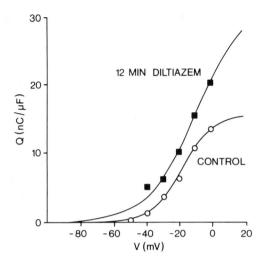

FIG. 25. (+)-*cis*-Diltiazem increases the amount of charge and shifts the voltage dependence in frog skeletal muscle. When a component of the charge, displaced on depolarization (Q_{on} at the beginning of a depolarization step), is measured, the steady-state distribution of charge depends on the holding potential as shown for the control curve. The curves were fit with the equation $Q = Q_{max}/(1 + \exp[-V - V/k])$. On exposure to 250 μM (+)-*cis*-diltiazem, Q_{max} increased from 15.5 to 31.6 nC/μF; k and V were 9.4 and -16.3 mV in the absence and 14.6 and -8.7 mV in the presence of (+)-*cis*-diltiazem, respectively. [From Walsh *et al.* (1987), *Pflügers's Arch.* **409**, 217–219, with permission.]

from -70 to 0 mV was applied. This was accompanied by a reduction in peak Ca^{2+} release by 37, 67, and 84%. In the presence of 0.1 μM nifedipine, interestingly, the amount of charge moved increased when a hyperpolarizing pulse from -100 to -170 mV was applied. As the peak of release flux was found to be directly proportional to the charge moved and effects on charge movement were cotemporal with effects on Ca^{2+} transients, the authors concluded that high affinity 1,4-dihydropyridine polypeptides are involved in excitation–contraction coupling.

3. 1,4-Dihydropyridine-Sensitive Slow Ca^{2+} Current Deficiency in Skeletal Muscle from Mice with Muscular Dysgenesis

Beam *et al.* (1986) have investigated Ca^{2+} currents from developing skeletal muscle cells of normal rats and mice. They found two kinetically distinct inward currents in myotubes held in primary culture, as well as in enzymatically dissected fibers of muscles from neonatal rats. One current was similar to the slow current in adult muscle (I_s)

whereas the fast current (I_f) was similar to the fast Ca^{2+} current recently observed in frog muscle (Cota and Stefani, 1986). Both currents were blocked by Cd^{2+}, although I_f was less sensitive. Only the I_s current was blocked by 5 μM nitrendipine. Knudson et al. (1986) later found that I_f decreased from 3.9 pA/pF (in fibers from 0- to 5-day-old animals) to unmeasurably low values after 25–50 days whereas I_s increased from 5.3 $\pm$ 1.1 to 18.8 pA/pF. Over the same time period the nonlinear charge movement increased from 6 to 25 nC/μF. Blocking of both currents with 1 mM Cd^{2+} did not prevent contractile responses to brief electrical stimuli or K^+ depolarization. Their conclusion that external Ca^{2+} entry is not involved in excitation–contraction coupling even in neonatal muscle is at variance with the findings on myotubes from Romey et al. (1986) (see below).

Having demonstrated the presence of I_f and I_s, Beam et al. (1986) studied Ca^{2+} currents in mice with muscular dysgenesis. This recessive, lethal autosomal mutation (mdg) is characterized by the complete lack of depolarization-induced contractions; however, Ca^{2+} release from the sarcoplasmic reticulum is normal, indicating that the defect is at the excitation–contraction coupling steps. They found two Ca^{2+} currents (I_f and I_s) in heart and nerve in wild-type animals as well as in cardiac myocytes and dorsal root ganglion neurons from mutant animals. I_s was completely lacking in skeletal muscle myotubes of dysgenic mice, whereas I_f was still detectable.

The lack of the slow calcium current (I_s) in dysgenic myotubes was also reported by Romey et al. (1986). In contrast to Beam et al. (1986), however, the latter authors could not detect I_f currents in myoballs grown from mdg/mdg skeletal muscle cells. Romey et al. (1986) also found that the mdg/mdg cells did not express (apamin-sensitive) Ca^{2+}-activated potassium channels, which were clearly identified in myotubes from nondysgenic mice. Replacement of external Ca^{2+} by Ba^{2+} led to a complete block of the contraction in (+/mdg?) myotubes from phenotypically normal littermates, suggesting that contractions in these cells are dependent on influx of Ca^{2+} via calcium channels.

Pincon-Raymond et al. (1985) reported that T-tubule–sarcoplasmic reticulum couplings were 6-fold fewer in diaphragm muscle from mutant mice. Whereas the maximum binding density of (+)-[^{3}H]PN 200-110 was reduced by factors of 3 to 5 for tongue, limb, or diaphragm muscle crude membranes from mdg/mdg mice, no significant difference in density of heart membrane 1,4-dihydropyridine binding sites was observed.

Taken together, the morphological defects, the lack of I_s, the reduction in 1,4-dihydropyridine binding site density, and the failure of excitation–contraction coupling suggest a T-tubular developmental effect in the *mdg* mutant. Although one conclusion would be that the mutation directly alters the gene for the slow calcium channel in skeletal muscle, other possibilities, suggested by Beam *et al.* (1986), are a defect in posttranslational processing and/or insertion of the channel protein and lack of cytosolic regulatory proteins for channel function. In this context it is interesting to note that a significant, albeit reduced, amount of high affinity (+)-[³H]PN 200-110 binding was still observed in skeletal muscle from mutant mice, although I_s was completely undetectable.

4. *The Skeletal Muscle Calcium Channel—A Potential-Dependent Ca^{2+} Release Structure?*

In the paragraphs above we have given a summary of the current hypotheses on excitation–contraction coupling and the effects of calcium channel drugs on charge movements, twitch responses, contractures, current flow, and the *mdg* mutation. Schwartz *et al.* (1985) carried out an important study on voltage-dependent binding of (+)-[³H]PN 200-110 to intact frog sartorius muscles. They found at −88 mV a binding site density of 26 pmol/g tissue with a K_D of 0.93 nM. One would expect that at −88 mV no high affinity binding of 1,4-dihydropyridine calcium channel blockers would be detectable; all other available data suggested only low affinity binding at these membrane potentials (Kokubun *et al.*, 1986). It is likely that damaged or dead cells contributed to the measured value; the whole tissue saturation analysis could not (for methodological reasons) detect 1,4-dihydropyridine sites in the low affinity state. This critique does not invalidate the important finding that depolarization to −15 mV (achieved by bathing the muscles in high K⁺ solution) increased (by about 50 pmol) the number of sites with a K_D of 1 nM to 79 pmol/g. The observed Ca^{2+} current was 102 ± 9 mA/ml fiber volume. Current flow through a single 1,4-dihydropyridine site calculated by Schwartz *et al.* (1985) was 2 fA. They concluded that there are many more 1,4-dihydropyridine binding sites in skeletal muscle than voltage-dependent calcium channels. In reconstituted purified calcium channel preparations from guinea pig skeletal muscle, however, different conductance levels (down to 1 pS) are observed, allowing the speculation that skeletal muscle current is conducted via a "true single" channel, whereas the usual L type is a cooperative aggregate of perhaps 20 such elementary channels (see Section VII,C).

From the results in Table VII, however, it is clear that calcium channel drugs, under certain experimental conditions, can have pro-

found effects on the charge movement, excitation–contraction coupling, Ca^{2+} transients, and threshold potential. So far no other structure has been identified in T-tubule membranes having stereoselective
receptors for the different classes of calcium channel drugs. Thus,
albeit indirect, this is a very strong argument for the identity of the
locus of action on charge movements, etc., and the structure now purified and reconstituted as a functional calcium channel from skeletal
muscle T-tubules. In addition, the magnitude of charge movement in
skeletal muscle appears to be directly correlated to the magnitude of
the slow Ca^{2+} current after birth. In Section III,B, we discuss one
unique feature of the calcium channel which distinguishes it from all
other known ionic channels, namely, its high affinity Ca^{2+} binding
sites.

The question arises whether the channel-bound Ca^{2+} functions in
excitation–contraction coupling. In order to give an idea of the quantitative aspects we have collected data on the density of 1,4-dihydro-
pyridine binding sites in skeletal muscle from different species (Table
VIII). In this table the number of feet, the calculated charged particles,
and the density of 1,4 dihydropyridine (nifedipine)-suppressed charges
are also summarized. The mean value for the density of 1,4-di-
hydropyridine sites is around 360 per μm^2 of T-tubular membrane,
which is identical to the number of nifedipine-suppressed charges per
μm^2 of T-tubule membrane. As discussed above, to raise the concentration of Ca^{2+} in the restricted volume extending from the T-tubule
membrane to the terminal cisternal membrane to 10 μM, one needs
the release of 120 molecules of Ca^{2+} per μm^2. Let us now assume that
the T-tubule calcium channel is the potential sensor identified by the
charge movement experiments. Perhaps, either by posttranslational
modification or some other constraint, the majority of membrane-
bound skeletal muscle T-tubule calcium channel polypeptides may not
allow inflow of ions. Nevertheless, the Ca^{2+} bound within the pore
could still be locally released. This would require that the conformational change of the pore structure, induced by depolarization, leads to
a drastic decrease in the affinity for Ca^{2+}, which diffuses to a Ca^{2+}
receptor on the ryanodine-sensitive release channel of the cisternae.
Only one-third of the T-tubule channel polypeptides need to partici-
pate in this release process if one 1,4-dihydropyridine site is equivalent to one bound Ca^{2+}. The other condition is that the pathway
between the Ca^{2+} receptor on the junctional sarcoplasmic reticulum
and the myoplasmic face of the channel is not permeable to Ca^{2+} from
other compartments of the myoplasm, including the Ca^{2+} released by

TABLE VIII

MEASURED DENSITIES OF 1,4-DIHYDROPYRIDINE RECEPTORS OF L-TYPE CALCIUM CHANNELS[a]

Tissue	Label	Absolute value	pmol cm^{-3}	Number of sites cm^{-3}	Number of sites (T-tubule membranes)		Ref.[b]
					cm^{-2}	μm^{-2}	
Guinea pig	(+)-[3H]PN 200-110	1.4 pmol mg^{-1} protein	220	1.3 × 10^{14}	0.59 × 10^{11}	590	a
Guinea pig	(±)-[3H]Nimodipine	0.66 pmol mg^{-1} protein	105	0.65 × 10^{14}	0.29 × 10^{11}	290	b
Rabbit	(±)-[3H]Nitrendipine	0.8 pmol mg^{-1} protein	130	0.78 × 10^{14}	0.35 × 10^{11}	350	c
Frog	(+)-[3H]PN 200-110	0.5 pmol mg^{-1} protein	79	0.48 × 10^{14}	0.22 × 10^{11}	220	d
All tissues (Mean)	—	—	134	0.8 × 10^{14}	0.36 × 10^{11}	360	

Feet density, density of charged groups, and nifedipine-suppressible charges in skeletal muscle

	Number of sites cm^{-3}	Number of sites (T-tubule membranes)		Ref.[b]
		cm^{-2}	μm^{-2}	
Charged groups	1.5 × 10^{14}	0.5 × 10^{11}	500–600	e
Feet	2.1 × 10^{14}	0.7 × 10^{11}	700	f
Nifedipine-sensitive charged groups	0.75 × 10^{14}	0.25 × 10^{11}	250–300	g

[a] Densities of 1,4-dihydropyridine receptors of L-type calcium channels were measured in skeletal muscle homogenates (Ref. a–c) or intact tissue (Ref. d). To convert pmol mg^{-1} homogenate protein to pmol cm^{-3}, 1 ml tissue volume was taken equivalent to 160 mg of protein (see also Ref. d); to convert cm^{-3} to cm^{-2} or μm^{-2} a value for T-tubule surface area of 0.22 μm^2/μm^3 (Mobley and Eisenberg, 1973) was used.

[b] Key to references: a, Glossmann et al. (1985b), J. Cardiovasc. Pharmacol. **7**, S20–S30; b, Glossmann et al. (1983b), Naunyn–Schmiedeberg's Arch. Pharmacol. **323**, 1–11; c, Fosset et al. (1983), J. Biol. Chem. **258**, 6086–6092; d, Schwartz et al. (1985), Nature (London) **314**, 747–750; e, Franzini-Armstrong (1970), J. Cell Biol. **47**, 488–499; f, Chandler et al. (1976b), J. Physiol. (London) **254**, 245–283; g, Lamb (1986b), J. Physiol. (London) **376**, 85–100.

the cisternae. One could imagine that Ca^{2+} shuttles between the T-tubule channel and the Ca^{2+} receptor of the cisternae (Fig. 26).

The general idea and the shortcomings of such models are discussed by Lüttgau et al. (1986). The model could explain the effects of calcium channel drugs (e.g., gallopamil) on excitation–contraction coupling in the absence of current flow, or with inflow channels blocked by Cd^{2+}. These drugs may shift the voltage dependence of Ca^{2+} binding and release from the pore.

Potentiation of twitch responses by (+)-cis-diltiazem, nifedipine, or gallopamil under certain experimental conditions could be due to drug-induced conformational changes in the channel proteins which in turn facilitate Ca^{2+} release. Alternatively, the slow Ca^{2+} current through those channels which are not part of the T-tubule shuttle mechanism could facilitate inactivation of the terminal cisternae calcium channels. Here the channel blockers would prolong the plateau of force development. However, for (+)-cis-diltiazem this cannot be the mechanism, since the inhibitory effect on channel current flow is found only at concentrations several orders of magnitude greater (see, however, Section VI,B) than needed for the potentiation effect on contracture. (+)-cis-Diltiazem bound to its receptor domain may facilitate Ca^{2+} release or perhaps recruit more channels to operate in the proposed Ca^{2+} shuttle mechanism. One would expect an increase in the charge movement rather than a decrease by such a mechanism, which was indeed found recently (Walsh et al., 1987). Finally, the proposed role for the majority of the skeletal muscle calcium channels is not necessarily contradictory to the effects of calcium channel drugs on contractures (Frank, 1984) or their effects on the second, slow component of the tension development reported, e.g., by Ildefonse et al. (1985) or in experiments where nifedipine blocked contractures (Lamb, 1986c).

5. Summary

We would like to suggest a combination of the charge movement with the trigger Ca^{2+} hypothesis wherein the voltage-dependent calcium channel in the T-tubule membrane could act as a potential-dependent binding site for Ca^{2+} and is the source of this chemical mediator. The Ca^{2+} acceptor would be on the Ca^{2+}-release channel of the sarcoplasmic reticulum, which is organized around the T-tubule channel in such a way that access of cytoplasmic Ca^{2+} is prohibited. The question of why the majority of the channels appear nonfunctional (with respect to ion permeation) in situ (as claimed by some authors) yet are functional after solubilization and purification remains to be answered. Perhaps it can be resolved when more information becomes

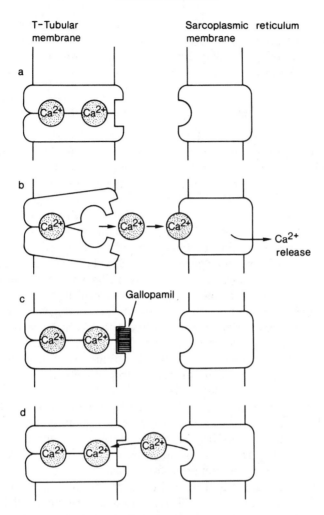

FIG. 26. Calcium channel polypeptides as potential sensors of excitation–contraction coupling in vertebrate skeletal muscle. In the resting state (a), the T-tubule channel polypeptides have Ca^{2+} bound, but the space between the T-tubule (left) and sarcoplasmic reticulum membranes has a Ca^{2+} concentration below 1 μM. In (b) a depolarization releases Ca^{2+}, which rapidly diffuses across the gap, binds to the calcium receptor of the release channel, and induces Ca^{2+} release from the sarcoplasmic reticulum as long as bound. In (c) a voltage-dependent calcium channel drug (e.g., gallopamil) binds to receptor site 2 of the T-tubule channel and blocks the release of Ca^{2+}. In (d) on repolarization the channel rebinds the Ca^{2+} and Ca^{2+} release from the sarcoplasmic reticulum is immediately blocked.

available on the tissue-specific subtypes of L-type calcium channels, when more ultrastructural data are obtained, and when coreconstitution experiments with ryanodine and 1,4-dihydropyridine receptors have been performed.

B. SENSITIVITY TO DRUGS IN ELECTROPHYSIOLOGICAL EXPERIMENTS

Almers and McCleskey (1984) and Almers *et al.* (1985) have investigated the drug sensitivity of frog skeletal muscle Ca^{2+} currents with voltage clamp techniques in fibers soaked with K_2EGTA and ATP. The $K_{0.5}$ values (half-maximal blockade) for nifedipine and methoxyverapamil (D-600) were 0.3 and 10 μM, respectively. Inorganic ions blocked in the order $Cd^{2+} > Co^{2+} = Ni^{2+} > Mn^{2+} > Mg^{2+}$. In a conventional two-electrode recording experiment with sartorius muscle from *Rana pipiens,* slow action potentials and their drug sensitivity were studied by Kerr and Sperelakis (1982). They could demonstrate that the Ca^{2+} current was abolished when fibers were detubulated by bathing them in high concentrations of glycerol (0.55 mOsm). Most importantly, they found that the effects of (±)verapamil and (±)bepridil were use dependent. Unless the fibers were electrically driven the drug effects were negligible. The cumulative dose–response curves did not obey simple mass law behavior, extending over three (instead of two) orders of magnitude. Drug effects were pronounced even at concentrations as low as 5 nM, and half-maximal inhibition in the range of the equilibrium dissociation constants of the skeletal muscle phenylalkylamine receptors (linked to calcium channels) measured by radioligand binding (compare data in Tables IX and XX).

Surprisingly, the rabbit skeletal muscle preparation, investigated by Walsh *et al.* (1985), did not show any sensitivity to the Ca^{2+} current with respect to the 1,4-dihydropyridine nitrendipine (up to 10 μM); the $K_{0.5}$ for (+)-*cis*-diltiazem was 63 μM, in good agreement with values for the constant obtained in voltage clamp experiments by Almers *et al.* (1984, 1985) in the frog. In the single study wherein a 1000-fold smaller $K_{0.5}$ value (50 nM) for inhibition of the Ca^{2+} current in frog muscle was found (Gonzales-Serratos *et al.,* 1982), the potentiation of the twitch response developed at similar concentrations (see Section VI,A).

Rat myoballs (obtained by addition of colchicine to primary cultures of thigh muscle of newborn rats) show two pharmacologically distinct types of calcium channels. One type (similar to the T type) was a low threshold calcium channel (activated at potentials of −65 mV), insensitive to 1,4-dihydropyridines, with a potential for maximal current amplitude around −30 mV (Cognard *et al.,* 1986b). The other 1,4-

TABLE IX
CALCIUM CURRENTS IN SKELETAL MUSCLE: SENSITIVITY TO ORGANIC AND INORGANIC CALCIUM CHANNEL DRUGS

Tissue	Species	Conditions	$K_{0.5}$ (μM)				Ref.[a]
			1,4-Dihydropyridines	Phenylalkylamines	Benzothiazepines	Others	
Semitendinosus muscle (single fibers)	*Rana temporiana*	Voltage clamp	Nifedipine, 0.9	Methoxyverapamil, 10	(+)-*cis*-Diltiazem, 80	Cd²⁺, 360; Co²⁺, 1,280; Ni²⁺, 1,280; Mn²⁺, 12,500; Mg²⁺, 36,600	a, b
Sternomastoid muscle (single fibers)	Rabbit	Voltage clamp (21–23°C)	(±)Nitrendipine, no effect up to 10 μM	(±)Verapamil, 10	(+)-*cis*-Diltiazem, 63	Cd²⁺, 500	c
Sartorius muscle	*Rana pipiens*	Conventional two-electrode recording technique	n.d.[b]	(±)Bepridil, 0.033; (±)verapamil, 0.033	n.d.	n.d.	d
Myoballs in culture	Rat	Whole cell patch clamp (20°C)	(+)PN 200-110, 0.0013 (at −90 mV); (+)PN 200-110, 0.00015 (at −65 mV); Bay K 8644 increases peak amplitude	(−)Desmethoxyverapamil, <1	n.d.	Fluspirilene, 0.0001– 0.0002	e, f
Sartorius muscle	Frog	Voltage clamp	(±)PN 200-110, 0.4	n.d.	n.d.	n.d.	g
Skeletal muscle	Frog	Voltage clamp	n.d.	n.d.	(+)-*cis*-Diltiazem, 0.050	n.d.	h

[a] Key to references: a, Almers *et al.* (1985), *In* "Calcium in Biological Systems" (R. P. Rubin, G. B. Weiss, and J. W. Putney, Jr., eds.), pp. 321–330, Plenum, New York; b, Almers and McCleskey (1984), *J. Physiol. (London)* **353**, 585–608; c, Walsh *et al.* (1985), *J. Pharmacol. Exp. Ther.* **236**, 403–407; d, Kerr and Sperelakis (1982), *J. Pharmacol. Exp. Ther.* **222**, 80–87; e, Cognard *et al.* (1986b), *Proc. Natl. Acad. Sci. U.S.A.* **83**, 1518–1522; f, Galizzi *et al.* (1986a), *Proc. Natl. Acad. Sci. U.S.A.* **83**, 7513–7517; g, Schwartz *et al.* (1985), *Nature (London)* **314**, 797–750; h, Gonzales-Serratos *et al.* (1982), *Nature (London)* **298**, 292–294.

[b] n.d., Not determined.

dihydropyridine-sensitive channel shows voltage-dependent blockade by (+)PN 200-110. At −90 mV (resting channel) the $K_{0.5}$ was 13 nM, whereas a 100-fold lower value was obtained at −65 mV (0.15 nM). Thus, the $K_{0.5}$ value is in very good agreement with the dissociation constant of radiolabeled (+)-[³H]PN 200-110 obtained with skeletal muscle T-tubule preparations from rats (0.22 nM) (see also Table XX). The calcium channel activator Bay K 8644 increased the inward Ca^{2+} current amplitude in these preparations. Maximal increase was seen near −25 mV, and Bay K 8644 slowed down the deactivation. Maximal effects of Bay K 8644 were found at 1 μM; thus the $K_{0.5}$ for activation must be in the high nanomolar range.

The most potent compound described so far for blockade of L-type calcium channels in skeletal muscle is the diphenylbutylpiperidine neuroleptic, fluspirilene. The interaction of this class of neuroleptics with the calcium channel was discovered by Gould *et al.* (1983a). The $K_{0.5}$ for blockade of Ca^{2+} currents in rat myoballs is around 0.1 nM. In contrast to the 1,4-dihydropyridines, fluspirilene was more active than (+)PN 200-110 in the resting state, indicating (almost) state-independent blockade by this compound. The $K_{0.5}$ value for blockade agrees well with the equilibrium dissociation constant measured with [³H]fluspirilene (Gallizi *et al.*, 1986a).

Summary

Electrophysiological studies with diverse techniques and tissues have yielded conflicting results for drug sensitivity of skeletal muscle calcium channels. In intact fibers sensitivity to the phenylalkylamines appears to be use dependent; some preparations are even devoid of the dihydropyridine effect, and effectiveness varies up to three orders of magnitude for (+)-*cis*-diltiazem. In the elegant studies on rat myoballs with whole cell patch clamp techniques, the data leave no doubt that in this preparation the action of 1,4-dihydropyridine channel blockers is voltage dependent and is observed over a concentration range in complete accord with direct binding studies on membrane fragments. In addition, a new class of calcium channel blockers has been characterized by both electrophysiological and binding techniques; fluspirilene is the most potent of such congeners.

C. Developmental and Regulatory Aspects

[³H]Nitrendipine was employed as a probe for calcium channel drug receptors in studies on development in chick skeletal myotubes by Schmid *et al.* (1984). Myoblasts fused into differentiated myotubes between days 1 and 2 of culture. High affinity 1,4-dihydropyridine binding appeared after 20 hours of culture and was maximal around 72 hours. Inhibition of fusion by either lowering extracellular Ca^{2+} (EGTA added) or blocking protein synthesis prevented the appearance of high affinity binding sites. The authors also investigated $^{45}Ca^{2+}$ influx as a function of resting membrane potential (E_m). For depolarized cells (E_m -25 mV) $^{45}Ca^{2+}$ influx (initial rates of uptake) in 3-day-old myotubes was increased 5-fold compared to -60 mV, and the uptake was inhibited by nitrendipine with a $K_{0.5}$ of 0.7 nM. This corresponded well to the K_D value of 0.4 $\pm$ 1 nM, measured in equilibrium binding experiments. In ovo the 1,4-dihydropyridine receptor is undetectable between 7 and 9 days. From days 10 to 17 before hatching, the B_{max} rises to 124 fmol/mg protein. Then the level of receptors rapidly increases to nearly 1 pmol/mg protein. The K_D value in the postnatal period immediately increases to 1.8 nM. After denervation of the sciatic nerve of one leg of 6- to 7-day-old chickens, the density of the 1,4-dihydropyridine receptors increased by 200% after 15 days, then returned to baseline around day 30. The appearance of 1,4-dihydropyridine binding sites in chick myoblasts in culture correlates well with the development of T-tubules as myoblasts are converted to myotubes; denervation may cause overproduction of (disorganized) T-tubules.

Most interesting is the change in K_D by a factor of 4 after hatching. As mentioned in Section IV,G, a characteristic of the skeletal muscle 1,4-dihydropyridine receptor is its lower K_D value for all 1,4-dihydropyridines investigated, compared to heart, smooth muscle, and brain. Stimulation of β-adrenoceptors in avian myotubes with isoproterenol enhances 1,4-dihydropyridine-sensitive $^{45}Ca^{2+}$ uptake 3-fold under depolarizing conditions (Schmid et al., 1985). Myotubes treated with this β-adrenergic agonist for 1–50 hours show no morphological changes, but B_{max} increases more than 3-fold with a decrease in affinity of the receptor for 1,4-dihydropyridine (K_D increased from 0.4 to 1.5 nM). The effect of isoproterenol was mimicked by agents that block cAMP phosphodiesterase or stimulate cAMP-dependent kinase. The authors also showed that short-term treatment (for 3 days) with the β-adrenoceptor blocker alprenolol or chronic catecholamine depletion by reserpine led to a decrease in the number of 1,4-dihydropyridine receptor sites and an increase in affinity. The K_D decreased from 1.8 to 0.4 nM. These results suggest that the development of the postnatal form of the 1,4-dihydropyridine receptor may be directly under the control of the cAMP system.

Summary

A direct functional correlation in myotubes in culture between 1,4-dihydropyridine receptor sites and $^{45}Ca^{2+}$ uptake has been found, and the switch from the prenatal to the postnatal form of the 1,4-dihydropyridine receptors can be initiated by β-adrenergic agonists (or agents which increase cAMP). The effect is reversed in (young) chicks by short-term treatment with β-adrenergic blockers or by blockade of catecholamine synthesis and secretion. These experiments suggest that posttranslational modification (phosphorylation of channel subunits?) and change of the membrane environment (or even expression of a different calcium channel gene) are under control of the cAMP system in skeletal muscle. However, Pauwels et al. (1987) could not reproduce the effects of β-adrenergic agonists in the myotube system with (+)-[³H]PN200-110 as ligand.

VII. STRUCTURE OF L-TYPE CALCIUM CHANNELS

A. TARGET SIZE ANALYSIS AND IRREVERSIBLE LABELING

Here we discuss structural information on L-type calcium channels obtained by means other than purification or immunochemical analysis (Section VII,B). Tables X to XIII give an overview. Data on target size analysis have been obtained from different laboratories with diverse tissues and ligands. Affinity or photoaffinity probes have been used to characterize the putative drug receptors of the L-type calcium channel in skeletal heart and smooth muscle. The radiation-sensitive mass of the 1,4-dihydropyridine receptor domain in different tissues has yielded molecular weights (target sizes) of between 136,000 and 278,000. The phenylalkylamine receptor target size in skeletal muscle T-tubule membranes is significantly smaller than that of the 1,4-dihydropyridine domain. Interestingly, the target sizes of 1,4-dihydropyridine receptors in three different tissues (brain, heart, and skeletal muscle) are identical. Interaction with the positive allosteric regulator (+)-cis-diltiazem induces an average apparent decrease in the radiation-sensitive mass by 75,000 mass units. Thus, in the presence of (+)-cis-diltiazem the molecular weight of the 1,4-dihydropyridine receptor is indistinguishable from that of the phenylalkylamine receptor (in skeletal muscle T-tubule membranes). The structural basis for the stereoselective effects of (+)-cis-diltiazem on the radiation-sensitive mass of the 1,4-dihydropyridine receptor has not been clarified although multiple interpretations have been offered (Goll et al., 1983a; Ferry et al., 1983b).

The target size analyses in general suggest that L-type calcium channels represent very similar structures in different tissues and are oligomeric in nature. Affinity and photoaffinity labeling experiments have yielded conflicting results, with two exceptions, namely, those obtained with [^{3}H]azidopine and a tritiated arylazide phenylalkylamine (vide infra). Most of this confusion arose because saturable sites for 1,4-dihydropyridines exist in crude membrane fractions which have no obvious relationship to the calcium channel. Figure 1 represents a particularly nice example. Different classes of these low affinity sites have been discriminated. Some of them are heat-stable, others are preferentially labeled by nimodipine (as is the nucleoside transporter), whereas nitrendipine recognizes a (mitochondrial?) site regulated by cations (and anions) (see Fig. 27 and Zernig et al., 1988). Peripheral benzodiazepine receptors and phosphodiesterases also show affinity for certain 1,4-dihydropyridines. Because these low affinity sites are abundant (often by several orders of magnitude) depending on tissue (see Table XIV) and will incorporate affinity or photoaffinity ligands, special attention must be paid to the choice and concentration of protecting ligand. Protecting ligands are usually competitive inhibitors that block (at saturating concentrations, i.e., $100K_D$) receptor labeling but still allow nonspecific incorporation. If the concentration of such a protecting ligand is in excess of that required for saturation of the receptor in question, incorporation into unrelated sites also may be reduced, and "pseudo-specific" irreversible labeling is observed (Bayley, 1983). For affinity probes the noncompetitive nature of inhibition in binding experiments with reversible ligands must be demonstrated, and functional data should support the irreversible inactivation of the receptor site.

Allosteric coupling of the distinct calcium channel drug receptors and stereoselective binding of molecules characterized by one or more asymmetric carbon atoms provide additional criteria. Protection of labeling should be stereoselective within the 1,4-dihydropyridine series. Blockers and channel activators (e.g., Bay K 8644) must yield similar results; allosteric regulators should affect irreversible labeling as well as reversible binding (Glossmann et al., 1987b). In some instances the "cold-trap" method appears to be useful. Ice-cold washes of membranes, prelabeled with the photoaffinity ligand, helps remove free label and label bound to non-channel-linked binding sites prior to photolysis.

Use of photoaffinity labeling throughout purification (preferably from crude homogenate to the final preparation) can be valuable in evaluating integrity of the receptor-carrying subunit of the calcium channel. The prerequisite for this powerful method is that postlabeling by ligands can be performed with the purified preparations. On the other hand, sufficiently high specific incorporation of a photoaffinity

Table X

RADIATION INACTIVATION DATA ON L-TYPE CALCIUM CHANNELS

Tissue (species)	Ligand	Target size	Comments	Ref.[a]
Skeletal muscle (rabbit)	(±)-[³H]Nitrendipine	210 kDa		a
Skeletal muscle (guinea pig)	(±)-[³H]Nimodipine	178 kDa; with (+)-cis-diltiazem, 115 kDa	The effect of (+)-cis-diltiazem is stereoselective	b
Skeletal muscle (guinea pig)	(±)-[³H]PN 200-110	136 kDa; with (+)-cis-diltiazem, 75 kDa	The effect of (+)-cis-diltiazem is stereoselective	c
Brain (guinea pig)	(±)-[³H]Nimodipine	185 kDa; with (+)-cis-diltiazem, 111 kDa	The effect of (+)-cis-diltiazem is stereoselective	d, e
Smooth muscle (guinea pig)	(±)-[³H]Nitrendipine	278 kDa		f
Heart (guinea pig)	(±)-[³H]Nimodipine	184 kDa; with (+)-cis-diltiazem, 106 kDa	The effect of (+)-cis-diltiazem is stereoselective	g, h

Tissue (species)	Ligand	M_r	Comments	Ref.
Heart (rat)	(+)-[^{3}H]PN 200-110	185 kDa		i
Skeletal muscle (guinea pig)	(±)-[^{3}H]Verapamil	110 kDa	The target size of receptor site II is significantly smaller than that of I	j
Skeletal muscle (guinea pig)	(−)-[^{3}H]Desmethoxyverapamil	107 kDa	This high affinity ligand for receptor site II gives the same M_r as (±)-[^{3}H]verapamil	k
Skeletal muscle (guinea pig)	(+)cis-[^{3}H]Diltiazem	131 kDa		k

[a] Key to reference: a, Norman et al. (1983), Biochem. Biophys. Res. Commun. 111, 878–883; b, Ferry et al. (1983b), EMBO J. 2, 1729–1732; c, Goll et al. (1983a), FEBS Lett. 157, 63–69; d, Ferry et al. (1983a), Naunyn–Schmiedeberg's Arch. Pharmacol. 323, 292–297; e, Glossmann et al. (1985a), Arzneim. Forsch. 35, 1917–1935; f, Venter et al. (1983), J. Biol. Chem. 258, 9344–9348; g, Goll et al. (1983b), Naunyn–Schmiedeberg's Arch. Pharmacol. 324, R178; h, Glossmann et al. (1985a), Arzneim. Forsch. 35, 1917–1935; i, Doble et al. (1985), Eur. J. Pharmacol. 119, 153–167; j, Goll et al. (1984b), Eur. J. Biochem. 141, 177–186; k, Goll et al. (1984a), FEBS Lett. 176, 371–377.

Table XI
AFFINITY LABELING OF 1,4-DIHYDROPYRIDINE RECEPTORS

Tissue (species)	Ligand	M_r of labeled peptides	Comments	Ref.[a]
Smooth muscle (guinea pig)	[³H]o-NCS-DHP	45,000 (35,000)	Affinity labeling performed in Tris buffer; labeling inhibited by 5 μM nifedipine or 10 nM unlabeled o-NCS-DHP	a
Heart (guinea pig)	[³H]o-NCS-DHP	45,000 (35,000)		
Heart (canine)	[³H]o-NCS-DHP	45,000, 42,000, 38,000	Affinity labeling performed in phosphate buffer; labeling partially protected by 50 μM nicardipine or 10 μM unlabeled o-NCS-DHP	b
Skeletal muscle (guinea pig)	[³H]o-NCS-DHP	—	[³H]o-NCS-DHP is a reversible ligand for the skeletal muscle Ca²⁺ channel	c
Heart (guinea pig)	[³H]o-NCS-DHP	39,000, 35,000	Unlabeled o-NCS-DHP or 50 μM (±)nicardipine partially protected labeling by [³H]o-NCS-DHP	d
Skeletal muscle (rabbit)	[³H]o-NCS-DHP	Several polypeptides	No specific protection of labeling reported	e

[a] Key to references: a, Venter *et al.* (1983), *J. Biol. Chem.* **258**, 9344–9348; b, Horne *et al.* (1984), *Biochem. Biophys. Res. Commun.* **121**, 880–898; c, Ferry *et al.* (1984b), *FEBS Lett.* **169**, 112–118; d, Ferry *et al.* (1987), *Biochem. J.* **243**, 127–135; e, Kirley and Schwartz (1984), *Biochem. Biophys. Res. Commun.* **123**, 41–49.

TABLE XII
PHOTOAFFINITY LABELING WITH NON-ARLAZIDE 1,4-DIHYDROPYRIDINES

Tissue (species)	Ligand	M_r of labeled peptide(s)	Comment	Ref.[a]
Heart (canine)	$(\pm)$-[³H]Nitrendipine	32,000	10 nM [³H]nitrendipine and high-intensity UV irradiation used; 20 μM nitrendipine, 20 μM nifedipine, 40 μM verapamil, 1 mM EDTA, or 10 mM ATP afforded partial protection	a
Skeletal muscle (rabbit)	$(+)$-[³H]PN 200-110	170,000	Reducing conditions in SDS PAGE; very weak photoincoporation; incorporation blocked by 0.3 μM $(+)$PN 200-110	b
Heart (calf), aorta (bovine), skeletal muscle (chicken)	¹²⁵I-Labeled 1,4-DHP (Bay P 8857)	33,000– 35,000	Reducing conditions in SDS–PAGE; photoincorporation partially blocked by 50 μM nicardipine	c

[a] Key to reference: a, Campbell et al. (1984), J. Biol. Chem. **259**, 5384–5387; b, Gallizi et al. (1986b), J. Biol. Chem. **261**, 1393–1397; c, Sarmiento et al. (1986), Life Sci. **39**, 2401–2409.

ligand in the membrane material will allow isolation of the labeled, receptor-carrying component even under denaturing conditions. Finally, in order to study (within the polypeptide chain) the respective receptor domains, photoaffinity probes are a prerequisite.

1. Affinity Labeling

a. The 1,4-Dihydropyridine Receptor. 2,6-Dimethyl-3,5-dicarboxymethoxy-4-(isothiocyanatophenyl)-1,4-dihydropyridine (o-NCS-dihydropyridine) was introduced as a tritiated putative affinity probe for calcium channel-linked 1,4-dihydropyridine receptors (Venter et al., 1983). Here membranes from guinea pig ileal smooth muscle were incubated with the tritium-labeled compound (specific activity 17.6 Ci/mmol) in 50 mM Tris–HCl buffer for 10 minutes at 25°C. Nonspecific incorporation was determined with added 5 μM nifedipine or

TABLE XIII
PHOTOAFFINITY LABELING WITH AZIDOPINE

Tissue (species)	Ligand	M_r of labeled peptides	Comments	Ref.[a]
Skeletal muscle (guinea pig)	$(\pm)$-[³H]Azidopine	145,000	Reducing conditions in SDS–PAGE	a
Skeletal muscle (guinea pig, rabbit, frog, chicken)	$(\pm)$-[³H]Azidopine	158,000	Nonreducing and reducing conditions in SDS–PAGE; lower and higher M_r bands identified in some species under nonreducing conditions	b
Skeletal muscle (rabbit)	$(\pm)$-[³H]Azidopine	170,000, 30,000	Excess nitrendipine blocked photoincorporation	c
Heart (canine)	$(\pm)$-[³H]Azidopine	185,000, 60,000	Excess nitrendipine blocked photoincorporation	c
Skeletal muscle, purified (guinea pig)	$(-)$-[³H]Azidopine	155,000	Nonreducing conditions in SDS–PAGE	d
Heart (guinea pig, chicken, rat)	$(-)$-[³H]Azidopine	165,000	Nonreducing conditions in SDS–PAGE	e

[a] Key to references: a, Ferry et al. (1984b), FEBS Lett. **169**, 112–118; b, Ferry et al. (1985), EMBO J. **4**, 1933–1950; c, Sharp et al. (1987), Biophys. J. **51**, 255a (Abstr.); d, Striessnig et al. (1986a), Eur. J. Biochem. **161**, 603–609; e, Ferry et al. (1987), Biochem. J. **243**, 127–135.

10 nM unlabeled o-NCS-dihydropyridine. The authors found a polypeptide of 45 kDa after SDS–PAGE which was specifically labeled in smooth muscle (and heart) membranes under reducing conditions. An additional peptide of 35 kDa (apparently a proteolytic product of the 45-kDa polypeptide) was occasionally observed, and under nonreducing conditions a higher molecular weight band was seen (however, no further data were given). It was concluded that the 45-kDa polypeptide was a component of the calcium channel.

It is worthwhile to analyze the results of Venter et al. (1983) in some detail. The "reversible" binding of the labeled affinity ligand and the affinity labeling were performed in Tris buffer. The authors later reported that the Tris adduct of o-NCS-dihydropyridine had been synthesized and shown to be a weak (K_i 1 μM), reversible inhibitor of [^{3}H]nitrendipine binding (Horne et al., 1984). One would expect that (by nucleophilic addition) the isothiocyanato group should be inactivated in Tris buffer. Apparently, this inactivation reaction was slow enough to allow an equilibrium saturation analysis and "specific" affinity labeling. Instead of testing for (noncompetitive) antagonism in a binding assay employing unlabeled o-NCS-dihydropyridine and a reversible ligand, e.g., [^{3}H]nitrendipine, the authors chose a functional assay. They incubated smooth muscle strips with unlabeled o-NCS-dihydropyridine or nifedipine and washed the preparation extensively. Whereas inhibition of the contractile response (using a muscarinic agonist as a stimulus) with nifedipine could be easily reversed by washing, that of o-NCS-dihydropyridine was not. With tissue homogenates or membranes, specific [^{3}H]nitrendipine binding was inhibited in muscle strips exposed to o-NCS-dihydropyridine but not to m-NCS-dihydropyridine or nifedipine. This was taken as an argument for irreversible inactivation of the 1,4-dihydropyridine receptor of the channel.

Kozlowski et al. (1986) found that [^{3}H]o-NCS-dihydropyridine binding to calcium channel drug receptors on cardiac membranes was completely reversible with a $t_{1/2}$ of 2.4 minutes at 37°C. They confirmed the result of Venter et al. (1983) that effects of o-NCS-dihydropyridine persisted in isolated perfused guinea pig hearts and in isolated ileal strips even after hours of washout. Similar findings were obtained with isolated guinea pig cardiac myocytes and measurements of the inward Ca^{2+} current under voltage clamp conditions. In the three biological systems, however, addition of the calcium channel activator Bay K 8644 caused a complete and rapid reversal of the inhibitory effects of o-NCS-dihydropyridine. Since the off-rate of the labeled ligand was rapid at 37°C but the nonspecific binding was a significant (>40%) fraction of the total binding, Kozlowski et al. (1986) concluded that o-NCS-dihydropyridine was only an apparent irreversible inhibitor in functional experiments because it was trapped as free drug in the membrane lipid compartment, thereby resisting removal by washout. The authors could not detect any specific incorporation of [^{3}H]o-NCS-dihydropyridine into guinea pig heart membranes using 1 μM o-NCS-dihydropyridine as a test for nonspecific binding. These results are in contrast to those of Horne et al. (1984) and Ferry et al. (1987) but can be explained, as shown below.

TABLE XIV

1,4-DIHYDROPYRIDINE BINDING SITES UNRELATED TO CALCIUM CHANNELS

Tissue (species)	Ligand	Results	Comments	Ref.[a]
Heart (guinea pig)	(±)-[^{3}H]Nitrendipine	$K_D = 67$ nM, $B_{max} = 35$ pmol/mg	Nonspecific binding definition was 20 μM nitrendipine; the sites did not discriminate between (−)- and (+)nitrendipine in buffer high ionic strength	a
Heart (guinea pig)	(±)-[^{3}H]Nitrendipine	(±)-[^{3}H]Nitrendipine binding ($K_D = 70$ nM) to low affinity sites increased by heating	Heated and unheated binding sites have the same affinity for the (+) enantiomer of nitrendipine; low affinity binding increased by anions ($NO_3^- > CF_3COO^- \gg PO_4^{-3}$) and cations ($Ca^{2+} > Mg^{2+} > K^+$)	b
Heart (rat), kidney, brain	(±)-[^{3}H]Ro 5-4864	B_{max} values 0.41 (brain), 8.16 (kidney), and 7.53 pmol/mg (heart)	Nifedipine and nitrendipine were apparently competitive inhibitors of nonneuronal benzodiazepine sites, with K_i values of 2 and 10 μM, respectively	c

Heart (canine)	(±)-[³H]Nitrendipine	$K_D = 166$ nM, $B_{max} = 20$ pmol/mg	B_{max} increased to 230 pmol/mg by heating; (±)Bay K 8644 was ineffective at the low affinity site	d
Heart (bovine)	(±)-[³H]Nimodipine	$K_D = 171$ nM, $B_{max} = 14$ pmol/mg	Binding to low affinity sites completely inhibited by nucleoside transport inhibitors	e
Heart (guinea pig)	(±)-[³H]Azidopine	$K_D = 25$ nM, $B_{max} = 22$ pmol/mg	Binding to low affinity sites not inhibited by nucleoside transport inhibitors; no discrimination between enantiomers of chiral 1,4-dihydropyridines; Bay K 8644 does not bind	f
Red blood cell ghost (human)	(±)-[³H]Nimodipine	$K_D = 52$ nM, $B_{max} = 10-20$ pmol/mg	Binding of (+)nimodipine to nucleoside transporters is completely inhibited by nitrobenzylthioinosine	g

[a] Key to references: a, Bellemann et al. (1981), Arzneim. Forsch. **31**, 2064–2067; b, Glossmann and Ferry (1983a), Drug Dev. **9**, 63–98; c, Cantor et al. (1984), Proc. Natl. Acad. Sci. U.S.A. **81**, 1549–1552; d, Vaghy et al. (1985), in "Cardiovascular Effects of Dihydropyridine-Type Calcium Antagonists and Agonists" (A. Fleckenstein, C. van Breemen, R. Gross, and F. Hoffmeister, eds.), pp. 156–184, Springer-Verlag, New York; e, Ruth et al. (1985), Eur. J. Biochem. **150**, 313–322; f, Ferry et al. (1987), Biochem. J. **243**, 127–135; g, Striessnig et al. (1985), Eur. J. Biochem. **150**, 67–77.

Horne *et al.* (1984) showed incorporation [^{3}H]o-NCS-dihydropyridine into canine heart membranes; incorporation was partially blocked by 50 μM nicardipine and 10 μM unlabeled o-NCS-dihydropyridine. Three polypeptides with molecular weights of 45,000, 42,000, and 33,000 were claimed to be specifically labeled. Interestingly, incorporation into the 45,000 protein was blocked not by o-NCS-dihydropyridine but by nicardipine, whereas nicardipine and o-NCS-dihydropyridine partially afforded protection against incorporation into the 42,000 and 33,000 species. Kirley and Schwartz (1984) attempted to affinity label rabbit skeletal muscle T-tubule 1,4-dihydropyridine receptors with [^{3}H]o-NCS-dihydropyridine. Their preparation displayed a specific density of 1,4-dihydropyridine sites in the range of 10–18 pmol/mg protein. Affinity labeling was performed at 37°C at pH 9.3 using amine-free buffer. No specific incorporation (inhibitable by 2 μM nimodipine) was observed, but the ligand incorporated nonspecifically into several polypeptides, the most prominent one of molecular weight 36,000.

(−)-[^{3}H]Azidopine binds with a K_D of 30 ± 7 pM to guinea pig heart membranes (Ferry *et al.*, 1987). This high affinity class of channel-linked receptors reveals a maximum density of 670 ± 97 fmol/mg protein. In addition, a second class of sites (B_{max} 21.6 ± 9 pmol/mg protein) was found at 30°C with a K_D of 25 ± 7 nM. The low K_D sites displayed typical calcium channel-specific binding inhibition profiles; the enantiomers of PN 200-110 showed an eudismic ratio greater than 100: (+)PN 200-110 gave a K_i of 60 pM, (−)PN 200-110, 7400 pM (Ferry *et al.*, 1987). An important tool to discriminate channel-linked receptors from low affinity binding sites is Bay K 8644, which does not bind to the low affinity sites. (−)-[^{3}H]Azidopine (in the presence of Bay K 8644 as a selective inhibitor of calcium channel-linked 1,4-dihydropyridine receptors) was then used to characterize the abundant high K_D sites (Table XV). Clearly, of all non-arylazide 1,4-dihydropyridines investigated, o-NCS-dihydropyridine showed the highest affinity (K_i 527 nM) whereas nicardipine was half as potent. (−)PN 200-110 was 2–3 times more potent than (+)PN 200-110 which is opposite to the calcium channel receptor. Photoaffinity labeling with (−)-[^{3}H]azidopine revealed that (in addition to a 165-kDa band representing the calcium channel α_1 subunit) 39- and 35-kDa bands incorporated the ligand. Whereas photoincorporation into the 165-kDa band was inhibited by very low concentrations of (+)PN 200-110 (10 or 20 nM), that of the two smaller polypeptides was not. Likewise, 100 nM o-NCS-dihydropyridine or 10 μM Bay K 8644 blocked the photoincorporation into the 165-kDa band but did not protect against photoincor-

TABLE XV

PHARMACOLOGICAL PROFILE OF CALCIUM CHANNEL-LINKED 1,4-DIHYDROPYRIDINE
RECEPTORS IN COMPARISON TO THE LOW AFFINITY SITES IN GUINEA PIG
HEART MEMBRANES[a]

| Ligand | Unlabeled competing drug | Control | | K_i (nM), 1 μM Bay K 8644 present |
		K_H (nM)	K_L (nM)	
[³H]Azidopine	(±)Nicardipine	0.31	898	923
	o-NCS-dihydropyridine	0.37	868	527
	(+)PN 200-110	0.06	7600	7400
	(−)PN 200-110	7.40	3000	2800
	(±)Nitrendipine	0.95	4600	6500
	(−)Bay K 8644	5.6	—	—
	(+)Bay K 8644	13.9	—	—
[³H]o-NCS-dihydropyridine	(+)PN 200-110	0.05	—	—
	(−)PN 200-110	7.90	—	—

[a] In control binding experiments (±)nicardipine defined the blank value, and displacement curves were biphasic with the exception of Bay K 8644. Data were fitted by nonlinear regression, and values for K_H (binding constant for channel-linked receptors) and K_L (binding constant for the low affinity site) were calculated. Identical experiments were performed in the presence of Bay K 8644 to block channel-specific binding. The displacement curves were monophasic, and K_L values are in good agreement with these K_i data. With Bay K 8644 as blank definition binding of [³H]o-NCS-dihydropyridine is stereoselective, indicating the channel-linked nature of the receptors characterized by this ligand. From Ferry et al. (1987), Biochem. J. 243, 127–135, with permission.

poration into the 39- or 35-kDa polypeptides. Fifty micromolar (±)nicardipine or 10 μM o-NCS-dihydropyridine, however, blocked the irreversible labeling of the 39- and 35-kDa polypeptides. These results strongly suggested that (−)-[³H]azidopine (bound to and) photoincorporated into low affinity 1,4-dihydropyridine sites that display preferential binding for o-NCS-dihydropyridine or nicardipine but do not recognize Bay K 8644.

[³H]o-NCS-dihydropyridine was a completely reversible ligand (K_D 0.35 nM) for guinea pig cardiac calcium channels (K_{-1} 0.2 minute^{-1}, $t_{1/2}$ 3.4 minutes at 30°C). [³H]o-NCS-dihydropyridine, like (−)-[³H]azidopine, incorporated into 39- and 35-kDa polypeptides but not into the 165-kDa polypeptide. Irreversible incorporation into the 39- and 35-kDa polypeptides was partially blocked by 50 μM (±)nicardipine or 10 μM o-NCS-dihydropyridine but not at all by 1 μM (−)Bay K 8644.

The lack of detection by Kozlowski et al. (1986) of "specific" incorporation (i.e., suppressed by unlabeled competitor) can be explained by the low concentrations of protecting o-NCS-dihydropyridine used. The K_D for the low molecular weight binding site is around 0.5 μM, and therefore at least 10 μM unlabeled affinity ligand must be employed to saturate these sites under such experimental conditions. Greenberg *et al.* (1985) and Ferry *et al.* (1987) tested o-NCS-dihydropyridine in competition experiments with (+)-[³H]PN 200-110 or [³H]nitrendipine. In brain as well as in heart membranes o-NCS-dihydropyridine was a pure competitive inhibitor (increase of apparent K_D of the labeled ligand, no reduction of B_{max}).

In summary, there is no evidence that o-NCS-dihydropyridine is an affinity ligand for the L-type calcium channel 1,4-dihydropyridine receptor. The remote possibility remains that it can be useful with purified channel preparations. On the other hand, [³H]o-NCS-dihydropyridine is a putative affintiy probe for a class of low affinity 1,4-dihydropyridine binding sites, often abundant in crude membrane preparations, that may represent additional targets for the pharmacological actions of certain 1,4-dihydropyridines.

    b. The Phenylalkylamine Receptor. 5-[3,4-(Dimethoxyphenethyl)-methylamine]-2-(3,4-dimethoxyphenyl)-2-isopropylpentylisothiocyanate was synthesized as a chemoaffinity ligand by Theodore *et al.* (1986). The compound competitively inhibited binding of [³H]gallopamil with an IC_{50} value of 0.3 μM, being approximately 20 times less potent than unlabeled gallopamil (16 nM), in rat myocardial membranes. The chemoaffinity ligand inhibited electrically stimulated myocardial strips in a concentration-dependent manner with an IC_{50} value of 4.6 μM (gallopamil, 1.95 μM). Homogenates were preincubated (after Venter *et al.*, 1983) with the putative chemoaffinity probe (or gallopamil) at a concentration of 10 μM and washed extensively. Whereas 68.5% of control binding was recovered with gallopamil in the preincubation, only 25% remained for the chemoaffinity probe. The authors concluded that gallopamil was not completely washed out but that the chemoaffinity probe irreversibly interacted with a portion of the calcium channel. Unfortunately, no saturation studies with [³H]-gallopamil were reported (to evaluate the noncompetitive nature of inhibition), and the usefulness of this probe remains to be established.

2. Photoaffinity Labeling with Non-Arylazides

    a. The 1,4-Dihydropyridine Receptor. Three non-arylazide 1,4-dihydropyridines have been employed to photolabel membranes containing 1,4-dihydropyridine receptors linked to calcium channels.

Irradiation of [^{3}H]nitrendipine bound to canine heart membranes with high intensity UV light causes incorporation of the labeled compound into a 32-kDa polypeptide (Campbell *et al.*, 1984). The photoincorporation conditions were as follows: 0.5 mg of membrane protein (~0.5 pmol of high affinity 1,4-dihydropyridine binding sites) was incubated with 10 nM labeled ligand in 0.15 M NaCl, 10 mM Tris–Cl buffer for 30 minutes at 37°C and subsequently irradiated for 25 seconds at 4°C with a 1000-W mercury arc lamp. Separation of the polypeptides was by SDS–PAGE under reducing conditions. Photolabeling was partially prevented by 20 μM unlabeled nifedipine, 40 μM verapamil, 1 mM EDTA, or 10 mM ATP. The latter was the most effective protecting agent. As proof for the photolabeling of a calcium channel component ryanodine-insensitive sarcoplasmic reticulum vesicles were used as a control; no 32-kDa band was photolabeled. Heating of the membranes (10 minutes at 65°C) and addition of La^{3+} (0.4 mM) also inhibited photolabeling. The concentration of [^{3}H]nitrendipine was 100 K_D [K_D for [^{3}H]nitrendipine, ~0.1 nM) and high ionic strength media were used. Under these conditions the occupancy of low affinity binding sites (which are abundant by orders of magnitude compared to calcium channel-linked receptors; see Table XIV) is significant. An example of two saturation isotherms of heart membranes in low and high ionic strength media is shown in Fig. 27. Experiments with the arylazide photoaffinity ligand (−)-[^{3}H]azidopine discussed below (Glossmann *et al.*, 1987b; Ferry *et al.*, 1987) make it very likely that the 32-kDa polypeptide photolabeled by Campbell *et al.* (1984) is not the 1,4-dihydropyridine receptor-carrying subunit of the L-type calcium channel.

Another (^{125}-labeled) ligand, Bay P 8857 [2-iodoethylisopropyl-1,4-dihydropyridine-2,6-dimethyl-4-(3-nitrophenyl)pyridine-3,5-dicarboxylate], with a specific activity of 2200 Ci/mmol, was used by Sarmiento *et al.* (1986) to photoaffinity label calf heart, bovine aorta, and chicken skeletal muscle T-tubule membranes. The nonspecific incorporation was defined by 50 μM nicardipine; 0.1 nM radiolabel and exposure to high intensity UV light (425 W) for 10 minutes were employed. Under these conditions there was affinity labeling of several bands in the 33–35 kDa region (separated by SDS–PAGE under reducing conditions). Surprisingly, the chicken T-tubule membrane (having a density of 1,4-dihydropyridine receptors two orders of magnitude greater than the heart membrane) showed only a minute incorporation into the 33–35 kDa region. This finding agrees, however, with the very low density of non-channel-linked 1,4-dihydropyridine receptors in skeletal muscle. It is therefore likely that the iodinated 1,4-dihydro-

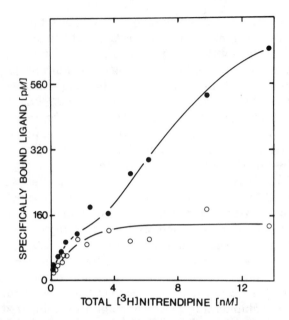

FIG. 27. High ionic strength reveals low affinity binding sites for 1,4-dihydropyridines in crude membranes. A particularly rich source of binding sites for 1,4-dihydropyridines which have no obvious relationship to calcium channels is guinea pig heart crude membranes. At low ionic strength (open circles) mainly the high affinity, stereoselective receptors on the calcium channel are labeled. If the ionic strength is increased by performing the binding experiment in the presence of 150 mM NaCl with 1 mM CaCl$_2$ (filled circles), low affinity binding is greatly enhanced whereas calcium channel receptor binding is not. The low affinity sites [with [^{3}H]nitrendipine as label] can be separated from channel-linked receptors by further purification of the membranes. These low affinity sites have confused researchers for almost 5 years as they can be photolabeled and were even believed to represent low-affinity states of the receptor for 1,4-dihydropyridines. [From Glossmann and Ferry (1983a), *Drug Dev.* **9**, 68–98, with permission.]

pyridine ligand identified the same polypeptides as seen by Campbell *et al.* (1984) and others.

(+)-[^{3}H]PN 200-110 was used by Galizzi *et al.* (1986b) to photoaffinity label rabbit skeletal muscle T-tubule membranes. To this end membranes (0.1 mg/ml, equivalent to 5 nM 1,4-dihydropyridine binding sites) were equilibrated with 2 nM of the labeled ligand (to reduce the concentration of free ligand), and nonspecific binding was defined by 0.3 μM unlabeled (+)PN 200-110. Exposure time was 12 seconds at 4°C with a 2000-W mercury lamp. After centrifugation the membranes were dissolved in SDS and 4% 2-mercaptoethanol, heated, and analyzed by SDS–PAGE under reducing conditions. Gels were then exposed to films for 30–40 days. A polypeptide migrating with an apparent molecular weight of 170,000 was thereby identified. The authors suggested that the 170-kDa polypeptide identified by photolabeling in the membranes was proteolytically degraded in a 142-kDa polypeptide purified from these membranes after solubilization (Borsotto *et al.*, 1984a, 1985; see also Section VII,B).

   b. Phenylalkylamine and Benzothiazepine Receptors. High intensity UV light was employed to photoincorporate (±)-[^{3}H]bepridil and (+)-*cis*-[^{3}H]diltiazem into a 170-kDa polypeptide in rabbit skeletal muscle T-tubule membranes. (±)-[^{3}H]Bepridil incorporation was blocked by (+)bepridil or (−)desmethoxyverapamil, and (+)-*cis*-[^{3}H]diltiazem labeling was protected by (−)desmethoxyverapamil or the unlabeled compound (Galizzi *et al.*, 1986b). The authors concluded that the receptors for these calcium channel blockers were located on the same polypeptide. It is not known whether these ligands are useful as photoaffinity probes to follow purification of the receptor or to prove which of the channel polypeptides carry the binding domain(s).

3. Photoaffinity Labeling with Arylazides

   a. The 1,4-Dihydropyridine Receptor. Arylazides are the most popular and widely used photoactivatable reagents (Bayley, 1983). They have the advantage of mild photolysis conditions (>300 nm); they are stable in the absence of UV light; and the singlet or triplet nitrene intermediates can react with C–H bonds, with amines to form azepines, or with benzyl rings containing electronegative substituents (Ruoho *et al.*, 1981). The only arylazides employed so far are (±)-[^{3}H]azidopine and the optically pure (−)-[^{3}H]azidopine. The properties of [^{3}H]azidopine are summarized in Table XVI. These ligands were used to characterize 1,4-dihydropyridine receptors in skeletal muscle T-tubule membranes as well as in heart and brain membranes from different species. Reversible binding characteristics of the photoaffinity ligand were studied extensively with skeletal muscle T-tubule membranes from guinea pigs (Ferry *et al.*, 1984b), with heart and hippocampus membranes from the same species (Ferry *et al.*, 1987; Striessnig *et al.*, 1988b) and with purified calcium channels from guinea pig skeletal muscle T-tubules membranes (Striessnig *et al.*, 1986a).

   An example of the pharmacological profile of (±)-[^{3}H]azidopine for skeletal muscle T-tubule calcium channels is shown in Fig. 28. Particularly noteworthy is the slow dissociation rate of the photoaffinity

TABLE XVI
PROPERTIES OF [³H]AZIDOPINE[a]

Specific radioactivity	High (>50 Ci/mmol)	
Stability in aqueous solvents	Good	
Binding ability	>40% for racemic ligand; >90% for (−)-[³H]azidopine	
Equipment needed	Inexpensive UV lamp (Phillips TL 40 W/08)	
Dissociation constants	(−)-[³H]Azidopine	(+)-[³H]PN 200-110
Skeletal muscle		
Particulate	0.35 nM	0.7 nM
Solubilized	0.70 nM	0.7 nM
Purified	3.1 nM	5–9 nM
Heart, particulate	0.03 nM	0.05 nM
Brain, particulate	0.09 nM	0.08 nM
Binding to low affinity, non-channel-linked, 1,4-dihydropyridine sites		
Skeletal muscle	Very low	
Heart	Yes (guinea pig ≫ rat = chicken)	
Optically pure enantiomers available for stereoselective photoaffinity labeling?	Yes, with identical specific activity	
Cold trap method possible?	Yes	
Specific photoincorporation		
Skeletal muscle		
Particulate	1.5%	
Solubilized	10%	
Purified	15%	
Heart, particulate	1.5%	
Brain, particulate	2.0%	
Antibodies against label available?	Yes	

[a] Binding ability of the ligand is defined as the fraction of total label which can be specifically bound by an excess of empty receptor sites. For this purpose partially purified T-tubule membranes from guinea pig skeletal muscle are employed (see Ferry and Glossmann, 1982b). The cold trap method is explained briefly in the text. Specific photoincorporation is that recovered in the 155 or 165 kDa (calcium channel) region after SDS–PAGE under nonreducing conditions, expressed as the percentage of specifically reversible bound photolabel using appropriate blank definitions. All K_D and photoincorporation data refer to guinea pig tissues. Particulate membranes are partially purified T-tubule membranes (B_{max} = 20–24 pmol of 1,4-dihydropyridine sites/mg protein), partially purified heart membranes (B_{max} = 0.7 pmol/mg protein), and hippocampus membranes from brain (B_{max} = 0.56 pmol/mg protein). The purified skeletal muscle T-tubule calcium channel has >1500 pmol/mg protein of 1,4-dihydropyridine binding sites by postlabeling.

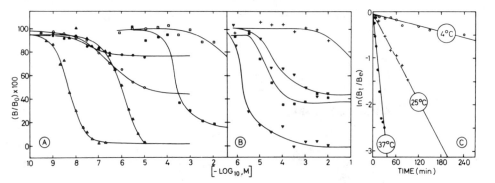

FIG. 28. Pharmacological profile of reversible [³H]azidopine binding to guinea pig skeletal muscle T-tubule membranes. (A) Drug and cation dependence of [³H]azidopine binding. [³H]Azidopine (0.4–0.6 nM) was incubated with 10–12 μg skeletal muscle membrane protein for 30 minutes at 25°C in a volume of 0.25 ml. B_0 is specific [³H]azidopine binding in the absence of added drug, and B the specific binding in its presence. The binding inhibition curves have been fitted to the general dose–response equation, and the following parameter estimates were made (± asymptotic SD): (+)PN 200–110 (△), $K_{0.5}$ = 5.8 ± 2.8 nM, slope factor = 1.3 ± 0.15; (−)PN 200–110 (▲), $K_{0.5}$ = 1400 ± 290 nM, slope factor = 0.96 ± 0.12; (−)verapamil (●), $K_{0.5}$ = 39 ± 18 nM, slope factor = 1.0 ± 0.43, maximal inhibition 33 ± 1.4%; (+)verapamil (○), $K_{0.5}$ = 340 ± 130 nM, slope factor = 0.62 ± 0.15, maximal inhibition, 56 ± 6%; Ca^{2+} (□), 3% inhibition at 10 nM; La^{3+} (■), $K_{0.5}$ = 200 ± 50 μM, maximal inhibition, 85 ± 5%. (B) Sulfhydryl reagent sensitivity of [³H]azidopine binding. The experiment was conducted as for (A), except that membranes were preincubated with sulfhydryl reagents for 30 minutes at 37°C prior to addition of [³H]azidopine. Dithiothreitol (■), $K_{0.5}$ = 55 ± 15 μM, slope factor = 1.6 ± 0.6, maximal inhibition 62 ± 3%; N-ethylmaleimide (▼), $K_{0.5}$ = 850 ± 110 μM, slope factor = 0.4 ± 0.4, maximal inhibition 65 ± 20%; p-chloromercuriphenylsulfonic acid (▽), $K_{0.5}$ = 3 ± 2 μM, maximal inhibition 95 ± 8%, iodoacetamide (+), 5% inhibition at 10 mM. (C) Dissociation kinetics of [³H]azidopine. Equilibrium populations of [³H]azidopine–calcium channel complexes were perturbed at t = 0 by addition of 0.01 ml of 25 μM unlabeled nimodipine, and then bound and free [³H]azidopine were separated at various times as indicated. B_e is specifically bound [³H]azidopine at t = 0, and B_t specifically bound [³H]azidopine at various times after addition of 1 μM unlabeled nimodipine. At 4°C (○) the dissociation rate constant (K_{-1}) is 0.002/minute, at 25°C (+) K_{-1} is 0.016/minute, and at 37°C (●) K_{-1} is 0.077/minute. [From Ferry et al. (1985b), EMBO J. 4, 1933–1940, with permission.]

ligand at low temperatures which allows the use of the "cold-trap" technique. Guinea pig skeletal muscle membranes (1–2 mg protein/ml, equivalent to 2.5–5 nM 1,4-dihydropyridine receptor) were preincubated at 25°C with 2.5 nM [³H]azidopine and subsequently washed twice by centrifugation (in the last step bovine serum albumin was included) at 2°C; irradiation of the preparation with UV light for 0–4 minutes afforded incorporation of the ligand into several bands.

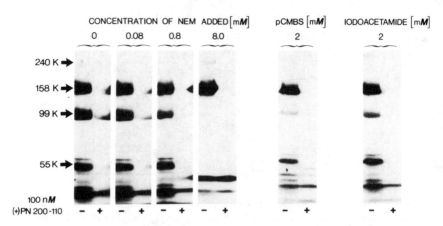

FIG. 29. Electrophoretic conditions influence the labeling pattern of calcium channel-linked 1,4-dihydropyridine receptors with the photoaffinity probe [³H]azidopine. A batch of guinea pig skeletal muscle T-tubule membranes was photoaffinity labeled with (±)-[³H]azidopine with (+) or without (−) (+)PN 200-110 (100 nM) as a protecting agent. The batches were solubilized with sodium dodecyl sulfate in the absence or presence of various sulfhydryl group blocking agents and separated by SDS–PAGE. Note that with 8 mM N-ethylmaleimide (NEM), p-chloromercuriphenylsulfonic acid (p-CMBS), or iodoacetamide the banding pattern is much cleaner. In contrast to guinea pig heart (see Fig. 34), nonspecific labeling (in the presence of the protecting agent) is much less pronounced. This correlates with the virtual absence of low affinity (non-channel-linked) 1,4-dihydropyridine binding sites in skeletal muscle T-tubule membranes. The autoradiogram of the SDS gel was obtained after a 3-week exposure of the gel impregnated with an enhancer at −70°C. For further details, see Ferry et al. (1985), EMBO J. 4, 1933–1940.

The molecular weights under mildly alkylating conditions (0.8 mM N-ethylmaleimide) were 240,000, 158,000, and 99,000; sometimes a 52,000–55,000 doublet was observed. Under reducing conditions a 158,000 band was the principal component. Two-dimensional electrophoresis indicated that the 158,000 band was linked to a 99,000 band by a disulfide bridge to form a 240,000 polypeptide. Not completely ruled out was the possibility of proteolysis on solubilization of the samples in SDS buffer; such might have been blocked by SH group alkylating reagents. Figure 29 shows an experiment in which increasing concentrations of N-ethylmaleimide, 2 mM p-chloromercuribenzosulfonic acid, iodoacetamide were added on solubilization for electrophoresis. Other than a faint 240,000 band, the 158,000 protein is the major specifically photolabeled moiety with 8 mM N-ethylmaleimide added. Similar results (with reduced amounts of 99,000 or 55,000 bands) were observed with the two other alkylating reagents.

This argues in favor of proteolytic cleavage, especially if one takes into account that the sum of 99,000 and 55,000 polypeptides approaches that of the molecular weight of the 158.000 band.

Skeletal muscle T-tubule membranes yielded labeled 240- and 99-kDa bands in guinea pig and rabbit but not in frog or chicken membranes. In all species, however, the 158-kDa band was the most prominent photolabeled polypeptide under nonreducing or reducing conditions (Ferry et al., 1985b).

T-tubule membrane preparations from guinea pig skeletal muscle solubilized with digitonin incorporate the (−) enantiomer of [^{3}H]aziodopine into several polypeptides, only one of which (155 kDa) was protected by unlabeled PN 200-110 (Striessnig et al., 1986a). The (+) enantiomer of [^{3}H]azidopine photoincorporated only to a minor extent into the 155-kDa polypeptide but showed identical photoincorporation into 100- and 45-kDa bands. This is an example of stereoselective photolabeling, although the eudismic ratio [K_D for the (−) enantiomer divided by the K_D of the (+) enantiomer] is not extremely high (15- to 20-fold). On purification the nonspecifically labeled 100- and 45-kDa polypeptides are apparently removed; only labeling in the 155-kDa region was then observed (Fig. 30).

The pharmacological profile of the purified guinea pig skeletal muscle calcium channel reversibly labeled by (−)-[^{3}H]azidopine is shown in Table XVII. The reversible binding characteristics are reflected by the irreversible incorporation profile. For example, (+)-cis-diltiazem, which stimulated the reversible binding of (−)-[^{3}H]azidopine, increased the photolabeling; La^{3+}, which blocked with an IC$_{50}$ value of 0.4 mM, afforded almost complete protection. Stereoselective protection of photolabeling is observed with the optical enantiomers of PN 200-110 (Fig. 31).

The specific photoincorporation of (−)-[^{3}H]azidopine is high in the purified calcium channel preparation, and after one photolysis approximately 10% of the reversibly bound ligand is irreversibly fixed. The label, which is exclusively found in the 155-kDa band, is stable to acid, heating, SDS, urea, and organic solvents. A significant fraction of the label, however, can be removed by nucleophilic agents, including dithiothreitol and 2-mercaptoethanol (Fig. 32). This appears to be a unique feature of (−)-[^{3}H]azidopine photoincorporation into the clacium channel α$_1$ subunit (see Section VII,B); specific photoincorporation into γ-globulin raised against 1,4-dihydropyridines is not sensitive to reduction (Fig. 33; see also Striessnig et al. (1988b).

(−)-[^{3}H]Azidopine has been employed to photoaffinity label the 1,4-dihydropyridine receptor in hippocampus and heart membranes from

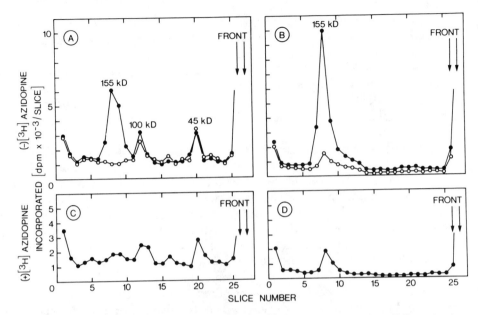

FIG. 30. Stereospecific photoaffinity labeling of the 1,4-dihydropyridine Ca^{2+} antagonist receptor with the tritiated enantiomers of azidopine in guinea pig skeletal muscle. $(-)$-[^{3}H]Azidopine (7.3 nM) was incubated with the digitonin extract (315 μg protein) (A) or purified calcium channel-linked receptor (2.8 μg protein) (B) in the absence (total binding lane) or presence (blank binding lane) of 3 μM ($\pm$)PN 200–110 for 40 minutes at 25°C. Aliquots of the incubation mixture were removed to measure total and reversibly bound ligand concentrations. One milliliter was transferred to plastic petri dishes (3.5 cm diameter) on ice and photolyzed for 3 minutes with a Philips TL 40 W/08 ultraviolet lamp at a distance of 10 cm. Irradiated samples were then dialyzed and lyophilized. After resuspension for electrophoresis in 0.2 ml of sample buffer containing 10 mM N-ethylmaleimide, the samples were heated for 3 minutes at 95°C. and 0.1 ml was applied to a 4–15% polyacrylamide gel. Lanes were cut into 3-mm strips and the radioactivity counted after 3 days of solubilization in Lipoluma/Liposolve liquid scintillation cocktail. (●) Radioactivity recovered from the total binding lane; (○) radioactivity recovered from the blank binding lane. $(+)$-[^{3}H]Azidopine (7.2 nM) was incubated with the digitonin extract (C) or the purified channel (D) under the same conditions as described for $(-)$-[^{3}H]azidopine. Only the radioactivity from the total binding lane is shown (●) since the blank lane was identical to the one shown for $(-)$-[^{3}H]azidopine. Specific binding after incubation for $(-)$-[^{3}H]azidopine was 1517 fmol/ml in digitonin extracts and 2370 fmol/ml in purified fractions. Values for $(+)$-[^{3}H]azidopine were 53 and 275 fmol/ml, respectively. Nonspecific binding was less than 9% of total binding in the case of $(-)$-[^{3}H]azidopine. Nonspecifically bound radioactivity did not differ between the two enantiomers of the photolabel. [From Striessnig et al. (1986a), Eur. J. Biochem. 161, 603–609, with permission.]

TABLE XVII
PHARMACOLOGICAL PROFILE OF REVERSIBLE $(-)$-[^{3}H]AZIDOPINE BINDING
TO PURIFIED CALCIUM CHANNELS BY Ca^{2+} ANTAGONIST DRUGS
OF DIFFERENT CHEMICAL CLASSES AND La^{3+a}

Compound	IC_{50} or K_i (nM)	Maximal inhibition or stimulation (%)
$(-)$Azidopine	3.6 $\pm$ 0.6	100 $\pm$ 9
$(+)$Azidopine	59.6 $\pm$ 14.8	100 $\pm$ 4
$(+)$PN 200-110	7.5 $\pm$ 4.4	100 $\pm$ 12
$(-)$PN 200-110	812 $\pm$ 261	100 $\pm$ 9
$(-)$Desmethoxyverapamil	126 $\pm$ 65	163 $\pm$ 14
$(+)$Desmethoxyverapamil	6600 $\pm$ 2200	6 $\pm$ 9
$(+)$-cis-Diltiazem	3470 $\pm$ 940	214 $\pm$ 10
$(-)$-cis-Diltiazem	>10000	98 $\pm$ 5
La^{3+}	3000 $\pm$ 15000	3 $\pm$ 8

a $(-)$-[^{3}H]Azidopine (0.9–1.2 nM) was incubated with 0.16–0.29 μg of purified channel protein. Data from two to three experiments were fitted to the general dose–response equation. IC_{50} or K_i values are given as means $\pm$ asymptotic SD. Percent maximal stimulation is defined as $100 \times B/B_0$ and maximal inhibition as $(1 - B/B_0) \times 100$. B_0 is specific binding of $(-)$-[^{3}H]azidopine in the absence, B in the presence of a saturating drug concentration. From Striessnig et al. (1986a), Eur. J. Biochem. 161, 603–609, with permission.

different species (Ferry et al., 1987; Striessnig et al., 1988b). The density of calcium channel-linked Ca^{2+} antagonist receptor sites is much lower in these tissues than in skeletal muscle T-tubule membranes. For example, with $(-)$-[^{3}H]azidopine, a B_{max} of 0.67 or 0.56 pmol/mg protein is found in guinea pig heart or brain membranes whereas in skeletal muscle T-tubules B_{max} is 28 pmol/mg protein (Ferry et al., 1984b). Moreover, the density of low affinity 1,4-dihydropyridine sites is much greater in, e.g., heart membranes compared to the T-tubule preparation. On the other hand, the K_D of $(-)$-[^{3}H]azidopine for the heart and brain receptor is 10 times lower than that of the T-tubule. Depending on species, K_D values between 350 and 990 pM are found for the latter (Ferry et al., 1985b). Figures 34 and 35 show autoradiographs from photolabeling experiments with guinea pig, chick, and rat heart membranes. A 165-kDa band is specifically labeled by $(-)$-[^{3}H]azidopine. Heart membranes (guinea pig >> rat = chicken) contain low affinity sites (39 and 35 kDa) that are also photolabeled and protected only with excessive concentrations of nicardipine but

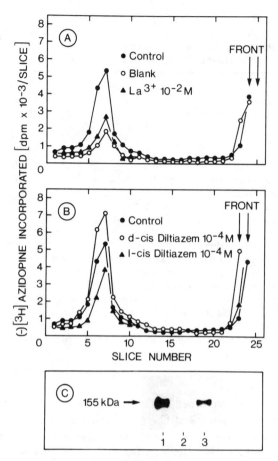

FIG. 31. The irreversible labeling profile of the purified 1,4-dihydropyridine receptor-carrying polypeptide is identical to the reversible binding characteristics of (−)-[³H]azidopine to purified calcium channels. In (A) and (B) photoaffinity labeling of the purified calcium channel from guinea pig skeletal muscle T-tubule membranes was performed in the presence of La³⁺ or (+)- or (−)-*cis*-diltiazem. After photolabeling and separation of the purified channel polypeptides by SDS–PAGE, gels were sliced and the incorporated radioactivity counted. The top of the gel is on the left. Note that the (+)-cis enantiomer of diltiazem stimulated photoincorporation whereas the (−)-cis enantiomer did not. In (C) an autoradiogram of a gel is shown in which the purified channel was photolabeled with no protecting agent present (lane 1), with 1 μ*M* (+)PN 200-110 (lane 2), or with 1 μ*M* (−)PN 200–110. This is an example of stereoselective protection: (+)PN 200-110 has a K_i of 7.5 n*M* but (−)PN 200–110 a K_i of 812 n*M* for the (−)-[³H]azidopine reversibly labeled purified calcium channel. [From Striessnig *et al.* (1986a), *Eur. J. Biochem.* **161**, 603–609, with permission.]

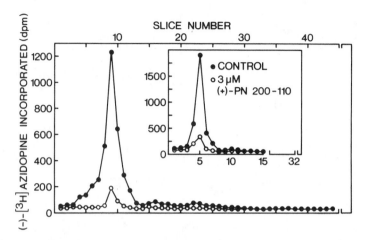

FIG. 32. The purified calcium channel α_1 polypeptide incorporates $(-)$-[³H]azidopine into bonds with differential sensitivity for nucleophilic agents. Using the same conditions for photolysis as in Fig. 33 (in which an antibody directed against 1,4-dihydropyridines is specifically labeled), the bond to the α_1 polypeptide is sensitive to nucleophilic reagents. In the example shown the purified channel was photolabeled and separated by SDS–PAGE under conditions where 2-mercaptoethanol (20 mM) was present (open circles) or 10 mM N-ethylmaleimide was added (filled circles). In the inset total labeling (filled circles) and nonspecific labeling (in the presence of a protecting ligand, open circles) are shown. With longer irradiation times a second type of bond is discovered (not shown) which is resistant to nucleophilic agents. All calcium channels isolated from different species display the same behavior.

not Bay K 8644. In guinea pig hippocampus a 190- to 195-kDa polypeptide was specifically labeled with $(-)$-[³H]azidopine. Thus the neuronal 1,4-dihydropyridine receptor is located on polypeptides slightly larger (by SDS–PAGE) than those found in heart or skeletal muscle.

In summary, results with the arylazides $(\pm)$-[³H]azidopine and $(-)$-[³H]azidopine show without doubt that a 155- to 158-kDa polypeptide, unchanged in mobility on SDS–PAGE with reduction, carries the 1,4-dihydropyridine receptor in skeletal muscle T-tubule membranes from diverse species. This polypeptide is now termed the α_1 subunit. The unique property of the α_2 subunit to change its apparent molecular weight by 30,000 on reduction discriminates the receptor-carrying α_1 subunit from this glycoprotein (vide infra). Evidence is cited below that the α_1 subunit also carries the phenylalkylamine receptor. Another satisfying result is that in three different tissues (representing different subtypes of calcium L channels) azidopine labeled poly-

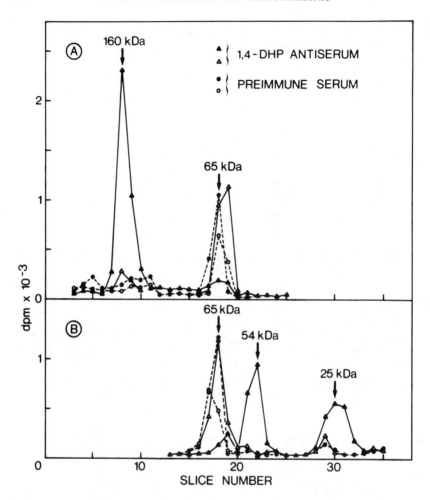

FIG. 33. Photoaffinity labeling of a 1,4-dihydropyridine antibody by (±)-[³H]azido-pine: stability of the bond to reducing agents. One microliter (in 1 ml of 50 m*M* Tris–HCl buffer, 150 m*M* NaCl, pH 7.4) of rabbit preimmune serum or rabbit anti-1,4-di-hydropyridine serum was incubated with 1.4 n*M* (±)-[³H]azidopine with (filled symbols) or without 10 μ*M* (±)PN 200-110 (open symbols) for 4 hours in the dark at 25°C. Samples were then photolabeled for 3 minutes and, after lyophilization, subjected to SDS–PAGE (4–15%) under alkylating conditions with 8 m*M* *N*-ethylmaleimide (A) or under reduc-ing conditions with 10% 2-mercaptoethanol (B). Gels were sliced, and the radioactivity was determined. The anti-1,4-dihydropyridine serum was raised against 1,4-di-hydro-2,6-dimethyl-4-(2-trifluoromethylphenyl)-3,5-pyridinecarboxylic 2-(aminoethyl) ethylester, coupled by 1-ethyl-3-(3-dimethylaminopropyl)carbodiimide–HCl to human serum albumin. Note that the label remains attached to the heavy and light chains (54 and 25 kDa) after reduction and that increased labeling of serum albumin (65 kDa) occurs in the presence of a saturating concentration of a protecting ligand (A).

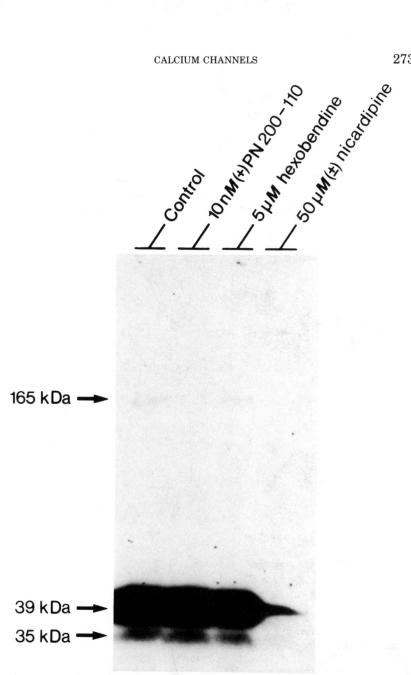

FIG. 34. Photoaffinity labeling of guinea pig heart membranes with (−)-[³H]azido-pine. Note that next to the calcium channel polypeptide (165 kDa) two polypeptides (39 and 35 kDa) are photolabeled which are protected only by excessive concentrations of nicardipine and not by 10 nM (+)PN 200-110. [From Ferry *et al.* (1987), *Biochem. J.* **243,** 127–135, with permission.]

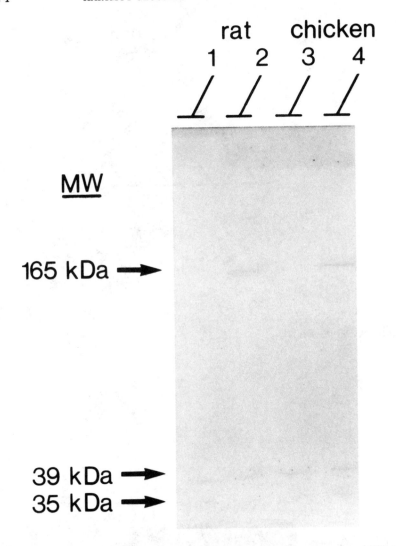

FIG. 35. Photoaffinity labeling of rat and chick heart membranes with $(-)$-[^{3}H]azido-pine. Note that in contrast to guinea pig heart (Fig. 34) far fewer low affinity sites are photolabeled. The protecting agent employed was 1 μM $(-)$Bay K 8644 (lanes 1 and 3). Here photolabeling of the 165-kDa polypeptide is completely protected, but photoaffinity labeling of the non-channel-linked binding sites (39 and 35 kDa) is not. [From Ferry *et al.* (1987), *Biochem. J.* **243**, 127–135, with permission.]

peptides of similar size, in accordance with target size analysis experiments.

b. The Phenylalkylamine Receptor. The tritiated arylazido, optically pure phenylalkylamine, [*N-methyl*-^{3}H]LU 49888, was introduced by Striessnig *et al.* (1987) as a specific photolabel for the phenylalkylamine receptor of the L-type calcium channel. Its properties are summarized in Table XVIII. The compound was selected out of a group of azido derivatives of verapamil on the basis of potent calcium antagonistic activity in different pharmacological test systems.

In reversible binding experiments with guinea pig skeletal muscle T-tubule membranes (performed in the dark) at 20°C, a K_{+1} of 0.072 ± 0.006 nM^{-1} minute^{-1} was found; the dissociation rate constant (after 80-fold dilution) was 0.179 ± 0.02 minute^{-1}. The compound labeled the phenylalkylamine receptors with a K_D of 2.0 ± 0.5 nM and a B_{max} 17 ± 0.9 pmol/mg protein, very similar to (−)-[^{3}H]desmethoxyverapamil (Goll *et al.*, 1984a). The reversible binding of the photoaffinity ligand was regulated in a stereoselective manner by the different classes of calcium channel drugs (see Table XIX). As observed for (−)-[^{3}H]desmethoxyverapamil (Striessnig *et al.*, 1986b), the dissociation constant for [*N-methyl*-^{3}H]LU 49888 increased approximately 30-fold on solubilization or purification of the guinea pig skeletal muscle calcium channel. Despite the decrease in affinity, photoaffinity labeling with the phenylalkylamine ligand was also satisfactory for the purified channel preparation. To this end Striessnig *et al.* (1987) incu-

TABLE XVIII

PROPERTIES OF THE PHENYLALKYLAMINE ARYLAZIDE,
[*N-Methyl*-^{3}H]LU 49888[a]

Specific activity (Ci/mmol)	>75
Optically pure enantiomer	Yes
Stability in aqueous buffers	Good
Binding ability (%)	>65
Dissociation constants (nM)	
Skeletal muscle	2.0 ± 0.4
Hippocampus	1.4 ± 0.3
Heart	n.d.
Antibody available	Yes
Irreversible labeling (%)	
Skeletal muscle membranes	>0.2
Purified channel (skeletal muscle)	>0.8
Hippocampus	>1.5

[a] All data refer to guinea pig tissues; n.d., not determined.

TABLE XIX
REVERSIBLE INTERACTION OF [N-methyl-³H]LU 49888-LABELED PHENYLALKYLAMINE
RECEPTORS WITH CALCIUM CHANNEL-ACTIVE DRUGS FOR MEMBRANE-BOUND AND PURIFIED
CALCIUM CHANNELS FROM GUINEA PIG SKELETAL MUSCLE T-TUBULE MEMBRANES[a]

	Membrane-bound channel		Purified channel	
Drug	K_i (*) or IC$_{50}$ (nM)	Maximum inhibition or stimulation (%)	K_i (*) or IC$_{50}$ (nM)	Maximum inhibition or stimulation (%)
(±)LU 49888	8.18 ± 2.6*	100	113.3 ± 48.1	100
(−)D 888	5.7 ± 1.0*	100	40.1 ± 12.5	100
(+)D 888	24.4 ± 3.2*	100	n.d.	—
(±)D 619	5600.2 ± 610 *	100	44000 ± 10780	100
(+)-cis-Diltiazem	163.6 ± 27.5	100	>3000	—
(−)-cis-Diltiazem	9140 ± 120	100	>3000	—
(+)PN 200-110	1.4 ± 0.2	46	21 ± 5	238 (+)
(−)PN 200-110	489 ± 105	100	>10000	—

[a] Results are means ± SD from at least three experiments. Binding inhibition is defined as 100 × (1 − B/B₀), and binding stimulation (+) as 100 × B/B₀. B and B₀ are specific binding in the presence and absence of added drug, respectively. K_i values are given in case of competitive inhibition as indicated (*). D 888, Desmethoxyverapamil; n.d., not determined. From Striessnig et al. (1987), FEBS Lett. **212**, 247–253, and Glossmann et al. (1987a). Ann. N.Y. Acad. Sci. (in press), with permission.

bated 15.1 nM of [N-methyl-³H]LU 49888 with 5.1 μg of purified channel protein and photoactivated with or without 3 μM (−)desmethoxyverapamil. Electrophoresis in 8% SDS gels allowed separation of the α₁ and α₂ subunits and proved the existence of the phenylalkylamine receptor domain on the α₁ subunit, which does not change its mobility on reduction (Fig. 36). In contrast to (−)-[³H]azidopine labeling of the 1,4-dihydropyridine receptor domain on the α₁ subunit, the incorporated label is completely stable to added nucleophilic reagents (e.g., 2-mercaptoethanol). As found with the 1,4-dihydropyridine photoaffinity ligand azidopine, several additional polypeptides were labeled in the membrane preparation employed as starting material for the purification (see Fig. 37). The most likely explanation is that fragments of the α₁ subunit, which are able to bind (and incorporate) the ligand, are removed on purification, but this remains to be tested more rigorously.

Together with (−)-[³H]azidopine, [N-methyl-³H]LU 49888 was used to photolabel high affinity phenylalkylamine drug receptors in guinea pig hippocampus. Both ligands specifically labeled a 190- to 195-kDa

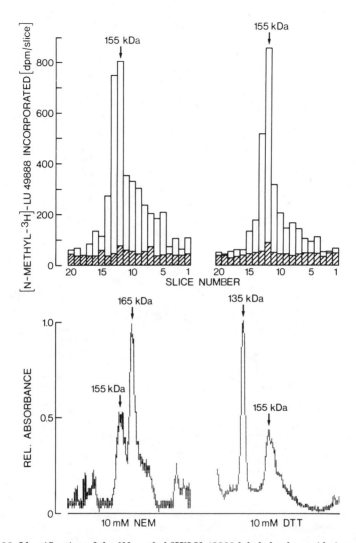

FIG. 36. Identification of the [*N-methyl-³H*]LU 49888-labeled polypeptide in purified calcium channel preparations from guinea pig skeletal muscle. Purified calcium channels (5.1 μg protein) were photoaffinity labeled, employing 15.1 nM of [*N-methyl-³H*]LU 49888. The irradiated samples were separated on a 8% polyacrylamide gel under alkylating (10 mM *N*-ethylmaleimide, NEM; left) and reducing conditions (10 mM dithiothreitol, DTT; right). The gel was stained with silver and scanned on a LKB Ultroscan Laserdensitometer. Gel lanes were subsequently cut into 2-mm slices, and the radioactivity was determined by liquid scintillation counting. Shown are the results from the top of the gel (slice number 1) to the 100-kDa region (slice 20). Incorporated radioactivity in the absence (open columns) and presence (hatched columns) of 3 μM (−)desmethoxyverapamil (top) is shown in comparison with the densitometric scan (bottom). Note that the photolabeled band (α$_1$ polypeptide) does not show a change in mobility and that the 165-kDa polypeptide (α$_2$ polypeptide) migrates as a 135-kDa band after reduction. [From Striessnig *et al.* (1987), *FEBS Lett.* **212,** 247–253, with permission.]

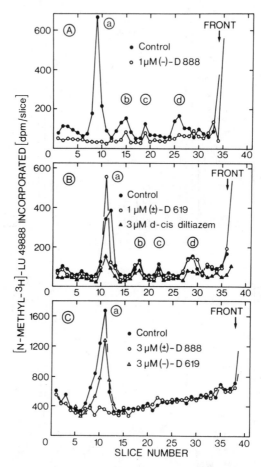

FIG. 37. Photolabeling of the phenylalkylamine receptor. Photoaffinity labeling of the membrane-bound (A, B) and purified calcium channel (C) from guinea pig skeletal muscle with (*N-methyl-*³H]LU 49888. [*N-methyl-*³H]LU 49888 (2.42 n*M*) was incubated with 0.62 mg of membrane protein for 45 minutes at 25°C. (A) 4.3 pmol was reversibly bound in the absence and 0.27 pmol in the presence of (−)desmethoxyverapamil prior to irradiation. (B) 3.9 pmol was reversibly bound in the absence of added drug, 3.8 pmol in the presence of 1 μ*M* (±)D 619, and 1.1 pmol in the absence of 3 μ*M* (+)-*cis*-diltiazem prior to irradiation. (+)D-619 has very low affinity for the phenylalkylamine receptor in reversible binding experiments and does not block photolabeling. (C) [*N-methyl-*³H]LU 49888 (17.8 n*M*) was incubated with 4.7 μg of purified calcium channel protein for 45 minutes at 25°C and irradiated with ultraviolet light. 2.6 pmol was specifically bound in the absence of added drug, 0.57 pmol in the presence of 3 μ*M* (−)desmethoxyverapamil, and 2.1 pmol in the presence of 3 μ*M* (±)D 619 prior to irradiation. [From Striessnig *et al.* (1987), *FEBS Lett.* **212,** 247–253, with permission.]

band, but only [N-methyl-³H]LU 49888 was incorporated into an additional 265-kDa polypeptide. Incorporation of [N-methyl-³H]LU 49888 into both bands occurred with a pharmacological profile typical of calcium channels and could be clearly distinguished from the labeling of calcium channel-unrelated low affinity binding sites (95, 60, and 35 kDa) (Striessnig et al., 1988b). It remains open whether the 265-kDa protein represents a calcium channel-related structure. One of the ω-CgTx-photolabeled polypeptides has virtually the same size in SDS–PAGE, which is an interesting result (see Section IV,E).

[N-methyl-³H]LU 49888 has also been used to characterize a neuronal high affinity binding site for phenylalkylamines in *Drosophila* head membranes. Unlike the phenylalkylamine receptors associated with L-type calcium channels, these binding sites are not allosterically coupled to 1,4-dihydropyridine receptors, and the affinity for tritiated phenylalkylamines is nearly an order of magnitude higher. The K_D values obtained for (−)-[³H]desmethoxyverapamil, (±)-[³H]verapamil, and [N-methyl-³H]LU 49888 were around 0.5 nM (Pauron et al., 1987; D. A. Greenberg et al., personal communication). In contrast to Pauron et al. (1987), Greenberg et al. also reported the presence of a low affinity binding site in *Drosophila* head membranes. The evidence for the presence of a low affinity binding site was as follows. First, [N-methyl-³H]LU 49888 binding was inhibited by the enantiomers of desmethoxyverapamil, methoxyverapamil, and verapamil with Hill slopes significantly smaller than unity. Second, two different time constants for dissociation of the [N-methyl-³H]LU 49888–binding site complex were determined in kinetic experiments (at 25°C, half lives were 0.5 and 20 minutes for the fast and slow component, respectively). Third, in a photoaffinity labeling experiments two polypeptides with apparent molecular masses of 120–130 kDa and 20–30 kDa were labeled by [N-methyl-³H]LU 49888. (−)Verapamil or (−)desmethoxyverapamil (10 nM) prevented incorporation into the large but not into the band representing the smaller polypeptide. When the concentration of the nonlabeled drugs was increased to 1 μM, incorporation into both bands was completely blocked. Furthermore, photolabeling of the 20- to 30-kDa polypeptide did not occur when the membranes were washed prior to irradiation in order to remove unbound [N-methyl-³H]LU 49888.

These experiments suggest that the low affinity binding site is localized on the 20- to 30-kDa polypeptide whereas the high affinity binding site is associated with the 120- to 130-kDa band, in accordance with the results of Pauron et al. (1987). However, in contrast to Pauron et al., Greenberg et al. (personal communication) could not confirm the extremely high eudismic ratios for the optical enantiomers of des-methoxyverapamil and verapamil in binding inhibition experiments. Although Ca^{2+} currents have been described in *Drosophila* flight muscle and embryonic neuronal cell cultures (Salkoff and Wyman, 1983) the physiological significance of these binding sites for phenylalkylamines is not yet known. If these sites were shown to be on calcium channels, this would strongly argue against the hypothesis that (+)-*cis*-diltiazem binds to the same receptor domain as verapamil, as has been claimed for, e.g., the skeletal muscle channel (Galizzi *et al.*, 1986b). The IC_{50} values for competition of (+)- and (−)-*cis*-diltiazem with the phenylalkylamine high affinity site in *Drosophila* head membranes are three orders of magnitude higher than for phenylalkylamines (Pauron *et al.*, 1987).

In summary, a high affinity arylazide phenylalkylamine allowed the unequivocal identification of the α_1 subunit as the receptor-carrying polypeptide in the purified skeletal muscle calcium channel preparation. Thus, both 1,4-dihydropyridine and phenylakylamine receptors are located on the same polypeptide chain in skeletal muscle and presumably in heart and brain. The discovery of a high affinity phenylalkylamine site in *Drosophila* head membranes is exciting. Further proof is required, however, for this site to be classified as a calcium channel-associated receptor.

B. PURIFICATION OF CALCIUM CHANNELS

Radioligand binding studies with high affinity ligands for the 1,4-dihydropyridine, phenylalkylamine, and benzothiazepine receptors allowed the identification of drug-sensitive calcium channels in several tissues (e.g., brain, skeletal muscle, smooth muscle, and cardiac muscle) with high sensitivity and a typical calcium channel pharmacological profile. Target size, photoaffinity labeling experiments, and basic biophysical and biochemical properties of the membrane-bound Ca^{2+} antagonist receptors were described (Glossmann and Ferry, 1985; Glossmann *et al.*, 1985a–c). These particular properties are very helpful in distinguishing calcium channel-related receptors from binding sites unrelated to calcium channels (see Section VII,A). Further investigation of the biophysics and biochemistry of calcium channel function and regulation (e.g., by phosphorylation) required purification.

Purification allowed cloning of the 1,4-dihydropyridine receptor gene and prediction of its amino acid sequence. Such analysis revealed structural and sequence similarities with the voltage-dependent sodium channel (Tanabe *et al.*, 1987). Purification, photoaffinity labeling, immunological, and reconstitution studies led to increased knowledge of the subunit structure of 1,4-dihydropyridine-sensitive calcium channels in different tissues. A critical overview is given in the following sections of this article.

1. *Skeletal Muscle*

a. *Solubilization of Calcium Channel-Related Drug Receptors.* Calcium channels from mammalian skeletal muscle T-tubule membranes contain the highest density of calcium antagonist receptors (Table XX) (Ferry and Glossmann, 1982b; Glossmann *et al.*, 1983b, 1982b; Fosset *et al.*, 1983; Glossmann and Ferry, 1985); thus, skeletal muscle T-tubule membranes are the most attractive source for channel purification. Table XXI shows the purification of guinea pig T-tubule membranes from skeletal muscle homogenates. After a simple differential centrifugation, which leads to a crude microsomal fraction (density of 1,4-dihydropyridine sites of >20 pmol/mg protein, measured under optimal conditions), a discontinuous sucrose gradient enriches in (the floating) fraction 4 T-tubule fragments. As can be seen the three directly measured calcium channel drug receptors copurify with the Na^+,K^+-ATPase (digitalis glycoside) binding site and the β-adrenoceptors. The sodium pump activity and adenylate cyclase activity coupled to β-adrenoceptors were first described by Brandt *et al.* (1980) and Caswell *et al.* (1978). With few exceptions the microsomal membrane preparation and not the purified T-tubule preparation has been used for solubilization and purification of the channel. The reasons are several. One is the ease by which the microsomal preparation can be isolated, the other may be that the more extensive the membrane preparation is the more degraded the receptor-carrying subunit of the channel becomes.

The first successful studies on solubilization and partial purification of 1,4-dihydropyridine receptors from guinea pig (Glossmann and Ferry, 1983b) and rabbit skeletal muscle (Kirley and Schwartz, 1984; Borsotto *et al.*, 1984b) employed the racemic 1,4-dihydropyridines [³H]nimodipine or [³H]nitrendipine as reversible labels. Solubilization was achieved with the detergents CHAPS [3-[(3-cholamidopropyl)dimethylammonio]-1-propanesulfonate] (10 or 16 mM), digitonin (0.25%), or deoxycholate. CHAPS- and digitonin-solubilized receptors showed reversible binding characteristics very similar to the membrane-bound receptor (Glossmann and Ferry, 1983b), whereas high nonspecific binding of radioligand was observed on solubilization with deoxycholate. It was shown (first by indirect drug competition studies) that the distinct receptors for calcium channel-active drugs were solubilized and that allosteric interactions described for particulate channels, albeit altered, were preserved.

TABLE XX

DENSITIES OF CALCIUM CHANNEL DRUG BINDING SITES IN SKELETAL MUSCLE PREPARATIONS

Receptor	Membrane	Species	Ligand	B_{max} (pmol/mg)	K_D (nM)	T	Ref.[a]
1,4-Dihydropyridine	Microsomal	Guinea pig	(±)-[^{3}H]Nimodipine	14.3 with (+)-cis-diltiazem	1.5; 1.0 with (+)-cis-diltiazem	37°C	a
	T-tubule	Guinea pig	(±)-[^{3}H]Nimodipine	35–60 with (+)-cis-diltiazem	1.5; 1.0 with (+)-cis-diltiazem	37°C	b
	Microsomal	Guinea pig	(±)-[^{3}H]PN 200-110	26 with (+)-cis-diltiazem	1.4	37°C	c
	Microsomal	Guinea pig	(±)-[^{3}H]PN 200-110	25.4	1.48	37°C	d
	T-tubule	Rabbit	(±)-[^{3}H]Nitrendipine	50.0	1.8	10°C	e
	T-tubule	Frog	(±)-[^{3}H]Nitrendipine	20.0	0.5	10°C	e
	Microsomal	Frog	(±)-[^{3}H]Azidopine	4.5	0.35		f
		Rabbit	(±)-[^{3}H]Azidopine	28.8	0.99	25°C	
		Chicken	(±)-[^{3}H]Azidopine	13	0.97		
		Guinea pig	(±)-[^{3}H]Azidopine	24	0.35		
	T-tubule	Rat	(±)-[^{3}H]PN 200-110	41	0.22	10°C	g
	T-tubule	Rabbit	(±)-[^{3}H]PN 200-110	85	0.2	10°C	h

	Preparation	Species	Ligand			Temp	Ref
	Microsomal	Rabbit	(+)-[³H]PN 200-110	15	0.2	4°C	i
		Chicken	(+)-[³H]PN 200-110	5	n.d.		
		Frog	(+)-[³H]PN 200-110	10	n.d.		
	T-tubule	Frog	(±)-[³H]Bay K 8644	2.2	1.8	20°C	j
Phenylalkylamine	Microsomal	Guinea pig	(±)-[³H]Verapamil	37	45	2°C	k
	Microsomal	Guinea pig	(−)-[³H]Desmethoxyverapamil	18	2.2	25°C	l
	T-tubule	Rabbit	(−)-[³H]Desmethoxyverapamil	70	1.5	10°C	m
	T-tubule	Rabbit	(±)-[³H]Bepridil	75	20	10°C	m
	T-tubule	Rabbit	(±)-[³H]Verapamil	50	27	10°C	n
Benzothiazepine	Microsomal	Guinea pig	(+)-cis-[³H]Diltiazem	11	39	2°C	o
	T-tubule	Rabbit	(+)-cis-[³H]Diltiazem	50	50	10°C	m
Others	T-tubule	Rabbit	[³H]Fluspirilene	80	0.1	25°C	p

[a] Key to references: a, Glossmann and Ferry (1982), *FEBS Lett.* **148**, 331–337; b, Glossmann et al. (1983b), *Naunyn–Schmiedeberg's Arch.* **323**, 1–11; c, Goll et al. (1983a), *FEBS Lett.* **157**, 63–69; d, Ferry et al. (1983a), *Nauyn-Schmiedeberg's Arch.* **323**, 276–277; e, Fosset et al. (1983), *J. Biol. Chem.* **258**, 6086–6092; f, Ferry et al. (1985b), *EMBO J.* **4**, 1933–1940; g, Cognard et al. (1986a), *Proc. Natl. Acad. Sci. U.S.A.* **83**, 1518–1522; h, Borsotto et al. (1984a), *Biochem. Biophys. Res. Commun.* **122**, 1357–1366; i, Borsotto et al. (1985), *J. Biol. Chem.* **260**, 14255–14263; j, Ildefonse et al. (1986), *Biochem. Biophys. Res. Commun.* **129**, 904–909; k, Goll et al. (1984b), *Eur. J. Biochem.* **141**, 177–186; l, Goll et al. (1984a), *FEBS Lett. B176*, 371–377; m, Galizzi et al. (1986b), *J. Biol. Chem.* **261**, 1393–1397; n, Galizzi et al. (1984b), *Biochem. Biophys. Res. Commun.* **118**, 239–245; o, Glossmann et al. (1983a), *FEBS Lett.* **160**, 226–232; p, Galizzi et al. (1986a), *Proc. Natl. Acad. Sci. U.S.A.* **83**, 7513–7517.

TABLE XXI

PURIFICATION OF T-TUBULE MEMBRANES FROM GUINEA PIG HIND LIMB SKELETAL MUSCLE[a]

	Calcium channel labels										Na+, K+, ATPase label: [3H]ouabain		β-Adreno-ceptor: (−)-[3H]di-hydroal-prenolol	
	Receptor site 1				Receptor site 2: (−)-[3H]Des-methoxy-verapamil		Receptor site 3: (+)-cis-[3H]diltiazem							
	(+)-[3H]PN 200-110		[3H]Nimo-dipine											
	Abs	Rel	Abs	Rel	Abs	Rel	Abs	Rel	Abs	Rel	Abs	Rel
Homogenate	1,440	1	460	1	700	1	91.5	1	109	1	12.9	
3,500 g pellet	2,557	1.8	831	1.8	1,149	1.64	144.4	1.6	364	3.3	34.0	
3,500 g supernatant	525	0.36	149	0.3	250	0.36	23	0.25	0	0	10.8	
45,000 g pellet	10,145	7.05	2,800	6.1	5,275	7.5	671	7.3	708	65	31	
45,000 g supernatant	21	0.01	27	0.05	391	0.6	24.9	0.27	427	3.9	2.8	
Sucrose gradient												
Fraction 1	12,278	8.5	3,564	7.7	7,063	10.0	1,099	12	759	6.9	76.8	
Fraction 2	15,971	11.0	3,418	7.4	7,352	10.5	1,026	11.2	717	6.5	125	
Fraction 3	5,069	3.5	1,394	3.03	2,197	3.0	318	3.5	1,011	9.28	93	
Fraction 4	32,500	22.5	7,868	17.1	12,973	18.0	2,124	23.2	2,079	19.1	189	

[a] The following radioligands were employed: [3H]ouabain (37.0 Ci/mmol at 49 nM), [3H]nimodipine (150 Ci/mmol at 2.9 nM), (+)-[3H]PN 200-110 (75 Ci/mmol at 4.8 nM), (+)-cis-[3H]diltiazem (83 Ci/mmol at 7.1 nM), (−)-[3H]dihydroalprenolol (102 Ci/mmol at 2.05 nM), and (−)-[3H]desmethoxyverapamil (83 Ci/mmol at 2.19 nM). Fraction 4 consists mainly of T-tubule membranes. Abs, Specific binding in fmol/mg protein; Rel, relative specific binding with respect to homogenate (=1). From Glossmann et al. (1985b), J. Cardiovasc. Pharmacol. 7, S20–S30, with permission.

The glycoprotein nature of the channel-associated proteins was discovered and conditions for effective absorption and biospecific elution from lectin affinity gels were described by Glossmann and Ferry (1983b). Seventeenfold purification of the CHAPS-solubilized 1,4-dihydropyridine receptor on concanavalin A–Sepharose was achieved. Sucrose gradient centrifugation allowed 2.5- (Borsotto *et al.*, 1984b) to 10-fold purification (Glossmann and Ferry, 1983b) and revealed a $s_{w,20}$ value of 13 S for the CHAPS–receptor complex. Binding activity of the solubilized material was stable at 4°C with a half-life greater than 60 hours in digitonin or CHAPS without the addition of exogenous lipids for stabilization. It was highly sensitive to α-chymotrypsin and phospholipases A and C and was immediately inactivated at higher temperatures, indicating lability of the structure (Glossmann and Ferry, 1983b).

b. *Ca²⁺-Antagonist Receptor Purification.* Several groups reported successful purification of the calcium channel drug receptors from rabbit or guinea pig skeletal muscle, using either CHAPS or digitonin for solubilization. A comparison of the basic findings is given in Table XXII. Curtis and Catterall (1984) claimed 330-fold purification employing a four-step purification procedure on WGA–Sepharose (30-fold), DEAE–Sepharose (4.2-fold), a second WGA–Sepharose (1.7-fold), and final sucrose gradient centrifugation (1.6-fold). In contrast to the CHAPS-solubilized receptor, [³H]nitrendipine binding activity migrated with a $s_{20,w}$ value of 20 S in the sucrose gradient. Nearly identical results were obtained by extensive hydrodynamic studies on cardiac receptors solubilized with these two detergents (Horne *et al.*, 1986; vide infra). A complete loss of binding activity was observed after solubilization. Therefore the approach was modified to solubilize after prelabeling with [³H]nitrendipine or later (+)-[³H]PN 200-110 in membranes. The receptor recovery was corrected for dissociated ligand after each purification step. As postlabeling of the purified receptor was impossible, no information could be obtained concerning its equilibrium binding characteristics and allosteric interactions with phenylalkylamines and benzothiazepines. Most importantly, this preparation did not allow photoaffinity labeling of the purified preparation.

After nonreducing SDS–PAGE (20 mM N-ethylmaleimide in the sample buffer) three major polypeptides with apparent molecular weights of 160,000, 53,000, and 32,000 (termed α, β, and γ "subunits") comigrated with [³H]nitrendipine binding activity in the sucrose gradient. Under reducing conditions, however. SDS–PAGE (20 mM dithiothreitol in the sample buffer) showed some microheterogeneity in the α subunit; an additional band could be identified in the high molecular weight region with an apparent molecular weight of 135,000.

TABLE XXII
Purification of Calcium Channels[a]

Species (tissue)	Detergent	Procedure	Purification (-fold)	Purified polypeptides (kDa)	Label	Pharmacological characterization	Phosphorylation substrate (kDa)	Photoaffinity labeling (kDa)	Antibodies (kDa)	Ref.[b]
Rabbit (skeletal muscle)	Digitonin	WGA, DEAE, WGA, SUC	330	R: 160, 135, 50, 33; NR: 160, 50, 33	PN, NTD	Not shown	160, 50	Not shown	Not shown	a
Rabbit (skeletal muscle)	CHAPS	DEAE, WGA, SEC	80	R: 142, 33, 32; NR: not shown	PN	Not shown	142	(170 in membranes)	Against 142 and 32	b
Guinea pig (skeletal muscle)	Digitonin	WGA, SUC	150	R: 155, 135, 65, 32; NR: 155, 65, 32	PN, AZD, DMV, LU	1,4-DHP, PA receptor	155	1,4-DHP and PA receptor (155)	Against 155 + 135	c
Rabbit (skeletal muscle)	Digitonin	WGA, DEAE, WGA, SUC	>200	R: 142, 122, 56, 31, 26, 22; NR: 142, 56, 31	PN	1,4-DHP receptor	142, 56	1,4-DHP receptor	Not shown	d
Rabbit (skeletal muscle)	Digitonin	WGA, SUC	—	R: 200, 143, 61, 33; NR: 220, 200, 61, 33	PN	Not shown	Not shown	Not shown	Against 200	e
Rabbit (skeletal muscle)	Digitonin	WGA, DEAE	—	R: 170, 150, 52, 32; NR: 175, 170, 52, 32	PN, AZD	Not shown	170, 52	1,4-DHP receptor (170)	Against 170	f

Rabbit (skeletal muscle)	Digitonin			R: 175, 143, 54, 30, 24–27; NR: 167, 54, 30	PN, AZD	Not shown	175	1,4-DHP receptor (175)	Against 175	g
Rabbit and guinea pig (skeletal muscle)	Digitonin	ᵛ GA, SUC; WGA, DEAE, WGA, SUC	150	R: 155–170, 135–150, 50–65, 30–35; NR: 160–190, 155–170, 50–65, 30–35	PN, AZD, DMV, LU	1,4-DHP, PA receptor	Not shown	1,4-DHP and PA receptor (155–170)	Not shown	h
Chicken (heart)	Digitonin	DEAE, Con A, WGA	900	R: 140	PN	Not shown	Not shown	Not shown	Against 140	i
Cow (heart)	Digitonin	Immunoprecipitation	—	R: 141; NR: 170	PN	Not shown	Not shown	Not shown	Against 170/141	j

[a] Abbreviations: AZD, (−)-[³H]azidopine; DMV, (−)-[³H]desmethoxyverapamil; LU, [*N-methyl*-³H]LU 49888; NTD, (±)-[³H]nitrendipine; PN, (+)-[³H]PN 200-110; R, reducing conditions; NR, nonreducing conditions; Con A, concanaval in A affinity chromatography; WGA, wheat germ agglutinin affinity chromatography; DEAE, DEAE ion-exchange chromatography; SEC, size exclusion chromatography; SUC, sucrose density gradient centrifugation; CHAPS, 3-[(3-cholamidopropyl)dimethylammonio]-1-propanesulfonate; 1,4-DHP, 1,4-dihydropyridine; PA, phenylalkylamine.

[b] Key to references: a, Curtis and Catterall (1984), *Biochemistry* **23**, 2113–2117, Curtis and Catterall (1985), *Proc. Natl. Acad. Sci. U.S.A.* **82**, 2528–2532; b, Borsotto *et al.* (1984a), *Biochem. Biophys. Res. Commun.* **122**, 1357–1366, Borsotto *et al.* (1985), *J. Biol. Chem.* **260**, 14255–14263, Galizzi *et al.* (1986b), *J. Biol. Chem.* **261**, 1393–1397; c, Striessnig *et al.* (1986a), *Eur. J. Biochem.* **161**, 603–609, Striessnig *et al.* (1987), *FEBS Lett.* **212**, 247–253, Glossmann *et al.* (1987), *Circ. Res.* **61**, I30–I36, Hymel *et al.* (1988), *Proc. Natl. Acad. Sci. U.S.A.* Glossmann *et al.* (1987), *Biomed. Biochim. Acta* **46**, S351–S356; d, Flockerzi *et al.* (1986a), *Nature (London)* **323**, 66–68, Flockerzi *et al.* (1986b), *Eur. J. Biochem.* **161**, 217–224, Sieber *et al.* (1987), *Eur. J. Biochem.* **167**, 117–122; e, Morton and Fröhner (1987), *J. Biol. Chem.* **262**, 11904–11907; f, Leung *et al.* (1987), *J. Biol. Chem.* **262**, 7943–7945; g, Takahashi *et al.* (1987), *Proc. Natl. Acad. Sci. U.S.A.* **84**, 5478–5482; h, Vaghy *et al.* (1987b), *J. Biol. Chem.* **262**, 14337–14342; i, Cooper *et al.* (1987), *J. Biol. Chem.* **262**, 509–512; j, Takahashi and Catterall (1987a), *Biochemistry* **26**, 5518–5526.

Together all three subunits comprised approximately 60% of the total silver stain intensity. Assuming a molecular weight of 210,000 for the 1,4-dihydropyridine receptor (and binding of 1 mol of dihydropyridine to 1 mol of receptor) one could estimate purity of 41–43% for this preparation (maximal specific activity assumed to be 2100 pmol/mg protein). The so-called β subunit was only a minor component when highly purified T-tubules were used as the starting material instead of rapidly prepared skeletal muscle microsomes (Glossmann and Ferry, 1982b; Ferry and Glossmann, 1983b). This was attributed to proteolysis of this polypeptide during T-tubule preparation even though protease inhibitors were used. However, it remained unclear which of the polypeptides carried the respective drug receptors and whether all three subunits are necessary for channel function.

Borsotto et al. (1985) did not find a β subunit after purification of channel drug receptors from rabbit skeletal muscle solubilized with CHAPS. Their procedure was much more complicated and time consuming so that proteolytic degradation of purified proteins may have been a factor. Although reversible binding activity was preserved after solubilization with CHAPS (Glossmann and Ferry, 1983b; Borsotto et al., 1984a, 1985), there was a loss of binding activity as determined with the convenient polyethylene glycol precipitation assay (Glossmann and Ferry, 1985) after one or more purification steps with this detergent (Borsotto et al., 1984a, 1985; Curtis and Catterall, 1986; H. Glossmann et al., unpublished results). A more complicated procedure for separation of bound and free ligand (column filtration) thus was required (Borsotto et al., 1985), precluding detailed pharmacological characterization. No ligand other than (+)-[^{3}H]PN 200-110 was used. Although methods were not detailed, reversible postlabeling of the 1,4-dihydropyridine receptor was apparently performed with (+)-[^{3}H]PN 200-110 throughout the purification. The increase in specific activity, determined from saturation analysis data, was approximately 80-fold. The affinity of (+)-[^{3}H]PN 200-110 for its receptor decreased from a K_D of 0.2 nM in the starting material to a K_D of 1.8 nM in the purified material. Disadvantages of this purification procedure were its duration (>20 hours) and the fact that high concentrations of detergent (~16 mM) were required to elute receptor activity from WGA–Sepharose, thereby inactivating a considerable amount of binding activity (Borsotto et al., 1984a, 1985).

The polypeptide pattern of the purified preparation revealed 142-, 33-, and 32-kDa bands under reducing conditions of SDS–PAGE (Borsotto et al., 1985). The 142-kDa band was found later to be covalently linked to the 30-kDa polypeptide via disulfide bonds (Schmid et al.,

1986a) and migrates with an apparent molecular weight of 170,000 under nonreducing conditions in polyacrylamide gradient gels. The 142-kDa polypeptide was phosphorylated (vide infra) by Ca^{2+}–calmodulin-dependent and cAMP-dependent protein kinases (Hosey et al., 1986). There is no direct evidence that these three polypeptides can form functional calcium channels. The same authors, interestingly, showed photoaffinity labeling of a 170-kDa band in T-tubule membranes with (+)-[³H]PN 200-110, (+)-cis-[³H]diltiazem, and [³H]bepridil after separation under reducing conditions of SDS–PAGE. Thus there is an apparent discrepancy of 30 kDa between the size of the membrane-bound (170 kDa) and purified (142 kDa) 1,4-dihydropyridine receptor.

This discrepancy can now be explained by the fact that two polypeptides (α_1 and α_2) of similar molecular weight comprise the so-called α subunit, which also provides an explanation for the microheterogeneity reported earlier by Curtis and Catterall (1984). Separation of these polypeptides under nonreducing conditions is not always successful. Better resolution can be achieved under reducing conditions (Flockerzi et al., 1986; Glossmann et al., 1987; Striessnig et al., 1987) as one of the two polypeptides (α_2) undergoes a change in molecular weight on reduction (Glossmann et al., 1987; Takahashi et al., 1987; Vaghy et al., 1987b). This is due to disulfide-linked 25- to 35-kDa polypeptides which are released on reduction (Schmid et al., 1986a,b). Several laboratories have confirmed this "subunit" composition, which is summarized in Table XXIII.

c. *Reversible Binding Characteristics of Purified Calcium Channels.* Photoaffinity labeling of the purified channel (see Section VII,A) is a direct method to identify polypeptide components of L-type calcium channels. As outlined above, reversible binding with the purified calcium channel preparation proved to be difficult (Borsotto et al., 1985) or impossible (Curtis and Catterall, 1984), precluding valid photoaffinity labeling. Striessnig et al. (1986b) described 150-fold purification of the calcium channel from guinea pig skeletal muscle with a rapid two-step procedure (affinity chromatography on WGA–Sepharose and subsequent sucrose gradient centrifugation) that allows reversible labeling of the 1,4-dihydropyridine as well as the phenylalkylamine receptor. Complete pharmacological characterization of the purified receptors was possible using (+)-[³H]PN 200-110, (−)-[³H]azidopine, (−)-[³H]desmethoxyverapamil, or [N-methyl-³H]-LU 49888 as reversible labels (Striessnig et al., 1986a,b, 1987).

Examples of the reversible binding of (−)-[³H]desmethoxyverapamil and (+)-[³H]PN 200-110 are shown in Figs. 38 and 39. It was shown

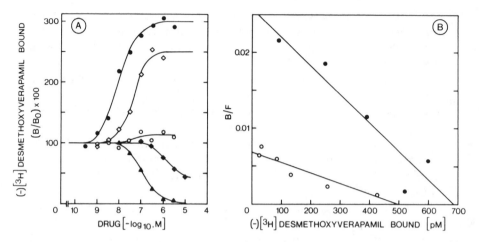

FIG. 38. Equilibrium binding properties of purified calcium channel from guinea pig skeletal muscle, labeled at the phenylalkylamine-selective receptor. (A) Stereospecific regulation of $(-)$-[^{3}H]desmethoxyverapamil binding by the enantiomers of PN 200-110 and 202-791. The competitive inhibition by unlabeled $(-)$desmethoxyverapamil is also illustrated. $(-)$-[^{3}H]Desmethoxyverapamil (6–10 nM) was incubated with 0.3–0.6 μg purified channel protein for 60 minutes at 25°C. Points are means from at least two to three experiments. IC$_{50}$ (or EC$_{50}$) values and apparent Hill slopes (n_H) ± asymptotic SD are as follows: (●) (+)PN 200-110, EC$_{50}$ = 7.0 ± 1.9 nM, n_H = 0.95 ± 0.23, maximal stimulation 201 ± 9%; (○) $(-)$PN 200-110, 10% stimulation at 3 μM; (◇) (R) 202-791, EC$_{50}$ = 44 ± 8 nM, n_H = 1.4 ± 0.3, maximal stimulation 151 ± 8%; (◆) (S) 202-791, EC$_{50}$ = 1.46 ± 0.48 μM, n_H = 1.5 ± 0.6, 58.1% maximal inhibition at 10 μM; (▲) $(-)$desmethoxyverapamil, EC$_{50}$ = 99 ± 18 nM, n_H = 1.01 ± 0.17, maximal inhibition 100%. (B) Mechanism of stimulation of $(-)$-[^{3}H]desmethoxyverapamil binding by (+)PN 200–110. Saturation experiments were performed with and without 1 μM (+)PN 200-110 in the incubation mixture. Scatchard transformation of the data of one typical experiment is shown. Best fits were obtained with the following parameter estimates: control (○), K_D = 73.7 ± 10 nM, B_{max} = 490.7 ± 42 pM; (+)PN 200-110 present (●), K_D = 26.4 ± 5.6 nM, B_{max} = 682 ± 51 pM. Note that the purified calcium channel discriminates between agonistic and antagonistic 1,4-dihydropyridines: agonists inhibit allosterically, and antagonists stimulate phenylalkylamine binding to the channel. [From Striessnig et al. (1986b), FEBS Lett. 197, 204–210, with permission.]

that the allosteric coupling of drug receptors was preserved throughout purification and was highly stereoselective. (+)-cis-Diltiazem, which stimulates the binding of 1,4-dihydropyridines to the membrane-bound channel in several tissues (Glossmann and Ferry, 1985), is required for maximal labeling of the solubilized and purified channel by (+)-[^{3}H]PN 200-110 or $(-)$-[^{3}H]azidopine. Interestingly, the extent of binding stimulation by (+)-cis-diltiazem increases on purification and is effected mainly via increasing the number of binding sites

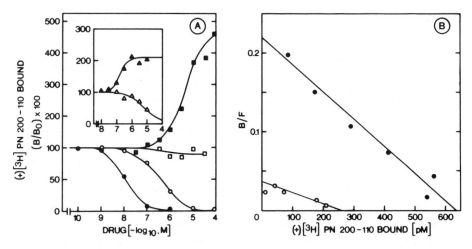

FIG. 39. Equilibrium binding properties of purified calcium channel from guinea pig skeletal muscle labeled at the 1,4-dihydropyridine-selective receptor with $(+)$-[^{3}H]PN 200-110. (A) Stereospecific regulation of $(+)$-[^{3}H]PN 200-110 binding by the disastereoisomers of diltiazem, the enantiomers of PN 200-110, and desmethoxyverapamil (inset). $(+)$-[^{3}H]PN 200-110 (2.0–3.5 nM) was incubated with 0.08–0.17 µg channel protein for 60 minutes at 20°C. B_0 is the specifically bound ligand in the absence, and B in the presence of unlabeled drug. IC_{50} (or EC_{50}) values and apparent Hill slopes (n_H) ± asymptotic SD are as follows: (●) $(+)$PN 200-110, IC_{50} = 12.3 ± 3.5 nM, n_H = 1.05 ± 0.1, maximal inhibition 100%; (○) $(-)$PN 200-110, IC_{50} = 434 ± 140 nM, n_H = 0.83 ± 0.20, maximal inhibition 100%; (■) $(+)$-cis-diltiazem, EC_{50} = 4.5 ± 1.7 µM, n_H = 1.0 ± 0.34, maximal stimulation 269 ± 40%; (□) $(-)$-cis-diltiazem, <10% inhibition at 10 µM; (▲) $(-)$desmethoxyverapamil, EC_{50} = 187 ± 113 nM, n_H = 2.2 ± 0.21, maximal stimulation 110 ± 16%; (△ $(+)$desmethoxyverapamil, 56% inhibition at 10 µM). (B) Saturation analysis of equilibrium binding in the absence or presence of $(+)$-cis-diltiazem. $(+)$-[^{3}H]PN 200-110 (0.4–30 nM) was incubated with 0.105 µg channel protein for 60 minutes at 25°C with (●) and without (○) 100 µM $(+)$-cis-diltiazem in the incubation mixture. Scatchard transformation of the data is shown. The following parameter estimates represent the best fit of the specific binding data to a monophasic saturation isotherm: $(+)$-cis-diltiazem absent, K_D = 7.2 ± 1.1 nM, B_{max} = 264.7 ± 14 pM (equivalent to 627 ± 33 pmol/mg protein); $(+)$-cis-diltiazem present, K_D = 2.87 ± 0.5 nM, B_{max} = 630 ± 35 pM (equivalent to 1500 ± 83 pmol/mg protein). [From Striessnig et al. (1986b), FEBS Lett. 197, 204–210, with permission.]

for 1,4-dihydropyridines rather than decreasing the dissociation constant. In contrast to the membrane-bound receptor, binding of $(-)$-[^{3}H]desmethoxyverapamil to the purified phenylalkylamine receptor is enhanced by antagonistic 1,4-dihydropyridines, [e.g., $(-)$ 202-791, $(+)$ Bay K 8644] and inhibited by their optical antipodes [i.e., agonistic 1,4-dihydropyridines, $(+)$ 202-791, $(-)$ Bay K 8644]. Thus $(-)$-[^{3}H]desmethoxyverapamil binding to the purified channel can be used as an *in vitro* test to determine "agonistic" or "antagonistic" properties of 1,4-dihydropyridines.

   d. Subunit Characterization with Photoaffinity Labeling, Phosphorylation, and Immunochemical Studies. $(-)$-[^{3}H]Azidopine and [*N-methyl*-^{3}H]LU 49888 are two highly potent photoaffinity ligands that selectively label 1,4-dihydropyridine and phenylalkylamine receptors in guinea pig and rabbit T-tubule membranes (see Section VII,A,3). Their reversible interactions with the purified channel were investigated (Striessnig *et al.*, 1986; Vaghy *et al.*, 1987b). Therefore these ligands are highly suitable photoaffinity labels for their respective receptors in the purification process. Studies with $(-)$-[^{3}H]azidopine first revealed that the large (α) subunit (see Curtis and Catterall, 1984) of the purified calcium channel preparation rather than the smaller subunits carried the 1,4-dihydropyridine binding domain (see Section VII,A,3). Resolution of the α polypeptide region (Figs. 36 and 40) into α_1 and α_2 later allowed the unequivocal identification of α_1 as the carrier of the calcium channel drug receptors (Glossmann *et al.*, 1987; Striessnig *et al.*, 1987; Vaghy *et al.*, 1987b).

   Thereafter several laboratories employed photoaffinity ligands for subunit characterization and confirmed the existence of two distinct α subunits (Sieber *et al.*, 1987; Sharp *et al.*, 1987; Takahashi *et al.*, 1987; Tanabe *et al.*, 1987). Takahashi *et al.* (1987) used a hydrophobic probe, [^{125}I]TID [3-(trifluoromethyl)-3-(*m*-iodophenyl)diazirine], to evaluate transmembrane domains. This photoreactive compound partitions into the detergent associated with major hydrophobic regions of solubilized integral membrane proteins and is irreversibly incorporated into these regions after photolysis. The α_1 and γ subunits were prominently labeled whereas α_2 showed only one-tenth of the α_1 labeling. The β subunit was not labeled at all. These data suggest that only the α_1 and γ subunits are transmembrane polypeptides of the complex that constitutes the purified calcium channel drug receptor preparation in SDS–PAGE.

   α_1 and α_2 subunits seem to be present in similar stoichiometric amounts. α_2 is coupled to a 25- to 35-kDa polypeptide (Schmid *et al.*, 1986a,b; Takahashi *et al.*, 1987) via disulfide bonds and is heavily glycosylated. As binding of wheat germ agglutinin or concanavalin A to α_1 is weak (H. Glossmann and J. Striessnig, unpublished observations) or absent (Takahashi *et al.*, 1987), copurification of α_1, β, and γ subunits on lectin columns occurs via an apparently strong, noncovalent association with the α_2 polypeptide. Dissociation of the peptides can be achieved only by exposure of the complex to detergents like Triton X-100 or sodium dodecyl sulfate but not CHAPS or digitonin.

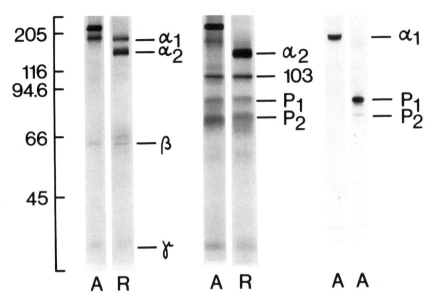

FIG. 40. The α_1 subunit of the purified calcium channel from skeletal muscle carries the 1,4-dihydropyridine receptor and is highly susceptible to proteolysis. Two silver-stained preparations of purified 1,4-dihydropyridine receptors (left, purified from fresh muscle, and middle, from previously frozen and thawed tissue) and a fluorogram (right) after SDS–PAGE are shown. A signifies alkylating conditions and R reducing conditions of electrophoresis. Note that for the frozen muscle preparation almost no intact α_1 is observed. α_1 does not change (see left-hand gels) its mobility under reducing conditions, whereas a large increase in mobility is observed for α_2. Two polypeptides above the so-called β subunit region are present in the frozen muscle preparation, termed P_1 and P_2. Although both purified 1,4-dihydropyridine–calcium channel preparations had a similar specific activity (~1.5 nmol of 1,4-dihydropyridine binding sites/mg protein), the fluorogram following $(-)$-[^{3}H]azidopine photoaffinity labeling reveals that only the fresh muscle receptors had an intact α_1 (left lane) whereas the frozen muscle calcium channel had none. P_1 and P_2 are labeled instead. Mobility of marker proteins (in kDa) is indicated.

Table XXIII summarizes the biochemical properties of the calcium channel polypeptides. It should be emphasized that only α_1 meets the criteria as a structural part of the L-type calcium channel: it carries the drug receptors, and its primary structure has striking similarities with the voltage-dependent sodium channel α subunit (Tanabe *et al.,* 1987). Moreover, it also is a major target for phosphorylation by protein kinase A (PKA), which regulates channel function in heart and skeletal muscle (see Sections III,C and VII,B). Earlier studies by Curtis and Catterall (1985) demonstrating phosphorylation of the (non-resolved) α and β subunits were recently confirmed (Hofmann *et al.,* 1987; Glossmann *et al.,* 1987; Hymel *et al.,* 1988b). The α_1 but not the

TABLE XXIII

SUBUNIT PROPERTIES OF PURIFIED SKELETAL MUSCLE CALCIUM CHANNEL PREPARATIONS[a]

Subunit	Molecular weight	Drug receptors	Glycoprotein	Phosphorylation	Proteolysis	Hydrophobic regions	Function
α_1	155,000–200,000 (R/NR)	DHP, PA, BT?	(+)	PKA +++, PKC +	Vaghy et al. (1987)	+++	Calcium channel?, voltage sensor?
α_2	165,000–175,000 (NR) 135,000–145,000 (R)	–	+	–	–	+	Unknown
β	55,000–65,000	–	–	PKA +, PKC +++	Curtis and Catterall (1984a)	–	Unknown
γ	30,000–35,000	–	+	–	–	+++	Unknown
δ	25,000–30,000	–	+	–	–	+	Disulfide linked to α_2

[a] Abbreviations: R and NR, SDS–PAGE under reducing and nonreducing conditions; DHP, 1,4-dihydropyridine receptor; PA, phenylalkylamine receptor; BT, benzothiazepine receptor; PKA and PKC, protein kinase A and C.

α_2 polypeptide was phosphorylated up to 0.7–1.8 mol phosphate per mole of 1,4-dihydropyridine receptor. Phosphorylation of the β subunit occurred with a slower time course (molar ratio of 1). In contrast, protein kinase C preferentially phosphorylated the β subunit (Hofmann et al., 1987). The physiological significance of this phosphorylation remains to be evaluated (see also Section III,C). Both α_1 and β subunits are also substrates for an intrinsic protein kinase in isolated triads (Imagawa et al., 1987a).

Experiments with polyclonal and monoclonal antibodies raised against *skeletal muscle* channel polypeptides emphasize that the two α subunits are distinct since they are immunologically unrelated. The two polypeptides have different amino-terminal amino acid sequences (α_1: Tanabe et al., 1987; Arnold Schwartz, personal communication; α_2: Nakayama et al., 1987). Antibodies against α_2 (Schmid et al., 1986a,b) were useful for the identification of its disulfide-linked 25- to 35-kDa component, which is only weakly stained by conventional silver stains. Immunoreactive polypeptides of similar size and electrophoretic behavior were found in immunoblots of brain, cardiac, and smooth muscle membrane proteins. In rabbit brain sections the distribution of α_2 immunoreactivity was similar to that of 1,4-dihydropyridine binding sites (Schmid et al., 1986b). This points to a structural association of α_2 with α_1 as shown for skeletal muscle. However, the conclusion drawn by the authors, namely, that the brain calcium channel drug receptors are localized on α_2, was misleading: recent photoaffinity labeling experiments have identified an α_1-like polypeptide (no change in the apparent molecular weight on reduction) in guinea pig hippocampus carrying the 1,4-dihydropyridine and phenylalkylamine receptors (Striessnig et al., 1988b).

Morton and Froehner (1987) used a monoclonal antibody for immunoaffinity purification of 1,4-dihydropyridine binding activity. Their purified preparation contained polypeptides with the properties of α_1, α_2, β, and γ. The antibody specifically recognized only one polypeptide in immunoblots namely, α_1. Assuming a functional role of the α_1 subunit, the effect of the antibody on channel function was tested using cultured muscle cells, BC3H1 myocytes. These cells express two types of calcium channels, corresponding to those found in skeletal muscle T-tubules: a fast-inactivating, low threshold, 1,4-dihydropyridine-insensitive channel and a slowly inactivating, high threshold, 1,4-dihydropyridine-sensitive channel (Morton and Froehner, 1987). Binding of the antibody to myocytes was associated with an attenuation of the high threshold Ca^{2+} current, whereas the fast current was unaffected. The inhibition was concentration dependent (50% inhibition of the maximum value of peak inward current at an antibody concentration of 60 nM) and did not occur with control antibodies. Sodium channels were also affected. Their activation threshold was shifted to more positive potentials, and the inactivation rate was slowed. This inhibition was explained by the structural similarity between the two channels (Tanabe *et al.*, 1987). These results further support the view that the α_1 subunit is the functionally important component of L-type calcium channels.

2. *Other Tissues*

The low density of calcium channels in nonskeletal muscle tissues makes purification from such sources more difficult. Only 100–980 fmol of (+)-[^{3}H]PN 200-110, [^{3}H]nimodipine, or (−)-[^{3}H]desmethoxy-verapamil receptor sites are labeled per milligram of protein in cardiac muscle membranes of several species (Bellemann *et al.*, 1981; Glossmann and Ferry, 1985; Ruth *et al.*, 1986; Rengasamy *et al.*, 1985; Goll *et al.*, 1986). Similarly low densities were found for 1,4-dihydropyridine and phenylalkylamine sites in smooth muscle and neuronal tissues (Bolger *et al.*, 1984; Glossmann *et al.*, 1985; Ferry *et al.*, 1985; Schmid *et al.*, 1986b). Assuming an identical molecular weight for the cardiac and skeletal muscle receptors, one projects that 3000-fold purification from other sources would be needed to approximate the 150-fold purification achieved from skeletal muscle T-tubules. Thus, purification can only be achieved employing efficient procedures with high receptor recovery for each step. Alternatively, membrane purification prior to solubilization must be much more extensive than for skeletal muscle. This has been achieved in some instances (Garcia *et al.*, 1986; Ehrlich *et al.*, 1986).

The hydrodynamic properties of the rat ventricular muscle 1,4-dihydropyridine receptor prelabeled with (+)-[^{3}H]PN 200-110 were investigated by Horne *et al.* (1986). The receptor was solubilized with a mixture of digitonin and Triton X-100; subsequently it was studied in several detergents (Tween 80, CHAPS, and digitonin). The stokes radius of the detergent–receptor complexes as determined by size exclusion chromatography was 8.6–8.7 nm, regardless of the detergent used for column equilibration. A Stokes radius of 7.1 nm was reported for the receptor–digitonin complex in skeletal muscle (Glossmann *et al.*, 1987c). In contrast the sedimentation coefficients measured were detergent dependent, being 12.4 in Tween 80, 15.4 in CHAPS, and 21 in digitonin. The values with CHAPS and digitonin are in close agreement with the data reported for the skeletal muscle channel (Glossmann *et al.*, 1983; Borsotto *et al.*, 1984b; Curtis and Catterall, 1984; Striessnig *et al.*, 1986a). Detergent exchange made it possible to determine the molecular weight of 370,000 for the detergent-free 1,4-dihydropyridine receptor–calcium channel complex.

Ruth *et al.* (1986) described the reversible labeling characteristics of the CHAPS (0.4%)-solubilized calcium channel from bovine cardiac sarcolemma. The affinity for [^{3}H]nimodipine and (−)-[^{3}H]desmethoxyverapamil (as in skeletal muscle) decreased on solubilization about 3- and 10-fold, respectively. The specific density was almost unaltered.

Rengasamy *et al.* (1985) reported the first attempt to purify the cardiac 1,4-dihydropyridine receptor–calcium channel complex prelabeled with (+)-[^{3}H]PN 200-110. They claimed 600-fold purification after chromatography of the digitonin-solubilized receptor on DEAE–, hexylamine–, and wheat germ agglutinin–Sepharose and subsequent sucrose gradient centrifugation. To determine the specific activities after each step the recovered receptor was corrected for dissociated ligand so that the true purification factors might be higher or lower than those calculated. In the silver-stained gels three polypeptides with apparent molecular weights of 60,000, 54,000, and 34,000 were enriched but no higher molecular weight polypeptide comigrated with (+)-[^{3}H]PN 200-110 binding activity. This is in contrast to photoaffinity labeling experiments which clearly show (−)-[^{3}H]azidopine bound to a 165 kDa polypeptide in heart membranes from several species, including chicken (see Section (VII,A).

In a more recent report the same authors (Cooper *et al.*, 1987) reported 900-fold purification of the 1,4-dihydropyridine receptor from chicken heart (see Table XXII). After chromatography of the digitonin-solubilized membranes on DEAE–, concanavalin A–, and wheat germ agglutinin–Sepharose, a single polypeptide with an apparent molecular weight of 170,000 (140,000 after reduction) was found on SDS–PAGE. No direct evidence was given that this band carries the calcium channel drug receptor sites. Their immunochemical analyses of skeletal muscle channels confirm that an α_2-like polypeptide not carrying drug receptors was preferentially isolated and characterized. Takahashi and Catterall (1987a,b) also characterized α_2-like polypeptides in heart and brain. Oeken and Schneider (1987) and Hofmann *et al.* (1987) reported a polypeptide composition for the heart calcium channel similar to that of skeletal muscle. A 180-kDa polypeptide was photolabeled by (±)-[^{3}H]azidopine and [*N-methyl*-^{3}H]LU 49888 in this preparation.

The isolation of intact calcium channel drug receptors from cardiac tissue is apparently difficult because the α_1 subunit is highly susceptible to proteolysis (H. Glossmann and J. Striessnig, unpublished observations). Transverse-tubule membranes obtained from previously frozen and thawed skeletal muscle yield a purified calcium channel preparation that is nearly completely devoid of intact α_1 subunits (Fig. 40). In these preparations several proteolytic degradation products of α_1 (60–90 kDa) were labeled with $(-)$-[^{3}H]azidopine and [N-methyl-^{3}H]LU 49888. Interestingly, this proteolysis did not alter the binding properties of calcium channel ligands nor destroy the calcium channel activity in reconstitution experiments (Vaghy et al., 1987b). Thus, neither reversible binding nor function assures the integrity of the α_1 subunit.

3. Summary

Purified skeletal muscle 1,4-dihydropyridine receptors which form functional calcium channels after reconstitution into artificial membranes (vide infra) consist of several tightly, noncovalently associated polypeptides, which are termed α_1, α_2, β, and γ. The 1,4-dihydropyridine and phenylalkylamine drug receptor sites are located on α_1. This subunit (together with the β subunit) is the substrate for protein kinases A and C as well as an intrinsic protein kinase from skeletal muscle triads. The α_1 subunit carries the regulatory sites for L-type calcium channel drugs and has a primary structure related to the α subunit of the voltage-dependent sodium channel. It is, by definition, a constituent of the L-type calcium channel. This view is supported by functional alterations of L-type calcium channels induced with monoclonal anti-α_1 antibodies. The role of the other so-called subunits (perhaps as modulators of channel function) is unknown. Data from purification or photoaffinity labeling studies using tissues other than skeletal muscle (heart, brain) suggest a similar subunit composition, the drug receptor-carrying α_1 subunit being slightly larger than in skeletal muscle.

C. RECONSTITUTION OF CALCIUM CHANNELS

Breaking of cells, destruction of the architecture of biological membranes, and subsequent reconstitution is a necessary approach for the study of soluble multienzyme systems. The first reconstitution of a complete enzyme pathway was accomplished with the enzymes of the reductive pentose phosphate cycle (see Racker, 1985). Our knowledge about membrane receptor function has grown considerably since the development of suitable reconstitution procedures. Reconstituted receptors can be studied in a relatively defined environment, and the molecular relationship between the receptor and its membrane environment (e.g., receptor–lipid interactions) can be investigated. These experiments can help to identify purified receptors as functional structures and to characterize mechanisms involved in signal transfer.

Among the membrane receptors reconstituted are the β-adrenergic receptor, the photoreceptor of the outer rod segment of the retina or channel receptors like the nicotinic acetylcholine receptor, and the tetrodotoxin-sensitive sodium channel (for a review, see Miller, 1986). Table XXIV summarizes successful reconstitutions of calcium channels from membranes or after purification. These studies should help to characterize the mechanisms of calcium channel regulation, identify the purified polypeptides necessary for L-, T-, or N-type calcium channel function, and could also help in channel purification as was shown for the sodium channel (Goldin et al., 1985).

In view of the wide use of calcium channel blockers in cardiovascular disease (see Fleckenstein, 1983) the channel in cardiac or smooth muscle is of great interest. Incorporation of the voltage-dependent calcium channel from cardiac tissue into planar lipid bilayers was reported by Ehrlich et al. (1986). Highly purified cardiac sarcolemmal vesicles were prepared and fused with planar lipid bilayers at the tip of a patch electrode pipet. The calcium channel activator Bay K 8644 was added to 0.3 μM in the solution bathing the bilayer to enhance the probability of identifying channel activity. Surprisingly, channel-like activity was sometimes observed in the absence of channel protein, probably due to lipid–glass interactions. This artificial activity, however, did not show properties typical of the observed calcium channel. Channel activity was voltage dependent and selective for divalent cations over anions ($Ba^{2+} > Ca^{2+} >> Mg^{2+}$). A mean channel conductance of 8 pS (with 0.1 M Ba^{2+}) was measured. Addition of 5 μM ($\pm$)nitrendipine blocked channel activity, and this blockade was antagonized by 5 μM Bay K 8644. Stereoselective inhibition by the enantiomers of gallopamil was also observed. After exposure to 1.6 μM (−)gallopamil channel activity was completely inhibited but recovered after equimolar substitution of the (−) enantiomer by the (+) enantiomer. The (+) enantiomer showed 25-fold lower affinity for the phenylalkylamine receptor and is 100-fold less potent than (−)gallopamil in producing negative inotropic effects in isolated heart muscle. Thus the properties of reconstituted cardiac calcium channels resemble those of drug-sensitive L-type calcium channels characterized with whole cell voltage clamp and patch clamp studies. It should be noted that, in contrast to the reconstitution experiments, L-type channels in excised patch clamp experiments undergo irreversible inactivation, a phenomenon yet to be explained.

Nelson et al. (1984) reconstituted voltage-dependent calcium chan-

TABLE XXIV

CALCIUM CHANNEL RECONSTITUTION INTO PLANAR LIPID BILAYERS OR LIPOSOMES (*)

Channel source	Single channel conductance (pS)	Regulation of channel activity[a]	Voltage dependence	Comment	Ref.[b]
Rat skeletal muscle T-tubule membranes	20 (100 mM Ba^{2+})	Bay K 8644 (3 μM), S; nitrendipine (10 μM), I; D 600 (IC_{50} 5 μM), I; D 890 (IC_{50} 3–75 μM), I	Yes	Assymmetry of D 890 inhibition	a, b, c
Purified calcium channel from rabbit skeletal muscle	—	Bay K 8644 (2 μM), S; PN 200-110 (IC_{50} 0.2 μM), I; D 600 (IC_{50} 1 μM), I; verapamil (IC_{50} 1.5 μM), I; La^{3+}, Cd^{2+}, Ni^{2+}, Mn^{2+}, I	—	Reconstitution into liposomes; uptake studies in liposomes with $^{133}Ba^{2+}$ and $^{45}Ca^{2+}$	d*
T-tubule membranes and purified calcium channel from rabbit skeletal muscle	20 (90 mM Ba^{2+})	Bay K 8644 (10 μM), S; D 600 (IC_{50} 14 μM), I	—	Phosphorylation prolonged open state, shortened shut intervals; α and β subunits were phosphorylated in experiments employing [^{32}P]ATP	e
T-tubule membranes and purified calcium channel from guinea pig skeletal muscle	1–48 (110 mM Ba^{2+})	Bay K 8644 (10 μM), S	Only for oligochannels	Association of monochannels to physiological aggregates (oligochannels)	f
T-tubule membranes and purified calcium channel from guinea pig skeletal muscle	12–14 and 22 (100 mM Ba^{2+})	Bay K 8644 (5 μM), S; nitrendipine (2 μM), I	Yes		g

Preparation	Conductance (pS)	Pharmacology	Single channel	Comments	Ref.
T-tubule membranes and purified calcium channel from guinea pig skeletal muscle	7 and 16 (80 mM Ba²⁺)	Bay K 8644 (6 μM), S; Cd²⁺ (2.5 μM), I; nifedipine (2 μM), I	—	Only 22 pS events blocked by Cd²⁺ and nifedipine	h
Bovine skeletal muscle	11 (100 mM Ba²⁺)	Bay K 8644 (1 μM), S	Yes		i
Bovine cardiac sarcolemma	23 (100 mM Ba²⁺)	Bay K 8644 (1 μM), S	Yes		i
Porcine cardiac sarcolemma	8 (100 mM Ba²⁺)	Bay K 8644 (0.3 μM), S; nitrendipine (5 μM), I; (−)D 600 (1.6 μM), I	Yes	Stereoselective effect by D 600 enantiomers	j
Rat brain calcium channel	5 (250 mM Ba²⁺)	La³⁺ (IC₅₀ 145 μM), I; Cd²⁺, Mn²⁺, I	Yes		k
Paramecium	30 (10 mM Ba²⁺, "large" conductance; 1.5–2 (50 mM Ba²⁺, "small" conductance)	—	Only "small" conductance	30 pS channel was slightly more permeable to Mg²⁺ than to Ba²⁺ (mechanoreceptor-related channel); 1.5–2 pS channel was more permeable for Ba²⁺ over Mg²⁺ (100:1, voltage-dependent calcium channel)	l

[a] I, Inhibition; S, stimulation of calcium channel activity.

[b] Key to references: a, Affolter and Coronado (1985), *Biophys. J.* **48**, 341–347; b, Affolter and Coronado (1986), *Biophys. J.* **49**, 767–771; c, Coronado and Affolter (1986), *J. Gen. Physiol.* **87**, 933–953; d, Curtis and Catterall (1986), *Biochemistry* **25**, 3077–3083; e, Flockerzi *et al.* (1986), *Nature (London)* **323**, 66–68, Pelzer *et al.* (1987), *Pflügers Arch.* **410**, R35 (Abstr.); f, Glossmann *et al.* (1987a), *Ann. N.Y. Acad. Sci.* (in press), Hymel *et al.* (1988b), *Proc. Natl. Acad. Sci. U.S.A.* (in press); g, Smith *et al.* (1987), *Biochemistry* **26**, 7182–7188; h, Talvenheimo *et al.* (1987), *Biophys. J.* **52**, 891–899; i, Rosenberg *et al.* (1986), *Science* **231**, 1564–1566; j, Ehrlich *et al.* (1986), *Proc. Natl. Acad. Sci. U.S.A.* **83**, 193–197; k, Nelson *et al.* (1984), *Nature (London)* **308**, 77–81; l, Ehrlich and Finkelstein (1984), *Science* **225**, 427–428.

nels from rat brain membranes. They found single channel currents selective for divalent cations with single channel conductances of 5, 8.5, and 5 pS for Ca^{2+}, Ba^{2+}, and Sr^{2+}, respectively. The channels displayed voltage dependence. No activity was found at -100 mV. Channels were more likely to be open at positive potentials; the channel open times increased and closed times (intervals between openings) decreased with more positive membrane potentials.

Calcium channel reconstitution from rat skeletal muscle T-tubule membranes was first reported by Affolter and Coronado (1985, 1986). Activity was blocked by ($\pm$)nitrendipine (10 μM) or racemic gallopamil (IC_{50} 5 μM) whether applied from the cis or the trans side (the cis side being equivalent to the intracellular side). However, D 890, a phenylalkylamine carrying a positively charged group (hence unable to diffuse through the bilayer), blocked with a IC_{50} of 3 μM when applied to the cis side; it was 25-fold less active when applied to the trans side. These experiments showed that the reconstituted T-tubule calcium channel inserted into the bilayer with the cytoplasmic end on the cis side. Sidedness can also be inferred from the fact that the frequency of the open channel and the fraction of open time increased with cis-positive potentials (Affolter and Coronado, 1985).

Curtis and Catterall (1986) reconstituted purified calcium channels into phosphatidylcholine vesicles. $^{133}Ba^{2+}$ and $^{45}Ca^{2+}$ uptake into these vesicles were compared to that of protein-free vesicles. $^{45}Ca^{2+}$ influx through calcium channels was blocked by the organic channel blockers PN 200-110 (IC_{50} 0.2 μM), D 600 (IC_{50} 1 μM), and verapamil (IC_{50} 1.5 μM). Blockage was induced by inorganic blockers ($La^{3+} >$ $Cd^{2+} > Ni^{2+} > Mg^{2+}$). Interestingly, the ions blocked in the absence of channel protein. They also calculated that less than 3% of their purified receptors were active as voltage-dependent pores.

Modulation of calcium channel function by cAMP-dependent protein kinase after reconstitution was identified by Flockerzi et al. (1986). They reconstituted the purified calcium channel from rabbit skeletal muscle T-tubules into phospholipid membranes at the tip of glass patch pipets. Single L-type channel currents with a "single" channel conductance of 20 pS (Ba^{2+}) were observed, but the channel was not voltage dependent. The activity was increased not only by addition of the calcium channel activator Bay K 8644 but also by cAMP-dependent phosphorylation. Phosphorylation increased the open channel lifetimes and shortened the closed intervals between open events.

Cavalie et al. (1987) reported that two functionally different divalent cation-selective calcium channels were present in bilayers containing reconstituted 1,4-dihydropyridine receptors derived from either T-tubule membranes or highly purified receptor preparations. A "large" channel (conductance 20 pS, 90 mM Ba^{2+}) and a "small" channel (conductance 10 pS) were distinguished. The large conductance was activatable by Bay K 8644 and inhibited by gallopamil (D 600). Further, it was activated by cAMP-dependent phosphorylation and showed a time-dependent "rundown" of activity. The small conductance was insensitive to L-type calcium channel drugs or phosphorylation and did not show rundown. Two conductances with very similar properties were also reported by Talvenheimo et al. (1987). In contrast, Smith et al. (1987) found only a 1,4-dihydropyridine-sensitive 12-pS channel after reconstitution of membrane-bound as well as purified 1,4-dihydropyridine receptor preparations.

The two calcium channel conductance levels could underlie the two components of macroscopic current (I_{slow} and I_{fast}; see Section VI,A,3) observed in cultured skeletal muscle cells. The question arises whether several conductance levels correspond to the opening of two structurally distinct calcium channels or are merely substates of one channel. It is puzzling that both conductances should copurify with the L-type Ca^{2+} antagonist receptor binding activity. Hymel et al. (1988b) provide an interesting model to explain these findings. Using the fast dilution method and the septum-supported, vesicle-derived bilayer technique (Schindler et al., 1984; Schindler, 1988) single, purified 1,4-dihydropyridine receptors were reconstituted into separate vesicles which were used to form bilayers for channel analysis (Hymel et al., 1988b). Conditions were such that on average 100 receptor sites were expected to be incorporated and randomly distributed in the plane of a bilayer. Just after bilayer formation, when the receptor molecules are expected to be singly distributed, clearly resolvable 0.9-pS channel events were observed. It was concluded that the channel controlled by the monomeric 1,4-dihydropyridine receptor has a conductance of 0.9 pS (in 100 mM BaCl$_2$, trace A1 and B1 in Fig. 41). The gating of this "monochannel" was independent of voltage. With increasing time after membrane formation higher conductance levels appeared as single events, whereas monochannels disappeared. These higher conductance levels often corresponded to even integer multiples of the monochannel conductance, predominantly 4, 8, 16, and multiples up to 64. Apparently, these resulted from oligomeric association of monochannels and were therefore termed "oligochannels." Most remarkably, oligochannels (in contrast to monochannels) showed clearly voltage-dependent gating. Further they displayed the following properties typ-

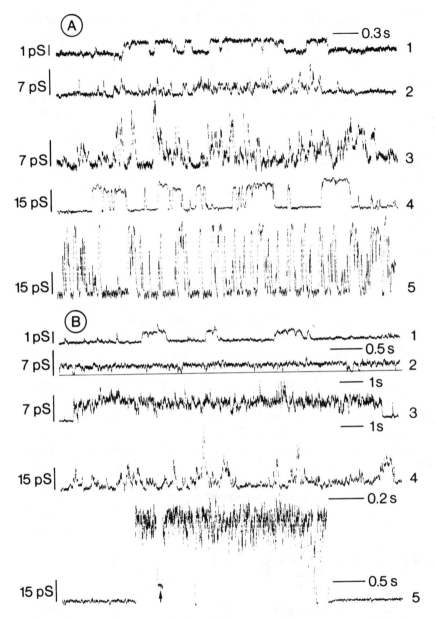

Fig. 41. Reconstitution of 1,4-dihydropyridine receptors from guinea pig skeletal muscle using the fast dilution technique and the septum-supported, vesicle-derived bilayer method of Schindler (Schindler 1980, 1988). Conditions were such that 100 1,4-dihydropyridine receptor sites were present in the bilayer. The smallest conductance level observed was 0.9 pS (100 mM BaCl$_2$, traces A1 and B1) independent of the source used

ical of ("L-type") calcium channels. (1) Their high conductivity for Na^+ was blocked by low Ca^{2+} concentrations. (2) Conductances were modulated by organic calcium channel-active drugs. (3) Activity was blocked by Cd^{2+} in the expected concentration range. (4) The channels responded to phosphorylation by the cAMP-dependent protein kinase which was absolutely required for channel function (see also Armstrong and Eckert, 1987).

From these results it was concluded that the L-type calcium channels observed in patch clamp studies represent oligomeric channels with strict functional coupling among associated monochannels. These findings are also consistent with the so far unexplained finding that 35–50 times more 1,4-dihydropyridine receptors than 20-pS calcium channels exist in intact skeletal muscle (Schwartz *et al.*, 1985; see Section VI). The sarcoplasmic reticulum Ca^{2+} release channel/ryanodine receptor was also identified as an oligochannel (Hymel *et al.*, 1988a). A close functional and structural interaction of these two oligomeric channels, working as coaligned, tetragonal arrays of, e.g., 16 channels each, could be the key to understanding excitation–contraction coupling in skeletal muscle (see Section VI).

Summary

Reconstitution of calcium channels into planar lipid bilayers from crude membranes or purified preparations has been successful. Varying conductance levels as well as voltage-independent and voltage-dependent gating have been observed. Drug sensitivity, stereoselective inhibition, or sidedness of drug effects confirm the findings from more classic work on calcium channels. Phosphorylation of the purified calcium channel from skeletal muscle alters function in a fashion similar to that observed for *in situ* channels from cardiac muscle. Reconstitution experiments with purified polypeptides must clarify if GTP-binding proteins involved in signal transfer regulate channel function as

---

(A, purified, B, T-tubule membrane-bound 1,4-dihydropyridine receptors). This elementary conductance was observed for only a short period of time after bilayer formation. These small conductances disappeared with time and were replaced by higher conductances, which occurred either in bursts (e.g., trace A3) or sometimes more stabilized events (e.g., trace A4, B5). The clearly resolvable substates were always *even* multiples of the elementary conductance (see text; traces 2–4). Hymel *et al.* (1988b) interpreted these results as the association of "monochannels" (0.9 pS) to form oligomeric channels with higher conductance levels ("oligochannels"). The reconstituted channel activity showed features typical for physiologically observed calcium channels (see text). Using this method, the number of functionally active molecules (e.g., per mole of 1,4-dihydropyridine receptor) can be estimated in purified preparations (see Hymel *et al.*, 1988b).

observed in neuronal and other membranes (see Brown and Birn-baumer, 1988). Differing conductance levels suggest a possibility never seriously discussed for calcium channels, namely, that the "single channel" (as defined by electrophysiologists) is a cooperative aggregate of perhaps 10 or 20 polypeptide chains with different properties dependent on aggregate size. Although it is highly likely that the α_1 subunit is a major (perhaps the only) L-channel polypeptide necessary for function, this remains to be vigorously tested in quantitative reconstitution experiments. To this end the so-called subunits must be separated under nondenaturating conditions. Such experiments could be decisive for the cloning (and expression) strategy.

D. CLONING AND EXPRESSION OF CALCIUM CHANNELS

Molecular biology provides the most powerful tool for structural characterization of ionic pores. Cloning of the different types of calcium channels will reveal the structural basis for their distinct electrophysiological properties and patterns of regulation by drugs, toxins, enzymes, and GTP-binding proteins.

The amino acid sequence of the rabbit skeletal muscle 1,4-dihydropyridine receptor/calcium channel α_1 subunit was recently deduced from sequence analysis of cDNA complementary to its mRNA (Tanabe et al., 1987). The polypeptide contains 1873 amino acids. The comparison with the voltage dependent sodium channel gave a surprising result: nearly one-third (29%) of the amino acids in corresponding positions are identical. The similarity is even greater (55%) if conservative residues (substitutions frequently made during the evolution of functionally similar proteins) are taken into account. In both channels four distinct internal repeats were identified which exhibit sequence similarity. Based on the hydropathy pattern (obtained by plotting the running average of the amino acid hydrophobicity scores against amino acid position), it was assumed that these four units span the membrane thus forming the channel pore. Each of them consists of five hydrophobic (termed S1, S2, S3, S5, and S6) and one (S4) hydrophilic segment. Each segment is thought to be a membrane-spanning α helix. Assuming a diameter of 0.6 nm for the calcium channel pore, its inner wall could be formed by one or two of the helical segments from each repeat. S4 is thought to form a positively charged spiral that could act as the voltage sensor. Not only voltage-dependent sodium and calcium channels but also a protein genetically identified as a potassium channel in Drosophila contain the S4 subregion (Alsobrook and Stevens, 1987).

At least two divalent cation binding sites are postulated for the L-type calcium channel based on electrophysiological and biochemical studies (see Sections III,B and V). One region in the α_1 subunit (assigned to the cytoplasmic side, residues 740–752) and the sequence of residues 155–164 (assigned mostly to the extracellular side) resembled the EF-hand (e.g., in calmodulin) and the consensus repeat of calcium-dependent membrane binding proteins, respectively. Two potential N-glycosylation sites (out of five) are present on the extracellular side, and all six potential cAMP-dependent phosphorylation sites are located on the cytoplasmic side in the model presented by Tanabe et al. (1987). An interesting difference exists between voltage-dependent sodium channels and the α_1 subunit: a large carboxy-terminal region (presumably oriented intracellularly), which is missing in sodium channels, has little secondary structure and is suspected to be involved in excitation–contraction coupling.

Unequivocal proof that the cloned α_1 subunit is the calcium channel must come from functional data obtained by expression of mRNA made in vitro. In case of the voltage-dependent sodium channel and acetylcholine receptor, Xenopus oocytes have been selected for such studies. These preparations provide a complete system for protein synthesis, posttranslational modification, and also assembly of multi-subunit proteins. Their size (1–1.2 mm) allows easy access for electrophysiological and even biochemical studies. Cardiac, brain, and skeletal muscle calcium channels have been already successfully expressed in oocytes after injection of total mRNA isolated from the respective tissues (Dascal et al., 1986; Leonard et al., 1987; Moorman et al., 1987).

Expression of cloned α_1 will be important for subsequent studies (e.g., site-directed mutagenesis, hybrid channels). As the α_2 polypeptide is cloned as well (A. Schwartz, personal communication), it is hoped that the question of whether or not the α_1-associated polypeptides have a functional role will be answered in the near future.

ACKNOWLEDGMENTS

The authors would like to thank Drs. Schwartz, Bryant, Vaghy, and Walsh (Cincinnati), Höltje (Bern, Berlin), Hofmann (Homburg/Saar), Kaczorowski (Rahway), Lüttgau (Dortmund), Miller (Chicago), Mir (Strasbourg), Porzig (Bern), Schultz (Berlin), Snyder (Baltimore), and Spedding (Edinburgh) for providing us with prepublication manuscripts. We are grateful to Drs. Hymel and Schindler (Linz) for their cooperation. C. Trawöger prepared the art work, and K. Hofer provided competent secretarial assistance.

The authors' work is supported by Fonds zur Förderung der wissenschaftlichen Forschung, Deutsche Forschungsgemeinschaft, Österreichische Nationalbank, and the Dr. Legerlotz Foundation. We pay tribute to Prof. Albrecht Fleckenstein (Freiburg), the scientific father of calcium antagonism.

REFERENCES

Abe, T., and Saisu, H. (1987). Identification of the receptor for ω-conotoxin in brain. *J. Biol. Chem.* **262,** 9877–9882.

Abe, T., Koyano, K., Saisu, H., Nishiuchi, Y., and Sakakibara, S. (1986). Binding of ω-conotoxin to receptor sites associated with the voltage-sensitive calcium channel. *Neurosci. Lett.* **71,** 203–208.

Affolter, H., and Coronado, R. (1985). Agonists Bay-K 8644 and GCP-28392 open calcium channels reconstituted from skeletal muscle transverse tubules. *Biophys. J.* **48,** 341–347.

Affolter, H., and Coronado, R. (1986). Sidedness of reconstituted calcium channels from muscle transverse tubules as determined by D600 and D890 blockade. *Biophys. J.* **49,** 767–771.

Almers, W. (1978). Gating currents and charge movements in excitable membranes. *Rev. Physiol. Biochem. Pharmacol.* **82,** 97–190.

Almers, W., and McCleskey, E. W. (1984). Non-selective conductance in calcium channels of frog muscle: Calcium selectivity in a single-file pore. *J. Physiol. (London)* **353,** 585–608.

Almers, W., McCleskey, E. W., and Palade, P. T. (1985). Calcium channels in vertebrate skeletal muscle. *In* "Calcium in Biological Systems" (R. P. Rubin, G. B. Weiss, and J. W. Putney, Jr., eds.), pp. 321–330. Plenum, New York.

Almers, W., McCleskey, E. W., and Palade, P. T. (1986). The mechanism of ion selectivity in calcium channels of skeletal muscle membranes. *Prog. Zool.* **33,** 61–73.

Alsobrook, J. P., and Stevens, C. F. (1987). Cloning the calcium channel. *Trends Neurosci.* **11,** 1–3.

Armstrong, C. M., and Eckert, R. (1987). Voltage-activated calcium channels that must be phosphorylated to respond to membrane depolarization. *Proc. Natl. Acad. Sci. U.S.A.* **84,** 2518–2522.

Armstrong, C. M., and Matteson, D. R. (1985). Two distinct populations of calcium channels in a clonal line of pituitary cells. *Science* **277,** 65–66.

Ashcroft, F. M., and Stanfield, P. R. (1982). Calcium and potassium currents in muscle fibres of an insect (*Carausius morosus*). *J. Physiol. (London)* **323,** 93–115.

Balwierczak, J. L., and Schwartz, A. (1987). Specific binding of [³H]*d-cis*-diltiazem to cardiac sarcolemma and its inhibition by calcium. *Eur. J. Pharmacol.* **116,** 193–194.

Balwierczak, J. L., Johnson, C. L., and Schwartz, A. (1987). The relationship between the binding site of [³H]*d-cis*-diltiazem and that of other non-dihydropyridine calcium entry blockers in cardiac sarcolemma. *Mol. Pharmacol.* **31,** 175–179.

Bayley, H. (1983). "Photogenerated Reagents in Biochemistry and Molecular Biology." Elsevier, Amsterdam.

Beam, K. G., Knudson, C. M., and Powell, J. A. (1986). A lethal mutation in mice eliminates the slow calcium current in skeletal muscle cells. *Nature (London)* **320,** 168–170.

Bean, B. P. (1984). Nitrendipine block of cardiac calcium channels: High-affinity binding to the inactivated state. *Proc. Natl. Acad. Sci. U.S.A.* **81,** 6388–6392.

Bean, B. P. (1985). Two kinds of calcium channels in canine atrial cells. *J. Gen. Physiol.* **86,** 1–30.

Bean, B. P., Cohen, C. J., and Tsien, R. W. (1983). Lidocaine block of cardiac sodium channels. *J. Gen. Physiol.* **81,** 613–642.

Bean, B. P., Sturek, M., Puga, A., and Hermsmeyer, K. (1986). Calcium channel in muscle cells isolated from rat mesenteric arteries: Modulation by dihydropyridine drugs. *Circ. Res.* **59,** 229–235.

Bellemann, P., Ferry, D., Lübbecke, F., and Glossmann, H. (1981). [³H]Nitrendipine, a potent calcium antagonist, binds with high affinity to cardiac membranes. *Arzneim. Forsch.* **31**, 2064–2067.

Belluzzi, O., Sacchi, O., and Wanke, E. (1985). Identification of delayed potassium and calcium currents in the rat sympathetic neurone under voltage clamp. *J. Physiol. (London)* **358**, 109–129.

Benson, M., Catterall, C., and Catterall, W. A. (1986). Reconstitution of the voltage-sensitive calcium channel purified from skeletal muscle transverse tubules. *Biochemistry* **25**, 3077–3083.

Berwe, D., Gottschalk, G., and Lüttgau, H. Ch. (1987). The effects of the Ca-antagonist gallopamil (D600) upon excitation–contraction coupling in toe muscle fibres of the frog. *J. Physiol. (London)* **385**, 693–707.

Blume, A. J., Lichtshtein, D., and Boone, G. (1979). Coupling of opiate receptors to adenylate cyclase: Requirement for Na⁺ and GTP. *Proc. Natl. Acad. Sci. U.S.A.* **76**, 5626–5630.

Bolger, G. T., Gengo, P., Klockowski, R., Luchowski, E., Siegel, H., Janis, R. A., Triggle, A. M., and Triggle, D. J. (1984). Characterization of binding of the calcium channel antagonist, [³H]nitrendipine, to guinea pig ileal smooth muscle. *J. Pharmacol. Exp. Ther.* **225**, 291–309.

Borsotto, M., Barhanin, J., Norman, R. I., and Lazdunski, M. (1984a). Purification of the dihydropyridine receptor of the voltage-dependent Ca^{2+} channel from skeletal muscle transverse tubules using (+)-[³H]PN 200-110. *Biochem. Biophys. Res. Commun.* **122**, 1357–1366.

Borsotto, M., Norman, R. I., Fosset, M., and Lazdunski, M. (1984b). Solubilization of the nitrendipine receptor from skeletal muscle transverse tubule membranes. *Eur. J. Biochem.* **142**, 449–455.

Borsotto, M., Barhanin, J., Fosset, M., and Lazdunski, M. (1985). The 1,4-dihydropyridine receptor associated with the skeletal muscle voltage-dependent Ca^{2+} channel. *J. Biol. Chem.* **260**, 14255–14263.

Bossert, F., and Vater, W. (1971). Dihydropyridine, eine neue Gruppe stark wirksamer Coronartherapeutika. *Naturwissenschaften* **58**, 578.

Bourne, H. R. (1986). One molecular machine can transduce diverse signals. *Nature (London)* **321**, 814–816.

Brandt, N. R., Caswell, A. H., and Brunschwig, J. P. (1980). ATP-energized Ca^{2+} pump in isolated transverse tubes of skeletal muscle. *J. Biol. Chem.* **255**, 6290–6298.

Breitwieser, G. E., and Szabo, G. (1985). Uncoupling of cardiac muscarinic and β-adrenergic receptors from ion channel by a guanine nucleotide analogue. *Nature (London)* **317**, 538–540.

Brown, A. M., and Birnbaumer, L. (1988). Direct G-protein gating of ion channels. *Am. J. Physiol.* **254**, H401–H410.

Brown, A. M., Kunze, D. L., and Yatani, A. (1986). Dual effects of dihydropyridines on whole cell and unitary calcium currents in single ventricular cells of guinea pig. *J. Physiol. (London)* **379**, 495–514.

Brum, G., Flockerzi, V., Hofmann, F., Osterrieder, W., and Trautwein, W. (1983). Injection of catalytic subunit of cAMP-dependent protein kinase into islated cardic myocytes. *Pflügers Arch.* **398**, 147–154.

Brum, G., Osterrieder, W., and Trautwein, W. (1984). β-Adrenergic increase in the calcium conductance of cardiac myocytes studied with the patch clamp. *Pflügers Arch.* **401**, 111–118.

Byerly, L., Chase, P. B., and Stimers, J. R. (1985). Permeation and interaction of divalent cations in calcium channels of snail neurons. *J. Gen. Physiol.* **85**, 491–518.

Cachelin, A. B., Peyer, J. E., Kokubun, S., and Reuter, H. (1983). Ca^{2+} channel modulation by 8-bromocyclic AMP in cultured heart cells. *Nature (London)* **304**, 462–464.

Campbell, K. P., Lipshutz, G. M., and Denney, G. H. (1984). Direct photoaffinity labeling of the high affinity nitrendipine-binding site in subcellular membrane fractions isolated from canine myocardium. *J. Biol. Chem.* **259**, 5384–5387.

Canfield, D. R., and Dunlap, K. (1984). Pharmacological characterization of amine receptors on embryonic chick sensory neurones. *Br. J. Pharmacol.* **82**, 557–563.

Cantor, H., Kenessey, A., Semenuk, G., and Spector, S. (1984). Interaction of calcium channel blockers with non-neuronal benzodiazepine binding sites. *Proc. Natl. Acad. Sci. U.S.A.* **81**, 1549–1552.

Carbone, E., and Lux, H. D. (1984a). A low voltage-activated, fully inactivating Ca^{++} channel in vertebrate sensory neurones. *Nature (London)* **310**, 501–502.

Carbone, E., and Lux, H. D. (1984b). A low voltage-activated calcium conductance in embryonic chick sensory neurons. *Biophys. J.* **46**, 413–418.

Casadei, J. M., Cordon, R. D., and Barchi, R. L. (1986). Immunoaffinity isolation of Na^+ channels from rat skeletal muscle. *J. Biol. Chem.* **261**, 4318–4323.

Caswell, A. H., Baker, S. P., Boyd, H., Potter, L. T., and Garcia, M. (1978). β-Adrenergic receptor and adenylate cyclase in transverse tubules of skeletal muscle. *J. Biol. Chem.* **253**, 3049–3054.

Cavalié, A., Pelzer, D., and Trautwein, W. (1986). Fast and slow gating behaviour of single calcium channels in cardiac cells. *Pflügers Arch.* **406**, 241–258.

Chad, J., and Eckert, E. (1985). Calcineurin, a calcium-dependent phosphatase, enhances Ca-mediated inactivation of Ca current in perfused snail neurons. *Biophys. J.* **47**, 266a.

Chandler, W. K., Rakowski, R. F., and Schneider, M. F. (1976a). Effects of glycerol treatment and maintained depolarization on charge movement in skeletal muscle. *J. Physiol. (London)* **254**, 285–316.

Chandler, W. K., Rakowski, R. F., and Schneider. M. F. (1976b). A non-linear voltage dependent charge movement in frog skeletal muscle. *J. Physiol. (London)* **254**, 245–283.

Cherubini, E., and North, R. A. (1984). Inhibition of calcium spikes and transmitter release by γ-aminobutyric acid in the guinea pig myenteric plexus. *Br. J. Pharmacol.* **82**, 101–105.

Cherubini, E., and North, R. A. (1985). μ- and κ-opioids inhibit transmitter release by different mechanisms. *Proc. Natl. Acad. Sci. U.S.A.* **82**, 1860–1863.

Cognard, C., Lazdunski, M., and Romey, G. (1986a). Different types of Ca^{2+} channels in mammalian skeletal muscle cells in culture. *Proc. Natl. Acad. Sci. U.S.A.* **83**, 517–521.

Cognard, C., Romey, G., Galizzi, J. P., Fosset, M., and Lazdunski, M. (1986b). Dihydropyridine-sensitive Ca^{2+} channels in mammalian skeletal muscle cell in culture: Electrophysiological properties and interaction with Ca^{2+} channel activator (Bay K 8644) and inhibitor (PN 200-110). *Proc. Natl. Acad. Sci. U.S.A.* **83**, 1518–1522.

Cooper, C. L., Vandaele, S., Barhanin, J., Fosset, M., Lazdunski, M., and Hosey, M. M. (1987). Purification and characterization of the dihydropyridine-sensitive voltage-dependent calcium channel from cardiac tissue. *J. Biol. Chem.* **262**, 509–512.

Cooper, R. H., Coll, K. E., and Williamson, J. R. (1985). Differential effect of phorbol ester on phenylephrine and vasopressin-induced calcium mobilization in isolated hepatocytes. *J. Biol. Chem.* **260**, 3281–3288.

Coronado, R., and Affolter, H. (1986). Insulation of the conduction pathway of muscle transverse tubule calcium channels from the surface charge of bilayer phospholipid. *J. Gen. Physiol.* **87,** 933–953.

Cota, G., and Stefani, E. (1986). A fast-activated inward calcium current in twitch muscle fibers of the frog *(Rana montezume) J. Physiol. (London)* **370,** 151–163.

Covarrubias, M., Prinz, H., Meyers, H.-W., and Maelicke, A. (1986). Equilibrium binding of cholinergic ligands to the membrane-bound acetylcholine receptor. *J. Biol. Chem.* **261,** 14955–14961.

Crowder, J. M., Norris, D. K., and Bradford, H. F. (1986). Morphine inhibition of calcium fluxes, neurotransmitter release and protein and lipid phosphorylation in brain slices and synaptosomes. *Biochem. Pharmacol.* **35,** 2501–2507.

Cruz, L. J., and Olivera, B. M. (1986). Calcium channel antagonists. *J. Biol. Chem.* **261,** 6230–6233.

Cruz, L. J., Johnson, D. S., and Olivera, B. M. (1987). Characterization of the ω-conotoxin target: Evidence for tissue-specific heterogeneity in calcium channel types. *Biochemistry* **26.** 820–824.

Curtis, B. M., and Catterall. W. A. (1984). Purification of the calcium antagonist receptor of the voltage-sensitive calcium channel from skeletal muscle transverse tubules. *Biochemistry* **23,** 2113–2117.

Curtis, B. M., and Catterall, W. A. (1985). Phosphorylation of the calcium antagonist receptor of the voltage-sensitive calcium channel by cAMP-dependent protein kinase. *Proc. Natl. Acad. Sci. U.S.A.* **82,** 2528–2532.

Curtis, B. M., and Catterall, W. A. (1986). Reconstitution of the voltage-sensitive calcium channel purified from skeletal muscle transverse tubules. *Biochemistry* **25,** 3077–3083.

Dascal, N., Snutch, T. P., Lübbert, H., Davidson, N., and Lester, H. A. (1986). Expression and modulation of voltage-gated calcium channels after RNA injection in *Xenopus* oocytes. *Science* **231,** 1147–1150.

Deisz, R. A., and Lux, H. D. (1985). γ-Aminobutyric acid induced depression of calcium currents of chick sensory neuron. *Neurosci. Lett.* **56,** 205–210.

De Pover, A., Grupp, I. L., Grupp, G., and Schwartz, A. (1983). Diltiazem potentiates the negative inotropic action of nimodipine in heart. *Biochem. Biophys. Res. Commun.* **114,** 922–929.

DeRiemer, S. A., Strong, J. A., Albert, K. A., Greengard, P., and Kaczmarek, L. K. (1985). Enhancement of calcium current in *Aplysia* neurones by phorbol ester and protein kinase C. *Nature (London)* **313,** 313–316.

Di Virgilio, F., Pozzan, T., Wollheim, C. B., Vicentini, L. M., and Meldolesi, J. (1986). Tumor promotor phorbol myristate acetate inhibits Ca^{2+} influx through voltage-gated Ca^{2+} channels in two secretory cell lines, PC 12 and RINm5F. *J. Biol. Chem.* **261,** 32–35.

Doble, A., Benavides, J., Ferris, O., Bertrand, P., Menager, J., Vaucher, N., Burgevin, M.-C., Uzan, A., Gueremy, C., and Le Fur, G. (1985). Dihydropyridine and peripheral type benzodiazepine binding sites, subcellular distribution and molecular size determination. *Eur. J. Pharmacol.* **119,** 153–167.

Dolphin, A. C., Forda, S. R., and Scott, R. H. (1986). Calcium-dependent currents in cultured rat dorsal root ganglion neurones are inhibited by an adenosine analogue. *J. Physiol. (London)* **373,** 47–61.

Dörrscheidt-Käfer, M. (1977). The action of D600 on frog skeletal muscle: Facilitation of excitation–contraction coupling. *Pflügers. Arch.* **369,** 259–267.

Drummond, A. H. (1985). Bidirectional control of cytosolic free calcium by thyrotropin-releasing hormone in pituitary cells. *Nature (London)* **315,** 752–755.

Dudel, J. (1983). Graded or all-or-nothing release of transmitter quanta by local depolarizations of nerve terminals on crayfish muscle? *Pflügers Arch.* **398**, 155–164.

Dunlap, K.,and Fischbach, G. D. (1981). Neurotransmitters decrease the calcium conductance activated by depolarization of embryonic chick sensory neurones. *J. Physiol. (London)* **317**, 519–535.

Ehara, T., and Kaufmann, R. (1978). The voltage- and time-dependent effects of (−)-verapamil on the slow inward current in isolated cat ventricular myocardium. *J. Pharmacol. Exp. Ther.* **207**, 49–55.

Ehrlich, B. E., and Finkelstein, A. (1984). Voltage-dependent calcium channels from paramecium cilia incorporated into planar lipid bilayers. *Science* **225**, 427–428.

Ehrlich, B. E., Schen, C. R., Garcia, M. L., and Kaczorowski, G. J. (1986). Incorporation of calcium channels from cardiac sarcolemmal membrane vesicles into planar lipid bilayers. *Proc. Natl. Acad. Sci. U.S.A.* **83**, 193–197.

Eisenberg, B. R. (1983). Quantitative infrastructure of mammalian skeletal muscle. *Handb. Physiol.* **10**, 73–112.

Eisenberg, R. S., McCarthy, R. T., and Milton, R. L. (1983). Paralysis of frog skeletal muscle fibres by the calcium antagonist D-600. *J. Physiol. (London)* **341**, 495–505.

Fabiato, A. (1985). Calcium-induced release of calcium from the sarcoplasmic reticulum of skinned fibers from the frog semitendinosus. *Biophys. J.* **47**, 195a.

Fatt, P. and Ginsborg, B. L. (1958). The ionic requirements for the production of action potentials in crustacean muscle fibers. *J. Physiol. (London)* **142**, 516–543.

Fatt, P., and Katz, B. (1953). The electrical properties of crustacean muscle fibers. *J. Physiol. (London)* **129**, 171–204.

Fedulova, S. A., Kostyuk, P. G., and Veselovsky, N. S. (1985). Two types of calcium channels in the somatic membrane of new-born rat dorsal root ganglion neurons. *J. Physiol. (London)* **359**, 431–446.

Ferguson, D. G., Schwartz, H. W., and Franzini-Armstrong, C. (1984). Subunit structure of junctional feet in triads of skeletal muscle: A freeze-drying, rotary-shadowing study. *J. Cell. Biol.* **99**, 1735–1742.

Ferry, D. R., and Glossmann, H. (1982a). Evidence for multiple receptor sites within the putative calcium channel. *Naunyn–Schmiedeberg's Arch. Pharmacol.* **321**, 80–83.

Ferry, D. R., and Glossmann, H. (1982b). Identification of putative calcium channels in skeletal muscle microsomes. *FEBS Lett.* **148**, 331–337.

Ferry, D. R., and Glossmann, H. (1983). Tissue-specific regulation of [^{3}H]nimodipine binding by the active isomer of diltiazem. *Br. J. Pharmacol.* **78**, 81.

Ferry, D. R., and Glossmann, H. (1984). ^{125}I-Iodipine, a new high affinity ligand for the putative calcium channel. *Naunyn–Schmiedeberg's Arch. Pharmacol.* **325**, 186–189.

Ferry, D. R., Goll, A., and Glossmann, H. (1983a). Differential labeling of putative skeletal muscle calcium channels by [^{3}H]nifedipine, [^{3}H]nitrendipine, [^{3}H]nimodipine and [^{3}H]PN 200-110. *Naunyn–Schmiedeberg's Arch. Pharmacol.* **323**, 276–277.

Ferry, D. R., Goll, A., and Glossmann, H. (1983b). Calcium channels: Evidence for oligomeric nature by target size analysis. *EMBO J.* **2**, 1729–1732.

Ferry, D. R., Goll, A., and Glossmann, H. (1983c). Putative calcium channel molecular weight determination by target size analysis. *Naunyn–Schmiedeberg's Arch. Pharmacol.* **323**, 292–297.

Ferry, D. R., Goll, A., Gadow, C., and Glossmann, H. (1984a). (−)-[^{3}H]Desmethoxyverapamil labelling of putative calcium channels in brain: Autoradiographic distribution and allosteric coupling to 1,4-dihydropyridine and diltiazem binding sites. *Naunyn–Schmiedeberg's Arch. Pharmacol.* **327**, 183–187.

Ferry, D. R., Rombusch, M., Goll, A., and Glossmann, H. (1984b). Photoaffinity labeling of Ca^{2+} channels with [^{3}H]azidopine. *FEBS Lett.* **169**, 112–118.

Ferry, D. R., Glossmann, H., and Kaumann, A. J. (1985a). Relationship between the stereoselective negative inotropic effects of verapamil enantiomers and their binding to putative calcium channels in human heart. *Br. J. Pharmacol.* **84**, 811–824.

Ferry, D. R., Kämpf, K., Goll, A., and Glossmann, H. (1985b). Subunit composition of skeletal muscle transverse tubule calcium channel evaluated with the 1,4-dihydropyridine photoaffinity probe, [^{3}H]azidopine. *EMBO J.* **4**, 1933–1940.

Ferry, D. R., Goll, A., and Glossmann, H. (1987). Photoaffinity labeling of the cardiac calcium channel. *Biochem. J.* **243**, 127–135.

Fill, M. D., and Best, P. M. (1986). Contracture of skinned skeletal muscle fibers induced by ionic substitution: Comparison of block by D-600 and nitrendipine. *Biophys. J.* **49**, 13a.

Fischmeister, R., and Hartzell, H. C. (1986). Mechanism of action of acetylcholine on calcium current in single cells from frog ventricle. *J. Physiol. (London)* **376**, 183–202.

Fleckenstein, A. (1983). "Calcium Antagonism in Heart and Smooth Muscle." Wiley, New York.

Flockerzi, V., Mewes, R., Ruth, R., and Hofmann, F. (1983). Phosphorylation of purified bovine cardiac sarcolemma and potassium-stimulated calcium uptake. *Eur. J. Biochem.* **135**, 131–142.

Flockerzi, V., Oeken, H. J., Hofmann, F., Pelzer, D., Cavalié, A., and Trautwein, W. (1986). The purified dihydropyridine-binding site from skeletal muscle T-tubules is a functional calcium channel. *Nature (London)* **323**, 66–68.

Forscher, P., and Oxford, G. S. (1985). Modulation of calcium channels by norepinephrine in internally dialyzed avian sensory neurons. *J. Gen. Physiol.* **85**, 743–763.

Forscher, P., Oxford, G. S., and Schulz, D. (1986). Noradrenaline modulates calcium channels in avian dorsal root ganglion cells through tight receptor–channel coupling. *J. Physiol. (London)* **379**, 131–144.

Fosset, M., Jaimovich, E., Delpont, E., and Lazdunski, M. (1983). [^{3}H]Nitrendipine receptors in skeletal muscle. *J. Biol. Chem.* **258**, 6086–6092.

Franckowiak, G., Bechem, M., Schramm, M., and Thomas, G. (1985). The optical isomers of the 1,4-dihydropyridine Bay K 8644 show opposite effects on the Ca-channel. *Eur. J. Pharmacol.* **114**, 223–226.

Frank, G. B. (1980). Commentary. The current view of the source of trigger calcium in excitation–contraction coupling in vertebrate skeletal muscle. *Biochem. Pharmacol.* **29**, 2399–2406.

Frank, G. B. (1984). Blockade of Ca^{2+} channels inhibits K$^+$ contractures but not twitches in skeletal muscle. *Can. J. Physiol. Pharmacol.* **62**, 374–378.

Franzini-Armstrong, C. (1970). Studies of the triad: Structure of the junction in frog twitch fibers. *J. Cell Biol.* **47**, 488–499.

Franzini-Armstrong, C., and Nunzi, G. (1983). Junctional feet and particles in the triads of fast-twitch muscle fiber. *J. Muscle Res. Cell Motil.* **4**, 233–252.

Freedman, S. B., Miller, R. J., Miller, D. M., and Tindall, D. R. (1984). Interactions of maitotoxin with voltage-sensitive calcium channels in cultured neuronal cells. *Proc. Natl. Acad. Sci. U.S.A.* **81**, 4582–4585.

Fukushima, Y., and Hagiwara, S. (1985). Current carried by monovalent cations through calcium channels in mouse neoplastic B lymphocytes. *J. Physiol. (London)* **358**, 255–284.

Galizzi, J.-P., Fosset, M., and Lazdunski, M. (1984a). Properties of receptors for Ca^{2+}-channel blocker verapamil in transverse-tubule membranes of skeletal muscle. *Eur. J. Biochem.* **144**, 211–215.

Galizzi, J.-P., Fosset, M., and Lazdunski, M. (1984b). [^{3}H]Verapamil binding sites in skeletal muscle transverse tubule membranes. *Biochem. Biophys. Res. Commun.* **118**, 239–245.

Galizzi, J.-P., Fosset, M., and Lazdunski, M. (1985). Characterization of the Ca^{2+} coordination site regulating binding of Ca^{2+} channel inhibitors d-cis-diltiazem, (±)bepridil and (−)desmethoxyverapamil to their receptor site in skeletal muscle transverse tubule membranes. *Biochem. Biophys. Res. Commun.* **132**, 49–55.

Galizzi, J.-P., Fosset, M., Romey, G., Laduron, P., and Lazdunski, M. (1986a). Neuroleptics of the diphenylbutylpiperidine series are potent calcium channel inhibitors. *Proc. Natl. Acad. Sci. U.S.A.* **83**, 7513–7517.

Galizzi, J.-P., Borsotto, M., Barhanin, J., Fosset, M., and Lazdunski, M. (1986b). Characterization and photoaffinity labeling of receptor sites for the Ca^{2+} channel inhibitors d-cis-diltiazem, (±)-bepridil, desmethoxyverapamil, and (+)-PN 200-110 in skeletal muscle tranverse tubule membranes. *J. Biol. Chem.* **261**, 1393–1397.

Galizzi, J.-P., Quar, J., Fosset, M., van Renterghem, C., and Lazdunski, M. (1987). Activation of calcium channels in smooth muscle cells by protein kinase C activators (diacylglycerol and phorbol esters) and by peptides (vasopressin and bombesin) that stimulate phosphoinositide breakdown. *J. Biol. Chem.* **262**, 6947–6950.

Galvan, M., and Adams, P. R. (1982). Control of calcium current in rat sympathetic neurons by norepinephrine. *Brain Res.* **244**, 135–144.

Garcia, M. K., King, V. F., Siegl, P. K. S., Reuben, J. P., and Kaczorowski, G. J. (1986). Binding of Ca^{2+} entry blockers to cardiac sarcolemmal membrane vesicles. *J. Biol. Chem.* **261**, 8146–8157.

Gilly, W. M. F., and Scheuer, T. (1984). Contractile activation in scorpion striated muscle fibers. *J. Gen. Physiol.* **84**, 321–345.

Gjörstrup, P., Harding, H., Isaksson, R., and Westerlund, C. (1986). The enantiomers of the dihydropyridine derivative H 160/51 show opposite effects of stimulation and inhibition. *Eur. J. Pharmacol.* **122**, 357–361.

Glossmann, H., and Ferry, D. R. (1982). *FEBS Lett.* **148**, 331–337.

Glossmann, H., and Ferry, D. R. (1983a). Molecular approach to the calcium channel. *Drug. Dev.* **9**, 63–98.

Glossmann, H., and Ferry, D. R. (1983b). Solubilization and partial purification of putative calcium channels labelled with [^{3}H]nimodipine. *Naunyn–Schmiedeberg's Arch. Pharmacol.* **323**, 279–291.

Glossmann, H., and Ferry, D. R. (1985). Assay for calcium channels. *In* "Methods in Enzymology" (L. Birnbaumer, ed.), Vol. 109, pp. 513–550. Academic Press, Orlando, Florida.

Glossmann, H., Ferry, D. R.. Lübbecke, F., Mewes, R., and Hofmann, F. (1982). Calcium channels: Direct identification with radioligand binding studies. *Trends Pharmacol. Sci.* **3**, 431–437.

Glossmann, H., Linn, T., Rhombusch, M., and Ferry, D. R. (1983a). Temperature-dependent regulation of [^{3}H]d-cis-diltiazem binding to Ca^{2+} channels by 1,4-dihydropyridine channel agonists and antagonists. *FEBS Lett.* **160**, 226–232.

Glossmann, H., Ferry, D. R., and Boschek, C. B. (1983b). Purification of the putative calcium channel from skeletal muscle with the aid of [^{3}H]nimodipine binding. *Naunyn–Schmiedeberg's Arch. Pharmacol.* **323**, 1–11.

Glossmann, H., Ferry, D. R., and Goll, A. (1984a). Molecular pharmacology of the calcium channel. *Proc. IUPHAR Int. Congr. Pharmacol. 9th,* pp. 329–336.

Glossmann, H., Ferry, D. R., and Rombusch, M. (1984b). Molecular pharmacology of the calcium channel: Evidence for subtypes, multiple drug-receptor sites, channel subunits, and the development of a radioiodinated 1,4-dihydropyridine calcium channel label, [^{125}I]iodipine. *J. Cardiovasc. Pharmacol.* **6,** 608–621.

Glossmann, H., Ferry, D. R., Goll, A., Striessnig, J., and Zernig, G. (1985a). Calcium channels and calcium channel drugs: Recent biochemical and biophysical findings. *Arzneim. Forsch.* **35,** 1917–1935.

Glossmann, H., Ferry, D. R., Goll, A., Striessnig, J., and Schober, M. (1985b). Calcium channels: Basic properties as revealed by radioligand binding studies. *J. Cardiovasc. Pharmacol.* **7,** S20–S30.

Glossmann, H., Ferry, D. R., Goll, A., Striessnig, J., and Zernig, G. (1985c). Calcium channels: Introduction to their molecular pharmacology. *In* "Cardiovascular Effects of Dihydropyridine-Type Calcium Antagonists and Agonists" (A. Fleckenstein, C. van Breemen, R. Gross, and F. Hoffmeister, eds.), pp. 113–139. Springer-Verlag, Berlin.

Glossmann, H., Striessnig, J., Hymel, L., and Schindler, H. (1987a). Purification and reconstitution of calcium channel drug receptor sites. *Ann. N.Y. Acad. Sci.* (in press).

Glossmann, H., Ferry, D. R., Striessnig, J., Goll, A., and Moosburger, K. (1987b). Resolving the structure of the Ca^{2+} channel by photoaffinity labeling. *Trends Pharmacol. Sci.* **8,** 95–100.

Glossmann, H., Striessnig, J., Ferry, D. R., Goll, A., Moosburger, K., and Schirmer, M. (1987c). Interaction between calcium channel ligands and calcium channels. *Circ. Res.* **61,** 130–136.

Godfraind, T., Miller, R., and Wibo, M. (1986). Calcium antagonism and calcium entry blockade. *Pharmacol. Rev.* **38,** 321–416.

Goldin, S. M., Rhoden, V., and Hess, E. J. (1985). Molecular characterization, reconstitution, and "transport-specific fractionation" of the saxitoxin binding protein/Na^+ gate of mammalian brain. *Proc. Natl. Acad. Sci. U.S.A.* **77,** 6884–6888.

Goll, A., Ferry, D. R., and Glossmann, H. (1983a). Target size analysis of skeletal muscle Ca^{2+}-channels. Positive allosteric heterotropic regulation by *d-cis*-diltiazem is associated with apparent channel oligomer dissociation. *FEBS Lett.* **157,** 63–69.

Goll, A., Ferry, D. R., and Glossmann, H. (1983b). Target size analysis reveals subunit composition of calcium channels in brain and skeletal muscle. *Naunyn–Schmiedeberg's Arch. Pharmacol.* **324,** 178.

Goll, A., Ferry, D. R., Striessnig, J., Schober, M., and Glossmann, H. (1984a). (−)-[^{3}H]Desmethoxyverapamil, a novel Ca^{2+} channel probe. Binding characteristics and target size analysis of its receptor in skeletal muscle, *FEBS Lett.* **176,** 371–377.

Goll, A., Ferry, D. R., and Glossmann, H. (1984b). Target size analysis and molecular properties of Ca^{2+}-channels labelled with [^{3}H]verapamil. *Eur. J. Biochem.* **141,** 177–186.

Goll, A., Glossmann, H., and Mannhold, R. (1986). Correlation between the negative inotropic potency and binding parameters of 1,4-dihydropyridine and phenylalkylamine calcium channel blockers in cat heart. *Naunyn–Schmiedeberg's Arch. Pharmacol.* **334,** 303–312.

Gonzales-Serratos, H., Valle-Aguilera, R., Lathrop, D. A., and Garcia, M. d. C. (1982).

Slow inward-calcium currents have no obvious role in muscle excitation–contraction coupling. *Nature (London)* **298**, 292–294.

Gould, R. J., Murphy, K. M. M., and Snyder, S. H. (1982). [³H]Nitrendipine-labelled calcium channels discriminate inorganic calcium agonists and antagonists *Proc. Natl. Acad. Sci. U.S.A.* **79**, 3656–3660.

Gould, R. J., Murphy, K. M. M.. Reynolds, I. J., and Snyder, S. H. (1983a). Antischizophrenic drugs of the diphenylbutylpiperidine type act as calcium channel antagonists. *Proc. Natl. Acad. Sci. U.S.A.* **80**, 5122–5125.

Gould, R. J., Murphy, K. M. M., and Snyder, H. (1983b). Tissue heterogeneity of calcium channel antagonist binding sites labeled by [³H]nitrendipine. *Mol. Pharmacol.* **25**, 235–241.

Gray, R., and Johnston, D. (1987). Noradrenaline and β-adrenoceptor agonists increase activity of voltage-dependent calcium channels in hippocampal neurons. *Nature (London)* **327**, 620–622.

Greenberg, D. A., Cooper, E. C., and Carpenter, C. L. (1985). Reversible dihydropyridine isothiocyanate binding to brain calcium channels. *J. Neurochem.* **44**, 319–321.

Gross, R. A., and MacDonald, R. L. (1987). Dynorphin A selectively reduces a large transient (N-type) calcium current of mouse dorsal root ganglion neurons in cell culture. *Proc. Natl. Acad. Sci. U.S.A.* **84**, 5469–5473.

Hagiwara, S., and Byerly, L. (1981). Calcium channel. *Annu. Rev. Neurosci.* **4**, 69–125.

Hamilton, S. L., Yatani, A., Hawkes, M. J., Redding, K., and Brown, A. M. (1985). Atrotoxin: A specific agonist for calcium currents in heart. *Science* **229**, 182–184.

Harris, K. M., Kongsamut, S., and Miller, R. J. (1986). Protein kinase C mediated regulation of calcium channels in PC-12 pheochromocytoma cells. *Biochem. Biophys. Res. Commun.* **134**, 1298–1305.

Hartzell, H. C., and Fischmeister, R. (1986). Opposite effects of cyclic GMP and cyclic AMP on Ca^{2+} current in single heart cells. *Nature (London)* **323**, 273–275.

Heizmann, C. W., and Berchtold, M. W. (1987). Expression of parvalbumin and other Ca^{2+}-binding proteins in normal and tumor cells: A topical review. *Cell Calcium* **8**, 1–41.

Hescheler, J., Kameyama, M., and Trautwein, W. (1986). On the mechanism of muscarinic inhibition of the cardiac Ca current. *Pflügers Arch.* **407**, 182–189.

Hescheler, J., Rosenthal, W., Trautwein, W., and Schultz, G. (1987). The GTP-binding protein, G_o, regulates neuronal calcium channels. *Nature (London)* **325**, 445–447.

Hess, P., and Tsien, R. W. (1984). Mechanism of ion permeation through calcium channels. *Nature (London)* **309**, 453–456.

Hess, P., Lansman, J. B., and Tsien, R. W. (1986). Calcium channel selectivity for divalent and monovalent cations. *J. Gen. Physiol.* **88**, 293–319.

Hidalgo, C., Carrasco, M. A., Magendzo, K., and Jaimovich, E. (1986). Phosphorylation of phosphatidylinositol by transverse tubule vesicles and its possible role in excitation–contraction coupling. *FEBS Lett.* **202**, 69–73.

Hille, B. (1984). "Ionic Channels of Excitable Membranes." Sinauer, Sunderland, Massachusetts.

Hille, B., and Schwarz, W. (1978). Potassium channels as multi-ion single-file pores. *J. Gen. Physiol.* **72**, 409–442.

Hirashawa, K., and Nishizuka, Y. (1985). Phosphatidylinositol turnover in receptor mechanism and signal transduction. *Annu. Rev. Pharmacol. Toxicol.* **25**, 147–170.

Hof, R. P., Rüegg, U. T., Hof, A., and Vogel, A. (1985). A stereoselectivity at the calcium channel: opposite action of the enantiomers of a 1,4-dihydropyridine. *J. Cardiovasc. Pharmacol.* **7**, 687–693.

Hofmann, F., Nastainczyk, W., Röhrkasten, A., Schneider, T., and Sieber, M. (1987). Regulation of the L-type calcium channel. *Trends Pharmacol. Sci.* **8**, 393–398.

Höltje, H.-D., and Marrer, S. (1987). A molecular graphics study on structure–action relationship of calcium antagonistic and agonistic 1,4-dihydropyridines. *J. Comput. Aid. Mol. Des.* **1**, 23–30.

Holz IV, G. G., Shefner, S. A., and Anderson, E. G. (1986a). Serotonin decreases the duration of action potentials recorded from tetraethylammonium-treated bullfrog dorsal root ganglion cells. *J. Neurosci.* **6**, 620–626.

Holz IV, G. G., Rane, S. G., and Dunlap, K. (1986b). GTP-binding proteins mediate transmitter inhibition of voltage-dependent calcium channels. *Nature (London)* **319**, 670–672.

Hondeghem, L. M., and Katzung, B. G. (1977). Time and voltage dependent interactions of antiarrhythmic drugs with cardiac sodium channels. *Biochim. Biophys. Acta* **472**, 373–398.

Horn, J. P., and McAfee, D. A. (1980). α-Adrenergic inhibition of calcium dependent potentials in rat sympathetic neurons. *J. Physiol. (London)* **301**, 191–204.

Horne, P., Triggle, D. J., and Venter, J. C. (1984). Nitrendipine and isoproterenol induce phosphorylation of A 42,000 dalton protein that co-migrates with the affinity labeled calcium channel regulatory subunit. *Biochem. Biophys. Res. Commun.* **121**, 890–898.

Horne, W. A., Weiland, G. A., and Oswald, R. E. (1986). Solubilization and hydrodynamic characterization of the dihydropyridine receptor from rat ventricular muscle. *J. Biol. Chem.* **261**, 3588–3594.

Horwitz, L. (1986). Pharmacology of calcium channels and smooth muscle. *Annu. Rev. Pharmacol. Toxicol.* **26**, 225–258.

Hosey, M. M., Borsotto, M., and Lazdunski, M. (1986). Phosphorylation and dephosphorylation of dihydropyridine-sensitive voltage-dependent Ca^{2+} channel in skeletal muscle membranes by cAMP- and Ca^{2+}-dependent processes. *Proc. Natl. Acad. Sci. U.S.A.* **83**, 3733–3737.

Hui, C. S., Milton, R. L., and Eisenberg, R. S. (1983). Charge movement in skeletal muscle fibers paralyzed by the calcium entry blocker D600. *Proc. Natl. Acad. Sci. U.S.A.* **81**, 2582–2585.

Huxley, A. F. (1971). The Croonian Lecture 1967. The activation of striated muscle and its mechanical response. *Proc. R. Soc. London Ser. B* **178**, 1–27.

Hymel, L., Inui, M., Fleischer, S., and Schindler, H. (1988a). Purified ryanodine receptor of skeletal muscle sarcoplasmic reticulum forms calcium activated oligomeric calcium channels in planar bilayers. *Proc. Natl. Acad. Sci. U.S.A.* **85**, 441–445.

Hymel, L., Striessnig, J., Glossmann, H., and Schindler, H. (1988b). Purified skeletal muscle 1,4-dihydropyridine receptor forms phosphorylation-dependent oligomeric calcium channels in planar bilayers. *Proc. Natl. Acad. Sci. U.S.A.* (in press).

Hymel, L., Inui, M., Striessnig, J., Fleischer, S., Glossmann, H., and Schindler, H. (1988c). *Ann. N.Y. Acad. Sci.* (in press).

Ildefonse, M., Jacquemond, V., Rougier, O., Renaud, J. F., Fosset, M., and Lazdunski, M. (1985). Excitation–contraction coupling in skeletal muscle: Evidence for a role of slow Ca^{2+} channels using Ca^{2+} channel activators and inhibitors in the dihydropyridine series. *Biochem. Biophys. Res. Commun.* **129**, 904–909.

Imagawa, T., Leung, A. T., and Campbell, K. (1987a). Phosphorylation of the 1,4-dihydropyridine receptor of the voltage-dependent Ca^{2+} channel by an intrinsic protein kinase in isolated triads from rabbit skeletal muscle. *J. Biol. Chem.* **262**, 8333–8339.

Imagawa, T., Smith, J. S., Coronado. R., and Campbell, K. P. (1987b). Purified ryanodine receptor from skeletal muscle sarcoplasmic reticulum is the Ca^{2+}-permeable pore of the calcium release channel. *J. Biol. Chem.* **262**, 16636–16643.

Inui, M., Saito, A., and Fleischer, S. (1987a). Purification of the ryanodine receptor and identity with feet structures of junctional terminal cisternae of sarcoplasmatic reticulum from fast skeletal muscle. *J. Biol. Chem.* **262**, 1740–1747.

Inui, M., Saito, A., and Fleischer, S. (1987b). Isolation of the ryanodine receptor from cardiac sarcoplasmatic reticulum and identity with the feet structures. *J. Biol. Chem.* **262**, in press.

Judd, A. M., Koike, K., Yasumoto, T., and MacLeod, R. M. (1986). Protein kinase C activators and calcium-mobilizing agents synergistically increase GH, LH, and TSH secretion from anterior pituitary cells. *Neuroendocrinology* **42**, 197–202.

Kameyama, M., Hescheler, J., Hofmann, F., and Trautwein, W. (1986). Modulation of Ca current during the phosphorylation cycle in guinea pig heart. *Pflügers Arch.* **407**, 123–128.

Kaumann, A. J., and Uchitel, O. D. (1976). Reversible inhibition of potassium contractures by optical isomers of verapamil and D 600 on slow muscle fibres of the frog. *Naunyn–Schmiedeberg's Arch. Pharmacol.* **292**, 21–27.

Kerr, L. M., and Sperelakis, N. (1982). Effects of the calcium antagonists bepridil (CERM-1978) and verapamil on Ca^{++}-dependent slow action potentials in frog skeletal muscle. *J. Pharmacol. Exp. Ther.* **222**, 80–86.

King, V. F., Garcia, M. L., Himmel, D., Reuben, J. P., Pan, J.-X., Lam, Y.-K. T., and Kaczorowski, G. J. (1988a). Interaction of tetrandrine with slowly inactivating calcium channels: Characterization of calcium channel modulation by an alkaloid of Chinese medicinal herb origin. *J. Biol. Chem.* **263**, 2238–2244.

King, V. F., Garcia, M. L., and Kaczorowski, G. J. (1988b). Interaction of fluspirilene with cardiac L-type calcium channels. *Biophys. J.* **53**, 557a.

Kirley, T. L., and Schwartz, A. (1984). Solubilization and affinity labeling of a dihydropyridine binding site from skeletal muscle: Effects of temperature and diltiazem on [^{3}H]dihydropyridine binding to transverse tubules. *Biochem. Biophys. Res. Commun.* **123**, 41–49.

Knaus, H.-G., Striessnig, J., Koza, A., and Glossmann, H. (1987). Neurotoxic aminoglycoside antibiotics are potent inhibitors of [^{125}I]-ω-conotoxin GVIA binding to guinea pig cerebral cortex membranes. *Naunyn–Schmiedeberg's Arch. Pharmacol.* **336**, 583–586.

Knudson, C. M., Jay, S. D., and Beam, K. G. (1986). Developmental increase in skeletal muscle slow calcium current. *Biophys. J.* **49**, 13a.

Koketsu, K., and Akasu, T. (1982). Modulation of slow inward Ca current by adrenaline in bullfrog sympathetic ganglia. *Jpn. J. Physiol.* **32**, 137–140.

Kokubun, S., Prod'hom, B., Becker, C., Porzig, H., and Reuter, H. (1986). Studies on Ca channels in intact cardiac cells: Voltage dependent effects and cooperative interactions of dihydropyridine enantiomers. *Mol. Pharmacol.* **30**, 571–584.

Kostyuk, P. G., Veselovsky, N. S., and Fedulova, S. A. (1981). Ionic current in the somatic membrane of rat dorsal root ganglion neurons—II. Calcium current. *Neuroscience* **6**, 2431–2437.

Kostyuk, P. G., Mironov, S. L., and Shuba, Ya. M. (1983). Two ion-selecting filters in the calcium channel of the somatic membrane of mollusc neurons. *J. Membr. Biol.* **76**, 83–93.

Kozlowski, R., Ehrhard, P., Fischli, W., Osterrieder, W., and Holck, M. (1986). *o*-Isothiocyanato-dihydropyridine (oNCS-DHP), a long-acting reversible inhibitor of the Ca^{++} channel. *J. Pharmacol. Exp. Ther.* **238**, 1084–1091.

Lai, F. A., Erickson, H. P., Rousseau, E., Liu, Q. Y., and Meissner, G. (1988). Purification and reconstitution of the calcium release channel from skeletal muscle. *Nature (London)* **331**, 315–319.

Lamb, G. D. (1986a). Components of asymmetric charge movement in contracting skeletal muscle fibers of the rabbit. *Biophys. J.* **49**, 12a.

Lamb, G. D. (1986b). Asymmetric charge movement in contracting muscle fibers in the rabbit. *J. Physiol. (London)* **376**, 63–83.

Lamb, G. D. (1986c). Components of asymmetric charge movement in rabbit skeletal muscle: Effects of tetracaine and nifedipine. *J. Physiol. (London)* **376**, 85–100.

Langs, D. A., and Triggle, D. J. (1984). Chemical structure and pharmacological activities of Ca^{2+} channel antagonists. *Proc. IUPHAR Int. Congr. Pharmacol., 9th* **2**, 323–328.

Langs, D. A., and Triggle, D. J. (1985). Conformational features of calcium channel agonist and antagonist analogs of nifedipine. *Mol. Pharmacol.* **27**, 544–548.

Lansman, J. B., Hess, P., and Tsien, R. W. (1986). Blockade of current through single calcium channels by Cd^{2+}, Mg^{2+}. and Ca^{2+}. *J. Gen. Physiol.* **88**, 321–347.

Lea, T. J., Griffiths, P. J., Tregear, R. T, and Ashley, C. C. (1986). An examination of the ability of inositol 1,4,5-trisphosphate to induce calcium release and tension development in skinned skeletal muscle fibres of frog and crustacea. *FEBS Lett.* **207**, 153–161.

Lee, H. R., Jaros, J. A., Roeske, W. R., Wiech, N. L., Ursillo, R., and Yamamura, H. I. (1985). Potent enhancement of [^{3}H]nitrendipine binding in rat cerebral cortical and cardiac homogenates: A putative mechanism for the action of MDL 12,330A. *J. Pharmacol. Exp. Therp.* **233**, 611–616.

Lee, K. S., and Tsien, R. W. (1983). Mechanisms of calcium channel blockade by verapamil, D600, diltiazem and nitrendipine in single dialysed heart cells. *Nature (London)* **302**, 790–794.

Leonard, J. P., Nargeot, J., Snutch, T.P., Davidson, N., and Lester, H. A. (1987). Ca channels induced in *Xenopus* oocytes by rat brain mRNA. *J. Neurosci.* **7**, 875–881.

Leung, A. T., Imagawa, T., and Campbell, K. P. (1987). Structural characterization of the 1,4-dihydropyridine receptor of the voltage-dependent calcium channel from rabbit skeletal muscle. Evidence for two distinct high molecular weight subunits. *J. Biol. Chem.* **262**, 7943–7946.

Levi, R., and DeFelice, L. J. (1986). Sodium-conducting channels in cardiac membranes in low calcium. *Biophys. J.* **50**, 5–9.

Lewis, D. L., Weight, F. F., and Luini, A. (1986). A guanine nucleotide-binding protein mediates the inhibition of voltage-dependent calcium current by somatostatin in a pituitary cell line. *Proc. Natl. Acad. Sci. U.S.A.* **83**, 9035–9039.

Linn, T., Ferry, D. R., and Glossmann, H. (1983). A novel phosphonate slow channel blocker is an allosteric regulator of 1,4-dihydropyridine binding. *Naunyn–Schmiedeberg's Arch. Pharmacol.* **324**, R45.

Lopez, J. R., Alamo, L., Caputo, C., and Dipold, R. (1983). Determination of ionic calcium in frog skeletal muscle fibers. *Biophys. J.* **43**, 1–4.

Luchowski, E. M., Yousif, F., Triggle, D. J., Maurer, S. C., Sarmiento, J. G., and Janis, R. A. (1984). Effects of metal cations and calmodulin antagonists on [^{3}H]nitrendipine binding in smooth and cardiac muscle. *J. Pharmacol. Exp. Ther.* **230**, 607–613.

Lüttgau, H. Ch., Gottschalk, G., and Berwe, D. (1986). The role of Ca^{2+} in inactivation and paralysis of excitation–contraction coupling in skeletal muscle. *Prog. Zool.* **33,** 195–204.

McAfee, D. A., Henon, B. K., Horn, J. P., and Yarowsky, P. (1981). Calcium currents modulated by adrenergic receptors in sympathetic neurons. *Fed. Proc., Fed. Am. Soc. Exp. Biol.* **40,** 2246–2249.

McCleskey, E. W. (1985). Calcium channels and intracellular calcium release are pharmacologically different in frog skeletal muscle. *J. Physiol. (London)* **361,** 231–249.

McCleskey, E. W., and Almers, W. (1985). The Ca channel in skeletal muscle is a large pore. *Proc. Natl. Acad. Sci. U.S.A.* **82,** 7149–7153.

McCleskey, E. W., Fox, A. P., Feldman, D., and Tsien, R. W. (1986). Different types of calcium channels. *J. Exp. Biol.* **124,** 177–190.

McCleskey, E. W., Fox, A. P., Feldman, D. H., Cruz, L. J., Olivera, B. M., Tsien, R.-W., and Yoshikami, D. (1987). ω-Conotoxin: Direct and persistent blockade of specific types of calcium channels in neurons but not muscle. *Proc. Natl. Acad. Sci. U.S.A.* **84,** 4327–4331.

MacDonald, R. L., and Werz, M. A. (1986). Dynorphin decreases voltage-dependent calcium conductance of mouse dorsal root ganglion neurones. *J. Physiol. (London)* **377,** 237–249.

MacDonald, R. L., Skerritt, J. H., and Werz, M. A. (1986). Adenosine agonists reduce voltage-dependent calcium conductance of mouse sensory neurones in cell culture. *J. Physiol. (London)* **370,** 75–90.

McDonald, T. F., Pelzer, D., and Trautwein, W. (1984). Cat ventricular muscle treated with D600: Characteristics of calcium block and unblock. *J. Physiol. (London)* **354,** 217–241.

MacVicar, B. A. (1984). Voltage-dependent calcium channel in glial cells. *Science* **226,** 1345–1347.

Mannhold, R., Höltje, H.-D., and Koke, V. (1986). Importance of nitrile substitution for the Ca antagonistic action of verapamil. *Arch. Pharmacol.* **319,** 990–998.

Mannhold, R., Bayer, M., Ronsdorf, M., and Martens, L. (1987). Comparative QSAR studies on vasodilatory and negative inotropic properties of ring-varied verapamil congeners. *Arzneim. Forsch.* **37,** 419–424.

Marchetti, C., Carbone, E., and Lux, H. D. (1986). Effects of dopamine and noradrenaline on Ca channels of cultured sensory and sympathetic neurons of chick. *Pflügers Arch.* **406,** 104–111.

Mathias, R. T., Levis, R. A., and Eisenberg, R. S. (1980). Electrical models of excitation–contraction coupling and charge movement in skeletal muscle. *J. Gen. Physiol.* **76,** 1–31.

Meissner, G. (1984). Adenine nucleotide stimulation of Ca-induced Ca release in sarcoplasmic reticulum. *J. Biol. Chem.* **259,** 2365–2374.

Melzer, W., Schneider, M. F., Simon, B. J.. and Szuges, G. (1986). Intramembrane charge movement and calcium release in frog skeletal muscle. *J. Physiol. (London)* **373,** 481–511.

Messing, R. O., Carpenter, C. L., and Greenberg, D. A. (1986). Inhibition of calcium flux and calcium channel agonist binding in the PC12 neural cell line by phorbol esters and protein kinase C. *Biochem. Biophys. Res. Commun.* **136,** 1049–1056.

Meyer, H., Wehinger, E., Bossert, F., Böshagen, H., Franckowiak, G., Goldmann, S., Seidel, W., and Stoltefuss, J. (1985). Chemistry of 1,4-dihydropyridines. *In* "Cardiovascular Effects of Dihydropyridine Type Calcium Antagonists and Agonists" (A. Fleckenstein, C. Van Breemen, R. Gross, and F. Hoffmeister, eds.), pp. 90–103. Springer Verlag, Berlin.

Miller, C. (1986). "Ion Channel Reconstitution." Plenum, New York.

Miller, R. J. (1985). How many types of calcium channels exist in neurones? *Trends Neurosci.* **8,** 45–47.

Miller, R. J. (1987). Multiple calcium channels and neuronal function. *Science* **235,** 46–52.

Mir, A. K., and Spedding, M. (1987). Calcium-antagonist properties of diclofurime isomers. II. Molecular aspects: Allosteric interactions with dihydropyridine recognition sites. *J. Cardiovasc. Pharmacol.* **9,** 469–477.

Mitchell, R. D., Saito, A.. Palade, P., and Fleischer, S. (1983). Morphology of isolated triads. *J. Cell Biol.* **96,** 1017–1029.

Mo, N., Ammari, R., and Dun, N. J. (1985). Prostaglandin E_1 inhibits calcium-dependent potentials in mammalian sympathetic neurons. *Brain Res.* **334,** 325–329.

Mobley, B. A., and Eisenberg, B. R. (1975). Sizes of components in frog skeletal muscle measured by methods of stereology. *J. Gen. Physiol.* **66,** 31–45.

Moorman, R. J., Zhou, Z., Kirsch, G. E., Lacerda, A. E., Caffrey, J. M., Lam, D. M.-K., Joho, R. H., and Brown, A. M. (1987). Expression of single calcium channels in *Xenopus* oocytes after injection of mRNA from rat heart. *Am. J. Physiol.* 253, H985–H991.

Morton, M. E., and Froehner, S. C. (1987). Monoclonal antibody identifies a 200-kDa subunit of the dihydropyridine-sensitive calcium channel. *J. Biol. Chem.* **262,** 11904–11907.

Murphy, K. M. M., Gould, R. J., Largent, B. L., and Snyder, S. H. (1983). A unitary mechanism of calcium antagonist drug action. *Proc. Natl. Acad. Sci. U.S.A.* **80,** 860–864.

Nagao, T., Sato, M., Iwasawa, Y., Takada, T., Ishida, R., Nakajima, H., and Kiyomoto, A. (1972). Studies on a new 1,5-benzothiazepine derivative (CRD-401). III. Effects of optical isomers of CRD-401 on smooth muscle and other pharmacological properties. *Jpn. J. Pharmacol.* **22,** 467–478.

Nakayama, N., Kirley, T. L., Vaghy, P. L., McKenna, E., and Schwartz, A. (1987). Purification of a putative calcium channel protein from rabbit skeletal muscle. *J. Biol. Chem.* **262,** 6572–6576.

Nelson, M. T. (1986). Interactions of divalent cations with single calcium channels from rat brain synaptosomes. *J. Gen. Physiol.* **87,** 201–222.

Nelson, M. T., French, R. J., and Krueger, B. K. (1984). Voltage-dependent calcium channels from brain incorporated into planar lipid bilayers. *Nature (London)* **308,** 77–80.

Neuhaus, R. (1986). The effect of nifedipine on slow Ca^{2+} inward current and force development in skeletal muscle fibers of the frog. *J. Physiol. (London)* **378,** 128P.

Nilius, B., Hess, P., Lansman, J. B., and Tsien, R. W. (1985). A novel type of cardiac calcium channel in ventricular cells. *Nature (London)* **316,** 443–446.

Nilius, B., Hess, P., Lansman, J. B., and Tsien, T. W. (1986). Two kinds of calcium channels in isolated ventricular cells from guinea pig heart. *Prog. Zool.* **33,** 75–82.

Noda, M., Takayuki, I., Suzuki, H., Takeshima, H., Takahashi, T., Kuno, M., and Numa, S. (1986). Expression of functional sodium channels from cloned cDNA. *Nature (London)* **322,** 826–828.

Norman, R. I., Borsotto, M., Fosset, M., and Lazdunski, M. (1983). Determination of the molecular size of the nitrendipine-sensitive Ca^{2+}-channel by radiation inactivation. *Biochem. Biophys. Res. Commun.* **111,** 878–883.

Norman, R. I., Burgess, A. J., Allen, E., and Harrison, T. M. (1987). Monoclonal antibodies against the 1,4-dihydropyridine receptor associated with voltage-sensitive

Ca^{2+} channels detect similar polypeptides from a variety of tissues and species. *FEBS Lett.* **212**, 127–132.

North, R. A., and Williams, J. T. (1983). Opiate activation of potassium conductance inhibits calcium action potential in rat locus coeruleus neurones. *Br. J. Pharmacol.* **80**, 225–228.

Nowycky, M. C., Fox, A. P., and Tsien, R. W. (1985a). Three types of neuronal calcium channel with different calcium agonist sensitivity. *Nature (London)* **316**, 440–443.

Nowycky, M. C., Fox, A. P., and Tsien, R. W. (1985b). Long-opening mode of gating of neuronal calcium channels and its promotion by the dihydropyridine calcium agonist Bay K 8644. *Proc. Natl. Acad. Sci. U.S.A.* **82**, 2178–2182.

Oeken, H. J., and Schneider, T. (1987). Purification of the dihydropyridine receptor from bovine cardiac muscle. *Naunyn–Schmiedeberg's Arch. Pharmacol.* **335**, R193.

Ogura, A., and Takahashi, M. (1984). Differential effect of a dihydropyridine to Ca^{2+} entry pathways in neuronal preparations. *Brain Res.* **301**, 323–330.

Olivera, B. M., Gray, W. R., Zeikus, R., McIntosh, J. M., Varga, J., Rivier, J., de Santos, V., and Cruz, L. J. (1985). Peptide neurotoxins from fish-hunting cone snails. *Science* **230**, 1338–1343.

Osterrieder, W., Brum, G., Hescheler, J., and Trautwein, W. (1982). Injection of subunits of cyclic AMP-dependent protein kinase into cardiac myocytes modulates Ca^{2+} current. *Nature (London)* **298**, 576–578.

Osugi, T., Imaizumi, T., Mizushima, A., Uchida, S., and Yoshida, H. (1986). 1-Oleoyl-2-acetyl-glycerol and phorbol diester stimulate Ca^{2+} influx through Ca^{2+} channels in neuroblastoma × glioma hybrid NG108-15 cells. *Eur. J. Pharmacol.* **126**, 47–51.

Paupardin-Tritsch, D., Hammond, C., Gerschenfeld, H. M., Nairn, A. C., and Greengard, P. (1986). cGMP-dependent protein kinase enhances Ca^{2+} current and potentiates the serotonin-induced Ca^{2+} current increase in snail neurones. *Nature (London)* **323**, 812–814.

Pauron, D., Qar, J., Barhanin, J., Fournier, D., Cuany, A., Pralavorio, M., Berge, J.-B., and Lazdunski, M. (1987). Identification and affinity labeling of very high affinity binding sites for the phenylalkylamine series of calcium channel blockers in the *Drosophila* nervous system. *Biochemistry* **26**, 6311–6315.

Pauwels, P. J., Van Assouw, H. P., and Leysen, J. E. (1987). Depolarization of chick myotubes triggers the appearance of $(+)$-[^{3}H]PN200-110-binding sites. *Mol. Pharmacol.* **32**, 785–791.

Peachey, L. P. (1965). The sarcoplasmic reticulum and transverse tubules of the frog's sartorius. *J. Cell Biol.* **25**, 209–231.

Peachey, L. D., and Franzini-Armstrong (1983). Structure and function of membrane systems of skeletal muscle cells. *Handb. Physiol.* **10**, 23–72.

Pelzer, D., Trautwein, W., and McDonald, T. F. (1982). Calcium channel block and recovery from block in mammalian ventricular muscle treated with organic channel inhibitors. *Pflügers Arch.* **394**, 97–105.

Pelzer, D., Cavalié, A., McDonald, T. F., and Trautwein, W. (1986). Macroscopic and elementary currents through cardiac calcium channels. *Prog. Zool.* **33**, 83–98.

Pelzer, D., Cavalie, A., Flockerzi, V., Hofmann, F., and Trautwein, W. (1987). Two types of calcium channels from skeletal muscle transverse tubule in lipid bilayers: Differences in conductance properties, gating kinetics, and chemical modulation. *Pflügers Arch.* **410**, R35 (Abstr.).

Pincon-Raymond, M., Rieger, F., Fosset, M., and Lazdunski, M. (1985). Abnormal transverse tubule system and abnormal amount of receptors for Ca^{2+} channel inhibitors of the dihydropyridine family in skeletal muscle from mice with embryonic muscular dysgenesis. *Dev. Biol.* **112**, 458–466.

Ptasienski, J., McMahon, K. K., and Hosey, M. M. (1985). High and low affinity states of the dihydropyridine and phenylalkylamine receptors on the cardiac calcium channel and their interconversion by divalent cations. *Biochem. Biophys. Res. Commun.* **129**, 910–917.

Qar, J., Schweitz, H., Schmid, A., and Lazdunski, M. (1986). A polypeptide toxin from the coral *Goniopora*. *FEBS Lett.* **202**, 331–336.

Qar, J., Galizzi, J.-P., Fosset, M., and Lazdunski, M. (1987). Receptors for diphenylbutylpiperidine neuroleptics in brain, cardiac and smooth muscle membranes. Relationship with receptors for 1,4-dihydropyridines and phenylalkylamines and with calcium channel blockade. *Eur. J. Pharmacol.* **141**, 261–268.

Racker, E. (1985). "Reconstitution of Transporters, Receptors and Pathological States." Academic Press, London.

Rane, S. G., and Dunlap, K. (1986). Kinase C activator 1,2-oleoylacetylglycerol attenuates voltage-dependent calcium current in sensory neurons. *Proc. Natl. Acad. Sci. U.S.A.* **83**, 184–188.

Rengasamy, A., Ptasienski, J., and Hosey, M. M. (1985). Purification of the cardiac 1,4-dihydropyridine receptor/calcium channel complex. *Biochem. Biophys. Res. Commun.* **126**, 1–7.

Reuter, H. (1983). Calcium channel modulation by neurotransmitters, enzymes and drugs. *Nature (London)* **301**, 569–574.

Reuter, H., and Scholz, H. (1977). The regulation of the calcium conductance of cardiac muscle by adrenaline. *J. Physiol. (London)* **264**, 49–62.

Reuter, H., Kokubun, S., and Prod'hom, B. (1986). Properties and modulation of cardiac calcium channels. *J. Exp. Biol.* **124**, 191–202.

Reynolds, I. J., Wagner, J. A., Snyder, S. H., Thayer, S. A., Olivera, B. M., and Miller, R. J. (1986a). Brain voltage-sensitive calcium channel subtypes differentiated by ω-conotoxin fraction GVIA. *Proc. Natl. Acad. Sci. U.S.A.* **83**, 8804–8807.

Reynolds, I. J., Snowman, A. D., and Snyder, S. H. (1986b). (−)-[^{3}H]Desmethoxyverapamil labels multiple calcium channel modulator receptors in brain and skeletal muscle membranes: Differentiation by temperature and dihydropyridines. *J. Pharmacol. Exp. Ther.* **237**, 731–738.

Rinaldi, M. L., lePeuch, C. J., and Demaille, J. G. (1981). The epinephrine-induced activation of the cardiac slow Ca^{2+} channel is mediated by the cAMP-dependent phosphorylation of calciductin, a 23,000 M_r sarcolemmal protein. *FEBS Lett.* **129**, 277–281.

Rios, E., and Brum, G. (1987). Involvement of dihydropyridine receptors in excitation–contraction coupling in skeletal muscle. *Nature (London)* **325**, 717–720.

Rios, E., Brum, G., and Stefani, E. (1986). E–C coupling effects of interventions that reduce slow Ca^{2+} current suggest a role of T-tubule Ca channels in skeletal muscle function. *Biophys. J.* **49**, 13a.

Rivier, J., Galyean, R., Gray, W. R., Azimi-Zonooz, A., McIntosh, J. M., Cruz, L. J., and Olivera B. M. (1987). Neuronal calcium channel inhibitors: Synthesis of ω-conotoxin GVIA and effects on ^{45}Ca uptake by synaptosomes. *J. Biol. Chem.* **262**, 1194–1198.

Romey, G., Rieger, F., Renaud, J. F., Pincon-Raymond, M., and Lazdunski, M. (1986). The electrophysiological expression of Ca^{2+} channels and of apamin sensitive Ca^{2+} activated K^+ channels is abolished in skeletal muscle cells from mice with muscular dysgenesis. *Biochem. Biophys. Res. Commun.* **136**, 935–940.

Rosenberg, R. L., Hess, P., Reeves, J. P., Smilowitz, H., and Tsien, R. W. (1986). Calcium channels in planar lipid bilayers: Insights into mechanisms of ion permeation and gating. *Science* **231**, 1564–1566.

Ruoho, A. E., Rashidbaigi, A., and Roeder, P. E. (1981). Approaches to the identification of receptors utilizing photoaffinity labelling. *In* "Membranes, Detergents and Receptor Solubilisation" (J. C. Venter and L. C. Harrison, eds.), pp. 119–160. Liss, New York.

Ruth, P., Flockerzi, V., von Nettelbladt, E., Oeken, J., and Hofman, F. (1985). Characterization of the binding site for nimodipine and (−)-desmethoxyverapamil in bovine cardiac sarcolemma. *Eur. J. Biochem.* **150**, 313–322.

Ruth, P., Flockerzi, V., Oeken, H. J., and Hofmann, F. (1986). Solubilization of the bovine cardiac sarcolemmal binding sites for calcium channel blockers. *Eur. J. Biochem.* **155**, 613–620.

Sagi-Eisenberg, R., Lieman, H., and Pecht, I. (1985). Protein kinase C regulation of the receptor-coupled calcium signal in histamine-secreting rat basophilic leukaemia cells. *Nature (London)* **313**, 59–60.

Sakman, B., and Neher, E. (1983). "Single Channel Recording." Plenum, New York.

Salkoff, L., and Wyman, R. (1983). Ion currents in *Drosophila* flight muscles. *J. Physiol.* **337**, 687–709.

Sandow, A. (1952). Excitation–contraction coupling in muscular response. *Yale J. Biol. Med.* **25**, 176–201.

Sandow, A. (1965). Excitation–contraction coupling in skeletal muscle. *Pharmacol. Rev.* **17**, 265–320.

Sanguinetti, M. C., and Kass, R. S. (1984). Voltage-dependent block of calcium channel current in the calf cardiac purkinje fiber by dihydropyridine calcium channel antagonists. *Circ. Res.* **55**, 336–348.

Sanguinetti, M. C., Krafte, D. S., and Kass, R. S. (1986). Voltage-dependent modulation of Ca channel current in heart cells by Bay K 8644. *J. Gen. Physiol.* **88**, 369–392.

Sarmiento, J. G., Epstein, P. M., Rowe, W. A., Chester, D. W., Smilowitz, H., Wehinger, E., and Janis, R. A. (1986). Photoaffinity labelling of a 33–35,000 dalton protein in cardiac, skeletal and smooth muscle membranes using a new ^{125}I-labelled 1,4-dihydropyridine calcium channel antagonist. *Life Sci.* **39**, 2401–2409.

Scherer, N. M., and Ferguson, J. E. (1985). Inositol 1,4,5-trisphosphate is not effective in releasing calcium from skeletal sarcoplasmic reticulum microsomes. *Biochem. Biophys. Res. Commun.* **128**, 1064–1070.

Scheuer, T., and Gilly, W. F. (1986). Charge movement and depolarization–contraction coupling in arthropod vs. vertebrate skeletal muscle. *Proc. Natl. Acad. Sci. U.S.A.* **83**, 8799–8803.

Schindler, H. (1980). Formation of planar bilayers from artificial or native membrane vesicles. *FEBS Lett.* **122**, 77–79.

Schindler, H. (1988). Planar lipid–protein membranes: Strategies of formation and of detecting dependencies of ion transport functions on membrane conditions. *In* "Methods in Enzymology" (in press). Academic Press, San Diego, California.

Schindler, H., Spillecke, F., and Neumann, E. (1984). Differential channel properties of torpedo acetylcholine receptor monomers and dimers reconstituted in planar membranes. *Proc. Natl. Acad. Sci. U.S.A.* **81**, 6222–6226.

Schmid, A., Renaud, J. F., Fosset, M., Meaux, J. P., and Lazdunski, M. (1984). The nitrendipine-selective Ca^{2+} channel in chick muscle cells and its appearance during myogenesis *in vitro* and *in vivo*. *J. Biol. Chem.* **259**, 11366–11372.

Schmid, A., Renaud, J.-F., and Lazdunski, M. (1985). Short-term and long-term effects of β-adrenergic effectors and cyclic AMP on nitrendipine-sensitive voltage-dependent Ca^{2+} channels of skeletal muscle. *J. Biol. Chem.* **260**, 13041–13046.

Schmid, A., Barhanin, J., Coppola, T., Borsotto, M., and Lazdunski, M. (1986a). Immunochemical analysis of subunit structures of 1,4-dihydropyridine receptors associated with voltage-dependent Ca^{2+} channels in skeletal, cardiac and smooth muscles. *Biochemistry* **25**, 3492–3495.

Schmid, A., Barhanin, J., Mourre, C., Coppola, T., Borsotto, M., and Lazdunski, M. (1986b). Antibodies reveal the cytolocalization and subunit structure of the 1,4-dihydropyridine component of the neuronal calcium channel. *Biochem. Biophys. Res. Commun.* **139**, 996–1002.

Schneider, M. F. (1981). Membrane charge movement and depolarization–contraction coupling. *Annu. Rev. Physiol.* **43**, 507–517.

Schneider, M. F., and Chandler, W. K. (1973). Voltage dependent charge movement in skeletal muscle: A possible step in excitation–contraction coupling. *Nature (London)* **242**, 244–246.

Schoemaker, H., and Langer, S. Z. (1985). [^{3}H]Diltiazem binding to calcium channel antagonists recognition sites in rat cerebral cortex. *Eur. J. Pharmacol.* **111**, 273–277.

Schramm, M., Towart, T. G., and Franckowiak, G. (1983). Novel dihydropyridines with positive inotropic action through activation of Ca^{2+} channels. *Nature (London)* **303**, 535–537.

Schramm, M., Bechem, M., Franckowiak, G., Towart, G. T., and Towart, R. (1986). Calcium antagonist and calcium agonist drugs. *Neurol. Neurobiol.* **20**, 213–225.

Schwartz, L. M., McCleskey, E. W., and Almers, W. (1985). Dihydropyridine receptors in muscle are voltage-dependent but most are not functional calcium channels. *Nature (London)* **314**, 747–750.

Scott, R. H., and Dolphin, A. C. (1986). Regulation of calcium currents by a GTP analogue: Potentiation of (−)-baclofen-mediated inhibition. *Neurosci. Lett.* **69**, 59–64.

Scott, R. H., and Dolphin, A. C. (1987a). Activation of a G protein promotes agonist responses to calcium channel ligands. *Nature (London)* **330**, 760–762.

Scott, R. H., and Dolphin, A. C. (1987b). Calcium channel currents and their inhibition by (−)-baclofen in rat sensory neurons: Modulation by guanine nucleotides. *J. Physiol.* **386**, 1–17.

Sharp, A. H., Imagawa, T., Leung, A. T., and Campbell, K. P. (1987). Identification and characterization of the dihydropyridine-binding subunit of the skeletal muscle dihydropyridine receptor. *J. Biol. Chem.* **262**, 12309–12315.

Sieber, M., Nastainczyk, W., Zubor, V., Wernet, W., and Hofmann, F. (1987). The 165 kDa peptide of the purified skeletal muscle dihydropyridine receptor contains the known regulatory sites of the calcium channel. *Eur. J. Biochem.* **167**, 117–122.

Smith, J. S., McKenna, E. J., Ma, J., Vilven, J., Vaghy, P. L., Schwartz, A., and Coronado, R. (1987). Calcium channel activity in a purified dihydropyridine-receptor preparation of skeletal muscle. *Biochemistry* **26**, 7182–7188.

Spedding, M. (1985). Activators and inactivators of Ca^{++} channels: New perspectives. *J. Pharmacol. (Paris)* **4**, 319–343.

Spedding, M., Gittos, M., and Mir, A. K. (1987). Calcium antagonist properties of diclofurime isomers. I. Functional aspects. *J. Cardiovasc. Pharmacol.* **9**, 464–468.

Stefani, E., and Chiarandini, D. J. (1982). Ionic channels in skeletal muscle. *Annu. Rev. Physiol.* **44**, 357–372.

Striessnig, J., Zernig, G., and Glossmann, H. (1985). Human red blood cell Ca^{2+} antagonist binding sites: Evidence for an unusual receptor coupled to the nucleoside transporter. *Eur. J. Biochem.* **150**, 67–77.

Striessnig, J., Moosburger, K., Goll, A., Ferry, D. R., and Glossmann, H. (1986a). Stereoselective photoaffinity labelling of the purified 1,4-dihydropyridine receptor of the voltage-dependent calcium channel. *Eur. J. Biochem.* **161**, 603–609.

Striessnig, J., Goll, A., Moosburger, K., and Glossmann, H. (1986b). Purified calcium channels have three allosterically coupled drug receptors. *FEBS Lett.* **197**, 204–210.

Striessnig, J., Knaus, H., Grabner, M., Moosburger, K., Seitz, W., Lietz, H., and Glossmann, H. (1987). Photoaffinity labelling of the phenylalkylamine receptor of the skeletal muscle transverse-tubule calcium channel. *FEBS Lett.* **212**, 247–253.

Striessnig, J., Meusburger, E., Grabner, M., Knaus, H.-G., Kaiser, J., Schölkens, B., Becker, R., Linz, W., Henning, R., and Glossmann, H. (1988a). Evidence for a distinct calcium antagonist receptor for the novel benzothiazinone compound HOE 166. *Naunyn–Schmiedeberg's Arch. Pharmacol.* **337**, 331–340.

Striessnig, J., Knaus, H.-G., and Glossmann, H. (1988b). Photoaffinity labelling of the calcium channel associated 1,4-dihydropyridine and phenylalkylamine receptor in guinea pig hippocampus. *Biochem. J.* (in press).

Strong, J. A., Fox, A. P., Tsien, R. W., and Kaczmarek, L. K. (1986). Phorbol ester promotes a large conductance Ca channel in *Aplysia* bag cell neurons. *Biophys. J.* **49**, 430a.

Strong, J. A., Fox, A. P., Tsien, R. W., and Kaczmarek, L. K. (1987). Stimulation of protein kinase C recruits covert calcium channels in *Aplysia* bag cell neurons. *Nature (London)* **325**, 714–717.

Takahashi, M., and Catterall, W.A. (1987a). Dihydropyridine-sensitive calcium channels in cardiac and skeletal muscle membranes: Studies with antibodies against the α subunits. *Biochemistry* **26**, 5518–5526.

Takahashi, M., and Catterall, W. A. (1987b). Identification of an α subunit of the dihydropyridine-sensitive calcium channels. *Science* **236**, 88–91.

Takahashi, M., Seagar, M. J., Jones, J. F., Reber, B. F. X., and Catterall, W. A. (1987). Subunit structure of dihydropyridine-sensitive calcium channels from skeletal muscle. *Proc. Natl. Acad. Sci. U.S.A.* **84**, 5478–5482.

Tanabe, T., Takeshima, H., Mikami, A., Flockerzi, V., Takahashi, H., Kangawa, K., Kojima, M., Matsuo, H., Hirose, T., and Numa, S. (1987). Primary structure of the receptor for calcium channel blockers from skeletal muscle. *Nature (London)* **328**, 313–318.

Talvenheimo, J. A., Worley, J. F., and Nelson, M. T. (1987). Heterogeneity of calcium channels from a purified dihydropyridine receptor preparation. *Biophys. J.* **52**, 891–899.

Theodore, L. J., Nelson, W. L., Zobrist, R. H., Giacomini, K. M., and Giacomini, J. C. (1986). Studies on Ca^{2+} channel agonists. 5-[(3,4-Dimethoxyphenethyl)methylamino]-2-(3,4-dimethoxyphenyl)-2-isopropylpentyl isothiocyanate, a chemoaffinity ligand derived from verapamil. *J. Med. Chem.* **29**, 1789–1792.

Thieleczek, R., and Heilmeyer, L. M. G., Jr. (1986). Inositol 1,4,5-trisphosphate enhances Ca^{2+}-sensitivity of the contractile mechanism of chemically skinned rabbit skeletal muscle fibres. *Biochem. Biophys. Res. Commun.* **135**, 662–669.

Trautwein, W., and Cavalie, A. (1985). Cardiac calcium channels and their control by neurotransmitters and drugs. *J. Am. Coll. Cardiol.* **6**, 1409–1416.

Triggle, D. J., and Swamy, V. C. (1983). Calcium antagonists. *Circ. Res.* **52**, 17–28.

Uematsu, T., Cook, N. S., Hof, R. P., Vozeh, S., and Follath, F. (1986). Effects of the enantiomers of the dihydropyridine derivative 202-791 on contractility, coronary flow and ischemia-related arrhythmias in rat heart. *Eur. J. Pharmacol.* **123,** 455–458.

Umbach, J. A., and Gundersen, C. B. (1987). Expression of an ω-conotoxin-sensitive calcium channel in *Xenopus* oocytes injected with mRNA from *Torpedo* electric lobe. *Proc. Natl. Acad. Sci. U.S.A.* **84,** 5464–5468.

Vaghy, P. L., Dube, G. P., Grupp, I. L., Grupp, G., Williams, J. S., Baik, Y. H., and Schwartz, A. (1985). A proposed pharmacological role for dihydropyridine binding sites in heart and coronary smooth muscle. *In* "Cardiovascular Effects of Dihydropyridine-Type Calcium Antagonists and Agonists" (A. Fleckenstein, C. van Breemen, R. Gross, and F. Hoffmeister, eds.), pp. 156–184. Springer-Verlag, Berlin.

Vaghy, P. L., Williams, J. S., and Schwartz, A. (1987a). Receptor pharmacology of calcium entry blocking agents. *Am. J. Cardiol.* **59,** 9–17.

Vaghy, P. L., Striessnig, J., Miwa, k., Knaus, H.-G., Itagaki, K., McKenna, E., Glossmann, H., and Schwartz, A. (1987b). Identification of a novel 1,4-dihydropyridine- and phenylalkylamine-binding polypeptide in a calcium channel preparation. *J. Biol. Chem.* **262,** 14337–14342.

Vandaele, S., Fosset, M., Galizzi, J.-P., and Lazdunski, M. (1987). Monoclonal antibodies that coimmunoprecipitate the 1,4-dihydropyridine and phenylalkylamine receptors and reveal the Ca^{2+} channel structure. *Biochemistry* **26,** 5–9.

Varsányi, M., Messer, M., Brandt, N. R., and Heilmeyer, L. M. G., Jr. (1986). Phosphatidylinositol 4,5-disphosphate formation in rabbit skeletal and heart muscle membranes. *Biochem. Biophys. Res. Commun.* **138,** 1395–1404.

Venter, J. C., Fraser, C. M., Schaber, J. S., Jung, C. Y., Bolger, G., and Triggle, D. J. (1983). Molecular properties of the slow inward calcium channel. *J. Biol. Chem.* **258,** 9344–9348.

Vergara, J., Tsien, R. Y., and Delay, M. (1985). Inositol 1,4,5-trisphosphate: A possible chemical link in excitation–contraction coupling in muscle. *Proc. Natl. Acad. Sci. U.S.A.* **82,** 6352–6356.

Vincentini, L. M., di Virgilio, F., Ambrosini, A., Pozzan, T., and Meldolesi, J. (1985). Tumor promotor phorbol 12-myristate-13-acetate inhibits phosphoinositide hydrolysis and cytosolic Ca^{2+} rise induced by the activation of muscarinic receptors in PC12 cells. *Biochem. Biophys. Res. Commun.* **127,** 310–317.

Volpe, P., and Stephenson, E. W. (1986). Ca^{2+} Dependence of transverse tubule-mediated calcium release in skinned skeletal muscle fibers. *J. Gen. Physiol.* **87,** 271–288.

Volpe, P., Salviati, G., Di Virgilio, F., and Pozzan, T. (1985). Inositol 1,4,5-trisphosphate induces calcium release from sarcoplasmic reticulum of skeletal muscle. *Nature (London)* **316,** 347–349.

Volpe, P., Di Virgilio, F., Pozzan, T., and Salviati, G. (1986a). Role of inositol 1,4,5-trisphosphate in excitation–contraction coupling in skeletal muscle. *FEBS Lett.* **197,** 1–4.

Volpe, P., Salviati, G., and Chu, A. (1986b). Calcium-gated calcium channels in sarcoplasmic reticulum of rabbit skinned skeletal muscle fibers. *J. Gen. Physiol.* **87,** 289–303.

Wagner, J. A., Snowman, A. M., and Snyder, S. H. (1987). Aminoglycoside effects on voltage-sensitive calcium channels and neurotoxicity. *N. Engl. J. Med.* **317,** 1669.

Walsh, K. B., Bryant, S. H., and Schwartz, A. (1984). Diltiazem potentiates mechanical activity in mammalian skeletal muscle. *Biochem. Biophys. Res. Commun.* **122,** 1091–1096.

Walsh, K. B., Bryant, S. H., and Schwartz, A. (1985). Effect of calcium antagonist drugs on calcium current in mammalian skeletal muscle fibers. *J. Pharmacol. Exp. Ther.* **236**, 403–407.

Walsh, K. B., Bryant, S. H., and Schwartz, A. (1987). Suppression of charge movement by calcium antagonists is not related to calcium channel block. *Pflüger's Arch.* **409**, 217–219.

Watson, S. P., and Lapetina, E. G. (1985). 1,2-Diacylglycerol and phorbol ester inhibit agonist-induced formation of inositol phosphates in human platelets: Possible implications for negative feedback regulation of inositol phospholipid hydrolysis. *Proc. Natl. Acad. Sci. U.S.A.* **82**, 2623–2626.

Williams, J. T, and North, R. A. (1985). Catecholamine inhibition of calcium action potentials in rat locus coeruleus neurones. *Neuroscience* **14**, 103–109.

Williams, J. T., Henderson, G., and North, R. A. (1985). Characterization of α_2-adrenoceptors which increase potassium conductance in rat locus coeruleus neurones. *Neuroscience* **14**, 95–101.

Worley, J. F., Deitmer, J. W., and Nelson, M. T. (1986). Single nislodipine-sensitive calcium channels in smooth muscle cells isolated from rabbit mesenteric artery. *Proc. Natl. Acad. Sci. U.S.A.* **83**, 5746–5750.

Yatani, A., Codina, J., Imoto, Y., Reeves, J. P., Birnbaumer, L., and Brown, A. (1987). A G protein directly regulates mammalian cardiac calcium channels. *Science* **238**, 1288–1292.

Yeager, R. E., Yoshikami, D., Rivier, J., Cruz, L. J., Miljanich, G. P. (1987). Transmitter release from presynaptic terminals of electric organ: Inhibition by the calcium channel antagonist ω-conotoxin. *J. Neurosci.* **7**. 2390–2396.

Zernig, G., and Glossmann, H. (1988). A novel 1,4-dihydropyridine-binding site on mitochondrial membranes from guinea-pig heart, liver and kidney. *Biochem J.* (in press).

Zernig, G., Moshammer, R., and Glossmann, H. (1986). Stereospecific regulation of [^{3}H]inositol monophosphate accumulation by calcium channel drugs from all three main chemical classes. *Eur. J. Pharmacol.* **128**, 221–229.

Index